Y0-AAA-914

ON WOMEN HEALTHSHARING

# on women
# healthsharing

edited by
**Enakshi Dua, Maureen FitzGerald,
Linda Gardner, Darien Taylor,
Lisa Wyndels**

women's
P R E S S

CANADIAN CATALOGUING IN PUBLICATION DATA

On women healthsharing
Collection of articles from Healthsharing.
ISBN 0-88961-201-3
1. Women – Health and hygiene. 2. Women – Health and hygiene – Political aspects. 3. Women – Health and hygiene – Canada. 4. Women – Health and hygiene – Political aspects – Canada. 5. Women's health services. 6. Women's health services – Political aspects. 7. Women's health services – Canada. 8. Women's health services – Political aspects – Canada.
I. Dua, Enakshi, 1958–

RA564.85.05     1994          362.1'082          C94-932510-4

Cover art & design: Beverly Deutsch
Proofreading: Nancy Chong

This book was produced by the collective effort of Women's Press. Women's Press gratefully acknowledges the financial support of the Canada Council and the Ontario Arts Council.

Printed and bound in Canada
1  2  3  4  5  1998  1997  1996  1995  1994

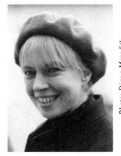

Photo: Diana Meredith

To the memory of Lina Chartrand.

And to all the women
who contributed to *Healthsharing*.

# contents

# introduction

When *Healthsharing: A Canadian Women's Health Quarterly* closed its doors in February 1994 many readers mourned its passing. For fifteen years, it had covered the issues set forward by an evolving women's health movement in Canada and the U.S. *Healthsharing* explored and debated these issues, keeping us up to date and connecting us with health activists, organizers and workers. Sometimes, in the best of magazine journalism, it sought to define the terms of an entirely new health debate.

As editors of this collection, we were in the fortunate position of revisiting *Healthsharing*. The five of us who worked on this book were brought together by our desire to participate in what we (then) thought would be a straightforward publishing project. Only Darien Taylor had actually written an article for *Healthsharing*, although all of us had experience as editors or writers. Some of us are organizers on women's health issues; some of us work as health care providers; all of us are consumers of the traditional and alternative health care systems. Once we got over the shock that the selection process was not going to be over in a weekend, we settled down to the requisite set of meetings. Our collective process was flexible and organic, allowing us to accomplish our task, at the same time as we remembered, gossiped and compared notes. As we met to whittle the manuscript down to size, we also enjoyed some far-reaching discussions of our own experiences with health and sickness, with organizing change and providing health services, with the contradictions in feminist organizing in Canada and elsewhere.

Every member of the founding *Healthsharing* collective probably has her own story about the magazine's beginnings. One version, believable in its banality, sees the impetus for launching a magazine developing from a discussion in a parking lot. From the outset, there were differences as to whether to produce a newsletter or a magazine. When, in 1979, *Healthsharing* was ready to go into print, it was simply called "a health quarterly."

The notion of a women's health newsletter seemed to imply a quick response to new and emerging issues, broader participation by more women including personal testimonials, a greater emphasis on collectivity, voluntarism, a consensual decision–making process, shorter articles, and, from the business end of things, cheaper production costs with a less "glossy" look. A magazine format, on the other hand, implied solicited material, including lengthier feature articles, paid and increasingly specialized work by staff, sustained debate on issues and a more complex structure around production and distribution.

The choice between these two options was never made. This tension persisted for the life of the magazine and gave *Healthsharing* a distinctive hybrid tone. Even in the last few years of its life, when the magazine had its most professional look, *Healthsharing* maintained and perhaps intensified its newsletter quality as many of the issues became regional reports, each with its own regional editor.

In the editorial group for *On Women Healthsharing*, we had our own guiding tensions which were similar and different from those of the original *Healthsharing* collective. We looked at the newsletter versus magazine debate from a formal perspective, and while we had considered including short pieces such as news updates, editorials, letters and selections from the "My Story, Our Story" section, in the end we chose to include feature articles almost exclusively for the greater analysis that they offered.

Particular to the project of putting together a retrospective, we struggled with the tensions between an accurate historical representation of the magazine, issues of current political relevance, appeal to a contemporary audience and our own personal interests and biases. It was instructive to look at what had, in the past fifteen years, been widely held feminist positions on certain topics and see how our construction of these issues had changed. By no means should this collection be regarded as our version of "the best" of *Healthsharing*. It is a selection that reflects the consensus of five individuals and for that reason there are gaps and omissions.

The single most defining feature of the *Healthsharing* approach was that most articles were written by activists and women who had experience with the topic they were writing about. Most of these women did not define themselves as writers and were able to get their ideas into print through working with *Healthsharing*'s editorial volunteers and staff.

Because of the commitment to have women speak for ourselves, *Healthsharing* never lost its connection with grassroots feminist issues. This meant that the magazine's own twists and turns were closely related to those of feminist organizing in Canada through the eighties and into the nineties. While *Healthsharing*'s organizational transition from a masthead with a list of collective members to one with a named managing editor and production coordinator was taking place, there was the added challenge of taking on in print the contradictions and tensions of current feminism.

*Healthsharing* made an ongoing attempt to balance analysis of health problems with specific strategies for organizing or suggestions of possible solutions. For example, *Healthsharing* waged a steady campaign against the use of the contraceptive Depo Provera, the promotion of which attested to complicity of the medical and pharmaceutical industries. Beyond this campaign in the pages of the magazine, *Healthsharing* was a steady advocate of a pan-Canadian women's health network which could lobby, strategize and advocate with a strong and diverse feminist voice on issues such as Depo Provera.

*Healthsharing* accommodated both the dominant medical model and alternative therapies. It never abandoned or jettisoned the results produced by allopathic treatments and it tended to portray alternative therapies as complementary to conventional medical practice. At the same time it sought to transform that practice to fully include the needs of women. This perspective is affirmed by the choices of the editorial group. For this reason *On Women Healthsharing*, like the magazine that preceded it, has a reformist, as distinct from a revolutionary, take on the subject of treatments.

In many ways *Healthsharing* was able to avoid assessing alternative and new therapies by emphasizing health. This emphasis posed a challenge to the medical model of illness and pathology. *Healthsharing* introduced and refined a holistic view of health for many of its readers. The Notes from the Collective in the first issue set out the definition of health that was to guide

*Healthsharing* throughout its history: "we refer to health in its broadest sense, to include a state of physical, mental, spiritual and social well–being. Thus, political, social and environmental conditions are all health issues. It is not enough to quit smoking, run five miles a day, eat only organic food if our environment remains polluted, our living and working conditions oppressive. Discussion of individual involvement and responsibility can be an empty exercise for a person who is struggling just to feed her children."

*Healthsharing*, like most feminist organizations until the late 1980s, tended to represent the experience of women as the experience of white middle–class, non-disabled heterosexual women. One of the notable aspects of *Healthsharing* was its lack of diversity, especially in the first ten years of its history. The presentation of health issues such as workplace health, poverty, mental health, reproductive technologies, abortion and menopause was as if they were universal, as if such information applied in the same ways to all women. While there were sporadic articles on the health of lesbian, disabled, First Nations and immigrant women, these articles tended to focus on the issue of access to health care. The underlying assumption was that except in the case of health care access, all women experienced their bodies, health and illness in similar ways.

The inability of *Healthsharing* to pioneer an analysis of diversity was disconcerting, since early issues do include notices of workshops, conferences and organizing by First Nations and immigrant women. The proceedings of these workshops were rarely reported in the first decade of *Healthsharing*. Nor did *Healthsharing* integrate the issues that were raised in these proceedings. In this, *Healthsharing* failed to reflect and record a vital part of the history of the Canadian women's health movement. Hopefully, these struggles have been recorded elsewhere. The absence of this record has perpetuated the image that there was only one health movement in Canada.

*Healthsharing* began to reevaluate its editorial policies in the mid–1980s. This process of self-criticism reflected changes in Canadian feminist organizing and discourse, as several feminist organizations had already begun to deal with issues of racism and diversity. At this point *Healthsharing* began to represent a more critical debate on racism. The attempt to be more inclusive at this time is also mirrored in the composition of *Healthsharing*'s staff, collective and contributors. The more inclusive character of Healthsharing contributed to a more integrated analysis of bodies, health and illness, one that included race.

Much work remains to be done. A truly integrated analysis of health, one that simultaneously incorporates issues of gender, race, disability, class, sexuality and age remains to be developed.

Finally *Healthsharing* is left with the question of whether its work and indeed the work of any women's health movement is able to reform or revolutionize health care practices and ideas or whether its ideas are merely absorbed, subsumed or co-opted by the medical establishment. *On Women Healthsharing* offers us a chance to reflect on the accomplishments of twenty years of thinking, debating and mobilizing. However, it also offers us the challenge of what remains to be done. The sad part is that we will have to go the next distance without *Healthsharing*.

Enakshi Dua, Maureen FitzGerald,
Linda Gardner, Darien Taylor, Lisa Wyndels

**Note**

The editorial collective thanks the Regional Women's Health Centre in Toronto for providing a meeting space. We also thank Heather Green, Shahnaz Stri and Shelley Tremain for their helpful advice on the collection.

# section one

# Formulating a Context

One of the tasks of feminism is to formulate a context through which *women* can understand and express our experiences of our bodies in health and in illness. The articles in this section explore the boundaries of what could constitute a feminist approach to health. These boundaries are shaped by a broad range of concerns, such as how western medicine defines illness, the ways in which science has shaped the social construction of knowledge, how women's health issues have been marginalized by conventional medicine, and the potentialities of both the "alternative" and allopathic health systems. Moreover, central to formulating a feminist framework on health is the acknowledgment that not all women experience health and the health care system in the same way. This has involved challenging systemic discrimination in both the mainstream health care system and in feminist knowledge on health and illness.

Rhonda Love and Patricia Kaufert both critique the disease focus of the conventional medical model. In "The Power of Science and Medicine," Love argues that the force of this model is based on the elevation of knowledge based on science rather than on experience. The resulting alliance of science with medicine has led medical practitioners to view our bodies as machines, to dehumanize the way in which both health and illness are dealt with, and to marginalize the social and economic basis for health and illness. While Love argues that we need to change the way in which we understand health, she warns against complete rejection of what science has to offer.

In "Through Women's Eyes: The Case for a Feminist

Epidemiology," Patricia Kaufert also believes that conventional medicine can be important for women. She maintains that political rhetoric is not enough for women to take control of their bodies. We need to integrate feminist politics with medicine, particularly by emphasizing research that is governed by a concern for women's health. For Kaufert, changing the focus and outcome of the medical research establishment must involve challenging where research gets funded, who conducts it and what methods are used. For Kaufert, developing links between researchers and women is paramount.

"Fighting Racism" and Robin Barnett's "Examining Lesbian Health" demonstrate the limitations of a universalizing feminist perspective. Both articles demonstrate that a feminist perspective on health needs to acknowledge the differences in how women experience health. "Fighting Racism" begins to look at how racism operates within the health care system. It points out that women of colour have unequal access to the health care system and if they work within the system they tend to be located in the lowest paid jobs. Importantly, this editorial also explores how racism has shaped the construction of feminist knowledge on health and illness within *Healthsharing*. "Examining Lesbian Health" raises similar issues regarding the feminist health movement. Barnett argues that the experiences of lesbians with homophobia and heterosexism within the health care system have been ignored by the various women's health movements. She argues that little is known about lesbian health issues and that more research, discussion and advocacy is needed to integrate lesbian health issues into health activism.

# The Power of Science and Medicine[*]

## Rhonda Love

The past decade has seen an increasing dissatisfaction with medicine and an increasing interest in finding alternatives that do not have the highly technological approaches to diagnosis and healing that characterize modern medicine. It is difficult, if not impossible, to gauge how many people have actually turned away from allopathy[1] and toward alternatives such as chiropractic, homeopathy, naturopathy or self-healing.

For people who are dissatisfied with allopathy, it can be difficult to find alternatives. Information is scarce and incomplete, practitioners are not readily available, and the costs of services are most likely not covered by insurance. It is especially difficult for many to change from just accepting what is easily available to trying an alternative because the economic, social and psychological supports for making changes are often not available or obvious. One major reason alternatives are not readily accessible and supported is that medicine and the medical model dominate the way we define health, illness and therapy and these definitions affect the choices that are made available and deemed legitimate.

The power that allopathic medicine has to dominate our thinking about health and fitness evolved as a result of its close tie with sciences such as biology, chemistry and physics which in the 20th century have been elevated to the lofty position once occupied by religion. We have put our faith in science to solve many of the health problems that plague us. One of the major results of putting so much faith in science is that only scientists and physicians who practise scientific medicine are seen to have answers.

[*] Reprinted from *Healthsharing* vol. 2 no.1 (Spring 1981): 9-12, with permission of the author.

It has also given one group of people, allopathic physicians, the power to discredit others who have skills which may help alleviate our suffering from ill health. This power has allowed allopathic medicine to label chiropractors and other non-allopathic healers as "quacks" and discredit as "unscientific" the knowledge and techniques of non-drug, non-surgical approaches to healing.

Medicine has not always been tied to science. The linkage of medicine and the laboratory sciences occurred at the turn of the century and has had far reaching effects. Before that time, as Ehrenreich and English describe in their *For Her Own Good, 150 Years of the Experts' Advice to Women*, the physician was "not yet a man of science [but was] a gentleman" who had studied, "Plato, Aristotle and Christian theology ... [and] merely saw any patents at all." Neither the nineteenth century's physicians' education nor experience had been scientific. However, in the late 19th century some segments of North America (particularly the middle class and professionals) were turning to science and expecting its experts to solve the pressing problems in housing, education, health and work. The social, moral and ethical dilemmas which were once the major domain of religion and its priests were now seen as problems to be solved by science and its scientists.

As Ehrenreich and English explain, many diverse groups of people supported the ascendance of science. Feminists of the day saw science as a way, to escape the influence of the oppressive, patriarchal social system. With science, there appeared to be objectivity instead of prejudice, discovery instead of doctrine and liberation instead of oppression. Many professionals also looked to science to lead the way for reform in other areas. There was not only scientific medicine but "scientific management, scientific public administration, scientific housekeeping, scientific child raising and scientific social work." In order to be considered experts, the professionals had to appear to be aligned with science. Medicine was no exception.

For medicine, its link with science was fortunate because there were some important discoveries in microbiology which helped to identify and isolate strains of bacteria and to develop agents to combat prevalent infections and contagious diseases. However, this focus on bacteria and drugs had some interesting ramifications for how allopathic physicians came to view health and illness.

Disease came to be seen as the result of an invasion by germs and germs were characterized as external agents attacking a vulnerable body. Germs and the diseases they caused became a target for a counterattack by physicians and their therapies. Thus, in allopathic medicine's terms, health was defined only in the negative. Health was the absence of clinical symptoms of disease; illness, the result of an attack by germs; and, treatment, a battle between the germs and the physicians' tools and skills.

In the 19th century, there were other healers (many of whom were women) who argued against so-called scientific medicine. They argued for a positive definition of health, challenged the theory that disease was primarily the result of an attack by germs and cautioned the practitioner not to be dazzled by the drama of success against some diseases. They cautioned the need to continue on a relatively unspectacular course to improve the living conditions and life situations which made their patients sick. These healers were not a homogenous group but seemed to share a belief that health was more than just the absence of disease. For them, the absence of disease was necessary as part of a definition of health but was not the only factor which determined health.

As Ehrenreich and English explain, "female lay healers did not have a rational theory of disease causation and therapy ... what they had was experience ... [they knew] patients as neighbors [and] the disappointments, the anxieties and the overwork that could mimic illness or induce it." Allopathic physicians did not consider disappointments, anxieties and overwork as causes of illness; these are hard to measure scientifically. They focused on the battle against germs, which could be seen in microscopes and fought illness with treatments "more powerful than the disease."

Interestingly, the so-called scientific physicians broke one of the major rules of any scientific adventure: they denied the evidence which had been accumulated through experience. The evidence favoured the healing power of herbs, the success of conservative treatment for most human ailments and the importance of the relationship between the healer and the sick. But much of this evidence had been compiled by supposedly non-scientific healers. For the physicians, any healing which could not be explained scientifically wasn't really healing.

This power to determine what would be considered as evidence of healing is one of the major results of medicine's tie to laboratory-based sciences. The reliance of medicine on the physical sciences fostered a dependence on laboratories, technology and tests. Instead of relying on the experience of the patient and the judgment of the practitioner to determine the diagnosis and treatment, medicine turned to the scientists to both pose the questions and form the solutions.

In addition to receiving the power to define the situation, medicine incorporated the world view of the physical sciences and applied it to the art of healing. This world view had its roots in the works of Galileo, Descartes and Newton who described the physical world as an entity separate and distinct from the human observer, an entity which could be quantified, predicted and controlled. The universe was described by these men, and all the scientists who followed them, as the Great Machine, a machine which could be figuratively disassembled for study and understood in total only when understood part by part.

Medicine adopted these predominantly mechanistic metaphors of the physical sciences. This use of the machine as metaphor was quite reasonable because in any expansion of human knowledge, the unknown must be understood in relation to the known. The machine was known; the human body was virtually unknown. The machine metaphors helped explain the body's functioning. For example, it is suggested that the invention of the pump hastened our understanding of the circulatory system.

However, all metaphors have limitations which must be recognized and understood. If the limitations are not explicated, then we see the unknown only as if it is an extension or reassembling of the known. But metaphors give us only partial knowledge: if the limitations of a metaphor go unchallenged, then what is *a truth* can come to be seen as *the* truth. Our bodies may function *as if* they are machines, but they *are not* machines. It is common for this distinction not to be made explicit. When this happens, a metaphor which could be used to increase our understanding could actually restrict our thinking.

It appears that conventional allopathic practitioners have often not recognized the limitations of mechanistic metaphors and have been severely criticized for treating their patients as if they were machines. This approach dehumanizes both practitioners and patients. Such dehumanization may result partly from the overzealous extension of metaphors and the uncritical acceptance of their partial truths. It demonstrates the power that metaphors may have over us. The "as if" becomes the "is."

It is possible for health practitioners to use mechanistic metaphors but not be dominated by them. For example, chiropractors, who certainly work with the machine-like aspects of the body, are less likely than are allopathic physicians to be accused of treating their patients like machines. In their book *Chiropractors: Do They Help?*, M. Kelner, O. Hall and I. Coulter report from their extensive study of Canadian chiropractic that chiropractors' patients praise the "personal care" which they receive where the "concern is for the whole person, not for the limb or the 'case.'" They say chiropractors are said to "approach their patients with a personal orientation and personalized attitudes." Chiropractors have seemingly found the way to use, but not be used by, mechanistic metaphors. By focusing on the human aspects of ill health and treatment, they put into practice their understanding of the limitations of the machine model.

The use of mechanistic metaphors is not allopathic medicine's only inheritance from its unquestioned embrace of the natural sciences. Allopathic medicine's tendency toward specialization reflects the reductionism of biology which studies the body by splitting it into numerous parts and then dividing these parts into their components. The study of the human body has become the study of systems such as the cardiovascular, respiratory and neurological systems and the study of structures such as the eye, the brain, the heart, and so on. Each system and structure has its own experts. For allopathic medicine, this has meant the decline in the number of general practitioners who understand the totality. Implicit in this sectioning of the knowledge of the human body is the idea that if we know all about the parts we can add all this knowledge together and have a complete understanding. It assumes that the whole is nothing more than the sum of its parts. But we know that being totally healthy is more than having a collection of healthy parts.

The aspects of allopathic medicine — reliance on laboratory science for diagnosis and cure, dehumanization and specialization — have all been criticized by feminists and other social critics. There has been both a demand for changing allopathic medicine and for creating alternatives. In this search for alternatives, many people have spoken of a holistic approach to healing. The definition of holistic health and medicine is not as simple as it is usually discussed. At minimum, a holistic approach must recognize that human beings are social, not clinical entities. It must practice this recognition by considering in both diagnosis and treatment that the social, political and economic network in which people live may either support their well being or contribute to their health problems.

If we are to seek an alternative we must rethink our ideas about health and curing. We must recognize that it is not only the allopathic practitioner who has worshipped at the altar of science, been careless with mechanistic metaphors and seen humans as a collection of parts. We too have been susceptible to the dominant images and ideologies of our day. Much of the struggle in women's health has been around the issues of reclaiming our bodies and discovering not only how we are dehumanized but also how we dehumanize ourselves. It is crucial to have the ability to recognize dehumanization and to know an alternative when we see it. We must also be able to know when an alternative is not really an alternative but merely masquerades as one.

Developing this ability is not always easy, but we could start by examining how we see our own bodies. Although it is less common than it once was, we may see ourselves as baby factories or domestic robots. We may refer to periodic examinations with terms appropriate to the servicing and maintenance of our cars or we may abuse our bodies with some hope that our parts can be replaced. We may think the social and political forces which affect our health can be counteracted with a few changes in our personal unhealthy habits. We may view illness as something to be cured with only a little chemical or physical realignment of our body parts. We may see our physical body as an entity distinct from our psyche with our body as a machine and our psyche as the force that drives it. If we have these images of ourselves we will not recognize when the images are used against us.

There was another major social consequence of medicine's link with the natural sciences which still affects much of our thinking. Because the answer to health problems was seen to lie in the physical sciences, medicine could retreat into the science laboratory and did not have to worry about the social conditions supporting diseases — poor nutrition, crowded housing, deplorable working conditions and polluted air. Instead of placing the blame for poor health where it belonged — in the organization of work and the politics of daily life — the experts placed the blame on workers who carried germs into the workplace and on wives and mothers who supposedly didn't maintain hygienic, germ-free homes. Now the individual, not society, is to blame — sickness is in the individual body, not the body politic.

Medicine was, of course, in some bind. It was charged with treating illness and illness did occur in individuals' bodies. Medicine argued its therapies were for individuals, not collectives, and, in the area of therapies for individual illnesses medicine did seem to have some successes. With the discoveries of antibiotics and improvement in surgical techniques, some assaults were made against the acute illnesses which killed so many people.

It has been debated though just how much of this success can be attributed to medicine. Numerous authors have made convincing cases that labour and housing reform had more positive effects on health than did any medical discoveries. But, social reform did not have the glamour of curative medicine and, of course, it always threatened those who made profits from sweatshops and slum housing. Social reform also did not have the tie to so-called objective science and was equated with politics which was seen by most people as having nothing to do with health and illness.

Today, it is in vogue to focus on lifestyle factors such as smoking, drug and alcohol abuse, nutrition and fitness and their effects on health. This so-called preventive approach has been hailed as an improvement over curative medicine which has not been as successful in treating chronic health problems as it has been in curing acute illness.

It is unquestionably important for people to reflect on how their own behaviour may damage their health and to attempt health changes. However, the lifestyle focus poses some real problems.

Just as the experts of the turn of the century blamed workers and not the work place for illness, the lifestyle approach can place the blame on the individual and may assume that the individual has total control over her lifestyle. For example, Victor Fuchs, a popular economist says in his book *Who Shall Live?*, "... the greatest potential for improving health lies in what we do and don't do for and to ourselves. The choice is ours."

Fuchs and experts like him are telling only one side of the story. That side does not seriously consider the social, political and economic basis of ill health and does not recognize the limits on individuals' choices. Fuchs and others are telling us to be relaxed and physically active when we live in a world of stress and the omnipresent automobile.

Although it is true that many of us have made and could make many healthy changes, it is important to recognize where the experts lay the blame, who they say should change and what changes they say should be made. For example, if your health problem is work-related stress, your allopathic physician may prescribe valium so you don't feel it anymore and your non-allopathic practitioner may teach you relaxation techniques to help you cope. Neither is likely to suggest that you try to find a job you like or that you organize or negotiate to get more control over your work situation. Neither is likely to do this even though a study from the U.S. Department of Health, Education and Welfare entitled "Work in America" found that work satisfaction, as measured by the amount of control workers had over their work, is the strongest predictor of longevity. The second best predictor was overall happiness. The findings also suggest that "diet, exercise, medical care and genetic inheritance may account for only 25 percent of the risk factors in heart disease, one of the major causes of death."

Of course, attempting to change your work situation may be exceedingly more difficult than changing your health habits. And changing your personal health habits is cheaper and puts less demand on those who provide health services. It may be, of course, an indicator of how unhealthy our society is when the forces that make us unhealthy are so difficult to change.

In attempting to make changes we must realize that our choices and judgments will be steeped in the predominant values of our society. These values will affect the kinds and numbers of alternatives that are available, influence our definitions of health, illness and healing, and influence our judgments of alternatives. There are few readily available answers to our questions but the process of questioning ourselves, our allopathic practitioners and those who purport to provide alternatives will bring about the redefinition of health which our society desperately needs.

In our search for alternatives, we must not make the mistake of totally rejecting the importance of science and the contributions scientists can make to healing. Our task should be to make science the liberating force that our foresisters in the feminist movement hoped it would be.

### Notes

I am indebted to Ian Coulter for the many discussions of the importance of metaphors in science and medicine. Any misinterpretations are, of course, my responsibility.

1. Allopathy is a method of treating disease with an agent which produces effects different than those of the disease. It usually implies suppression of symptoms. Allopathy is a term commonly used to describe today's conventional medicine.

RHONDA LOVE teaches community health in Toronto.

# Through Women's Eyes
## The Case for a Feminist Epidemiology[*]

### Patricia Kaufert

In April of 1987, Health and Welfare Canada hosted a sympo-
sium — Changing Patterns of Health and Disease in Canadian
Women — in Ottawa. Researchers, scientists, policy makers,
health care workers and activists and government representatives came from across Canada to share information and
ideas. The focus of the conference was women's health from an
epidemiological perspective: participants examined factors determining the frequency and distribution of diseases which
affect women.

Sociologist Patricia Kaufert presented a paper on the importance of developing a more woman-centred approach within
medical research. Kaufert broadens our definition of epidemiology to look not only at the distribution and causes of disease
but to examine what within a disease is important to us as
women.

This essay is a slightly reworked version of Kaufert's speech
which she entitled "Ensuring Our Voice is Heard: Knowledge,
Coping and Caring."

The papers at this conference show how important epidemiology
is to women. For it is this discipline which can provide us with
the information and the facts we need when making decisions
about our health or our health care. If women are to take control
over our bodies, political rhetoric is no longer enough; we must
become better informed. This conference is unusual in that most
of the epidemiologists here are women, although like other
branches of medical science, epidemiology is essentially hierarchical and patriarchal in structure and orientation. Experts speak

[*]  Reprinted from *Healthsharing* vol. 10 no. 1 (Winter 1988): 10-13, with
permission of the author.

and women listen, even when the discourse is about women, their health and disease.

What would happen if the pathway of communication was reversed? What if women spoke back to the researchers, demanded to participate in the research process, demanded their rights to choose the problems to be investigated, demanded to have the results presented in an accessible form? We have feminist lawyers, philosophers, psychiatrists, sociologists and anthropologists; I want to advocate the emergence of a feminist epidemiology.

As a discipline, epidemiology is concerned with the distribution and causes of disease, but its focus is on the general population rather than the individual. For example, epidemiologists do not treat endometriosis, but they can tell us what proportion of women share the same condition; they do not treat pelvic inflammatory disease (PID), but they have pointed to the association between PID and using an IUD (intrauterine device). Epidemiologists can tell women the odds on becoming pregnant through in vitro fertilization, or on developing cancer after taking Depo-Provera. It is epidemiologists who have calculated the risks for coronary heart disease among women clerical workers under occupational stress.

I confess to choosing examples which are under-researched, but of critical importance to significant groups of women. As earlier speakers at the conference noted, research in occupational epidemiology has focused on men at work rather than women. Research on the risk factors for coronary disease have been similarly male-oriented. In the medical excitement about in vitro fertilization scant attention has been paid to the psycho-social cost/benefit analysis which must be performed by the individual woman and for which she needs facts. Only a fraction of total research dollars has gone to projects investigating the long-term effects of any contraceptive and only a trivial portion of that amount has been spent on the risks associated with the long-acting injectable contraceptives. PID and endometriosis, while creating misery for women, do not attract major quantities of research money.

The choice of research topics might better reflect the needs of women if more women were epidemiologists. But a new direction in epidemiological research requires more than the recruitment of women scientists; these women must have power to bring about change, and this must include playing a larger role in making research policy and allocating research monies. (The importance of increasing both the representation of women on the Medical Research Council and the amount of money spent on research pertinent to women's health was subsequently discussed at the conference. It was a first step in recognizing the importance of epidemiological research and exerting pressure to ensure it reflected women's needs.)

Yet, good scientists with adequate funding doing good research on issues affecting the health of women are not enough. We need a new feminist consciousness among researchers, a willingness to ground research in the experience of women and to treat other women not as objects of research but as participants.

We need a feminist epidemiology which is defined by a new willingness to take experiential knowledge, women's own knowledge of their situation, into account at all stages in the research process. Experiential knowledge is the sort of knowledge in which we all share; it comes from our direct experience of our bodies and from sharing vicariously in the experience of other women. Medical researchers tend to downgrade the value of knowledge based on experience, treating it as subjective data of dubious validity or reliability. My criticism of this approach is that the experience of women gets left out of the research process, with serious results for both women and epidemiology. Let me take an example from my own research on menopause. The medical literature generally advises that menopausal women should be given hormone replacement therapy as protection against osteoporosis. This advice is based on the assumption that women will take estrogen for as long as prescribed by a physician. In my own research in Manitoba and in another study in Massachusetts by Sonia McKinlay, we found that women taking hormone therapy do so only intermittently. They start, stop for a few months, may restart, only to stop again. The consequences of this "on-off, on-off" use pattern for bone loss have not been investigated, partly because epidemiologists assume compliance; if they see a physician has prescribed a hormone, they presume it is being taken.

In a feminist epidemiology this sort of mistake would not be made, because women would not be seen as passive patients, but as autonomous actors. Once the perspective on women changes, then a researcher would not presume compliance, but would ask women not only what they do, but why they are reluctant to take hormones continuously.

As a general rule, epidemiologists prefer to take their data from medical records rather than talk to women. They also prefer "hard" data to soft, the objective, quantifiable "fact" to the subjective, qualitative experience. The result (as in the hormone replacement example) can be bad science, because it is based on an inadequate understanding of how things actually work in the real world of women.

Due to the same unwillingness to start from the experience of women, epidemiology can be very narrow in its definition not only of what is data, but also of what the problem is to be investigated. I am currently working on a project in Keewatin which is looking at the evacuation of Inuit women for childbirth to hospitals in the South. Going through the reports and published papers describing obstetric policy in the area over the past 15 years, I found a relatively substantial body of epidemiological research describing perinatal mortality and morbidity rates, obstetric risk factors and outcome measures, the number of women evacuated each year, where they were sent, for how long and so forth. I also found occasional references to the objections that Inuit women had made against a policy which forced them to leave their families, particularly when they have young children. No one looked at the consequences of the stress of separation to the children left in the communities. No one looked at the stress of being alone in a strange hospital for women in childbirth. No one listened to what women were saying about the dangers of leaving community nursing stations without nurse midwives (one of the effects of the evacuation policy). In sum, no one had listened to women nor defined the problem to be researched by the concerns they expressed. For me, the contrast between current standard epidemiology and a new feminist epidemiology would be primarily in a willingness to take the experiences and voices of women seriously. Rather than making women the objects of research, they would participate in the research process.

Participation must mean women having a say in determining what problems are researched, how they are defined and what information is collected from whom! But a feminist epidemiology would also mean that the results of research are returned to women in a useable form. To illustrate the relationship between women and research as it presently exists, I have taken an example from an interview with a woman who describes the problem of trying to find out from her physicians whether to rest or exercise: "I don't know where to begin, you see if they told me in words of one syllable I could adjust accordingly, but at the moment I'm completely in the dark." This woman had suffered from arthritis for many years; she "knew" her arthritis in the experiential sense, but she also wants to "know" it in the sense of having medical labels for it, a medical history and prognosis. She was asking for access to scientific knowledge, but in a form she can use to make sense out of her condition. Simply providing data is not enough; it must be in language she can understand.

Having medical information (whether to exercise or not to exercise) is important to this woman's ability to actively participate in the management of her arthritis. Research on the relative value of exercise or rest may not be the most trendy in terms of grant getting from the Medical Research Council (MRC). Communicating results to women with arthritis is not as prestigious as publishing in the *New England Journal of Medicine*. Questions such as whether exercise or rest is best for arthritis may not lie at the frontier of medical knowledge, but they are critical to women who are trying to cope with this disease. I do not decry the MRC grant, the prestigious publication or the pursuit of knowledge, but I do want a feminist epidemiology which sees the needs of women as a legitimate priority for scientific endeavour.

The critical problem is to create a linkage between the world as seen by epidemiologists and the world of women. Women have always shared knowledge among themselves. They have exchanged tales about giving birth, about how to avoid, achieve or end a pregnancy, or how to sooth the aches and pains of old age or sickness. The constant thread running through my interviews with menopausal women was the comparisons they made between their own experiences and those of other women. Comparison and sharing experience are the basis of self-help workshops for menopausal women run at the Women's Health Clinic in Winnipeg. Similar exchanges take place through the pages of the newsletter for menopausal women, *A Friend Indeed*. Such comparisons serve partly as a validation of the normalcy — or else the extraordinariness — of one's own experience relative to that of other women. A feminist epidemiology would be similarly rooted in the real experience of women, but would allow sharing on a larger scale than the local self-help group.

If we want participation in the research process and want a more feminist epidemiology, then we have to make our voices heard. Again I would look to the example of self-help groups. There is a particular form of strength and support which develops only between those who share the same experience. Self-help groups may originate in the search for shared experience, but out of the processes of sharing often comes a new consciousness and a new set of definitions of the common and critical problems. From being collectors and disseminators of information, groups such as DAWN (DisAbled Women's Network) and the Alzheimer's Society become lobbyists, pursuing goals defined out of group experience and priorities. They are demanding improved services, new medical programs and research, housing, transport, educational programs and employment.

My suggestion is that there is much to be learned from groups like DAWN and the Alzheimer's Society about networking, about making the voice of the group audible to the research community and the funding agencies, about demanding that research should be from the perspective which takes the needs and experiences of the group into account and that information comes back to the group. The Coalition on Depo-Provera which formed to challenge a move to license that drug as a contraceptive for use in Canada is an example of the way in which women's groups can coalesce and organize around an issue important to the health of the women's community.

I do not know what the next coalition should be about, but whatever it is, it will depend on the same things; that is, networking between women, collaboration, a combination of political activism, expertise, and the willingness to be a public nuisance until we are heard. This conference is a rare opportunity. It is more than the sum of its formal sessions, but is providing the opportunity for researchers, policy makers and practitioners to meet and discuss the priorities in women's health, always thinking, however, of how women themselves define them. I want to close with a quotation from Adrienne Rich.

I know no woman — virgin, mother, lesbian, married or celibate, whether she earns her keep as a housewife, a cocktail waitress, or a scanner of brain waves — for whom her body is not a fundamental problem; its clouded meanings, its fertility, its desire, its so-called frigidity, its bloody speech, its silences, its changes and mutilations, its rapes and ripenings. There is for the first time today a possibility of converting our physicality into both knowledge and power.

**PATRICIA KAUFERT** is an associate professor in the Department of Community Health Sciences at the University of Manitoba.

# Fighting Racism

## Notes from the Collective[*]

Susan Elliott, Deirdre Gallagher,
Amy Gottlieb, Alice Grange, Ruth Kidane,
Diana Majury, Lisa McCaskell, Katie Pellizzari

In recent years Women of Colour have been raising their voices in the women's movement, dramatically initiating a new women's politics. Pivotal to their call for change has been the establishment of the fight against racism as a priority for the women's movement. In their struggle to broaden and strengthen Canadian feminism, Women of Colour have had to confront institutionalized racism and racist prejudice within the women's movement.

Racism like all prejudice and bigotry is a sickness as well as a system of exploitation and oppression. If you are Black and poor in this country you have less access to health services and if you work in the health care system you are likely to have the lowest paid jobs and worst working conditions. Racism against Native women is deep and abiding. Native women are mistreated in the health care system in an especially pernicious way. Tuberculosis is still a serious disease, women are often forced to leave their home communities to give birth, and Native healing is not understood or supported in the health care system.

But this reality has not been represented or reflected in the pages of *Healthsharing* over the past ten years. We must ask ourselves why.

Women Healthsharing arose out of the women's health movement — a movement which has been and continues to be dominated by white middle class women. The Healthsharing collective and the volunteers who produce the magazine have largely reflected these origins. While we have, over the years, acknowledged to ourselves the narrowness of our view, whatever we

* Reprinted from *Healthsharing* vol. 9 no. 4 (Fall 1988): 3.

have done in an attempt to have the magazine reflect the concerns of all women, has not been enough.

Collective members remain overwhelmingly white, and articles usually represent the experience of white middle class women as the experience of all women. The appearance and functioning of our magazine and our organization has acted as a barrier to involvement by many women. This exclusion represents a tremendous loss, for everyone. Not only have Women of Colour been denied the opportunity to speak and organize through the pages of *Healthsharing*, white women have missed the chance to broaden their understanding of women's issues. These divisions along lines of class and race are increasingly becoming an area of struggle within the Canadian women's movement.

White feminists are being challenged and we hear this as a challenge to *Healthsharing*. It may be difficult for white women to recognize that we have gained from being white in this society. Confronting our privilege is a first step in the process of taking up the challenge, educating ourselves and making change.

It is undeniable that white feminists have had in *Healthsharing* an important vehicle for anger and concerns around the health care system. And *Healthsharing* has been a tool for organizing to control our bodies and all aspects of our health. As in other organizations within the women's movement, we have had access to the resources of, been published by, been on staff of and been supported by *Healthsharing*. The time to share these resources, to change our method of functioning to include a diversity of women, is long overdue.

*Healthsharing* is in the process of change. As a first step we have decided to enlist the help of a facilitator to assist us in developing a plan to overcome the barriers that exist within our organization to the participation of Women of Colour and to help us find the means to make our magazine more truly reflective of the varied and different experiences of women in this country.

We recognize that we need to take on the responsibility of ensuring that all our articles contain an anti-racist perspective and a consciousness around racism. This involves not only working closely with women who write for *Healthsharing* but also developing clear written guidelines for all our contributors. The collective acknowledges that we have a responsibility to take on racism and develop a deeper understanding of ourselves.

Usually *Healthsharing* has not paid writers or illustrators/photographers. But as part of our first step in changing, *Healthsharing* has decided to pay for articles and illustrations from Women of Colour in recognition of the specific obstacles they encounter in writing for the magazine and to encourage women to work with *Healthsharing* to make it relevant in their communities. We see this as the beginning of sharing the resources that Healthsharing has built up over the past ten years. While we are making this a top priority, it is also our intention to share our resources equitably with other women who face barriers in writing for the magazine.

We want change at *Healthsharing*. We will continue our discussions but we also want to take action. We recognize that this process will be one that will redefine *Healthsharing* — who participates, who writes and illustrates, who works on staff — whose voices *Healthsharing* represents. We know that *Healthsharing* and the women's health movement will be strengthened. And by creating a stronger movement we will be able to fight the sexism and racism in the health care system more effectively.

# Examining Lesbian Health*

## Robin Barnett

The feminist health movement has highlighted the misogynist training of doctors and the anti-woman bias of much modern medicine. Women do not experience an equal relationship with doctors since knowledge has power. The high status of doctors in this society gives them power — chosen or assigned — over their patients. Nearly all women have difficulty dealing with doctors and choices about treatments. Is this situation any different for lesbians?

Yes, the difference results from homophobia and heterosexism. Lesbians cannot forget that this society operates from a heterosexual perspective. Many lesbians are cautious about revealing their lifestyle because they never know when coming out will have negative consequences. They face discrimination in every part of society. Heterosexual relationships and the nuclear family are standards in our society by which all are judged. Lesbians are always making decisions about whether to come out or to pass as heterosexual. Lesbians' interactions with the health care system are no different than with other parts of their lives. Lesbians are vulnerable in any given health situation because they never know what to expect, sometimes even if they have known a health worker for years. An incorrect or awkward statement made by a health worker may be made in ignorance of a client's sexuality or it may be made from bias or fear. Going to a doctor may be more stressful for a lesbian than living with whatever ailment she has. Inadequate or hostile treatment by medical professionals may prevent lesbians from seeking care. Stories of misdiagnosis and voyeuristic health care workers abound in the lesbian community.

Heterosexism and homophobia aside, lesbians may be less

* Reprinted from *Healthsharing* vol. 6 no. 2 (Spring 1985): 7-10, with permission of the author.

likely to see health professionals simply because they are less likely to use birth control than heterosexual women. Statistics show that women consult medical professionals more than men. Key reasons are contraceptive, gynecological and reproductive concerns; and most routine gynecological screening is handled in conjunction with birth control or prenatal visits. Even sexually active heterosexual women, with good reasons for having birth control check-ups would often rather put off seeing the doctor. For lesbians, this tendency is easier to act upon.

Current lack of knowledge about lesbian health matters and ensuing ignorance promotes and perpetuates myths about lesbians, and makes it difficult for lesbians to get accurate and thorough information about their health. Medical studies about lesbian health problems are almost nonexistent. Indeed under homosexuality — read male — the few articles mentioning lesbians mostly focus on hormonal studies and mental health, I suspect intent upon finding abnormalities with lesbians. Alternative health practices and research appear to fare no better. Moreover, health training for doctors, nurses and alternative health practitioners rarely introduces matters relevant specifically to lesbians. Generally, only when lesbians or gay men in these programs raise the issue of homosexuality does the topic get mention.

Most health workers assume that every woman is heterosexual, that sexuality means intercourse and that all women need birth control. In this context, lesbianism represents a deviation from the norm. Many lesbians tell me they dread hearing from an unfamiliar health worker, "What kind of birth control do you use?"

Different types of sexuality must be acknowledged by the health professions; assumptions cannot be made. For instance, some self-identified lesbians have sexual encounters with men, or a woman may be celibate. A suggestion I find useful is for the birth control question to be phrased more sensitively, such as "Do you have need of birth control?" Sometimes the question should not be raised in an initial meeting with a client.

Even some health workers who try to be supportive of lesbians may make assumptions or generalizations about the sexual practices of lesbians based on limited knowledge. This could have serious repercussions. For instance, a woman I know arrived in the hospital emergency department with severe abdominal pain.

Several months before she had come out to her doctor, who seemed supportive. While she was under anesthetic her doctor told the specialist about her "gay lifestyle." The specialist ruled out pelvic inflammatory disease (PID) based on this knowledge; her normal appendix was removed. She was not asked how long she had been a lesbian or whether she had sex with men. Later, following further consultation, she was diagnosed with PID and treated for it, and she had had to suffer the effects of major surgery for the appendectomy.

Finding a sympathetic health worker can be difficult. Lesbian information centres or feminist health centres, where available, can be valuable sources for practitioners names. Many lesbians depend on word-of-mouth referrals, but this is easiest for lesbians in contact with a lesbian community. Access is a problem, especially for rural women, who may have no choice but to depend on the available health practitioner. I know of many women in rural British Columbia who travel hours to see a sympathetic or supportive doctor.

## Coming Out
Women have different needs when shopping for health care workers. Some are interested in personality, some in qualifications or attitudes. Where choice is available, many lesbians seek health workers who understand the societal pressures on lesbians. Some seek lesbian health practitioners. Others choose heterosexual male workers. Given the range of choice, it is difficult to offer guidelines about how and when to come out. What works with one woman in a particular situation may not work for another woman.

I feel the issue of coming out to professionals is complex and variable. A woman should not feel compelled to come out; the decision is personal. I find it depends on a woman's rapport with her health worker, and how she assesses her own health needs and risks. It may also depend on a woman's willingness to raise issues with her health worker and their ability to build a relationship of trust and respect. A woman told me of her conversation with her male doctor regarding artificial insemination. He was uncomfortable with the idea and tried to talk her out of it, ostensibly concerned about his own legal liability. She had known him for several years and he was aware of her lesbianism. She did not accept his recommendations, and she continued to pursue the possibility of artificial insemination. After several more visits he was helpful and working with her.

I urge a woman who chooses to come out to clarify with her health care worker what information is to be documented and the future use of information in order to ensure security. Notation is especially important in the case of emergency medical care and hospitalization where hospital staff have access to a woman's medical records. Despite a public commitment to confidentiality among the medical and health professions, in my experience many health workers talk among themselves about clients' medical problems and personal lives.

Lesbian identification — verbal or documented — can have serious delayed consequences. I can envision a horrible scenario: a woman's sexual orientation is noted in her medical chart; years later her medical records are subpoenaed by the courts in a child custody casè in which she is hiding her lesbianism; she loses custody of her children. I do know of one case where information about a woman's lesbianism was passed from a sympathetic worker to one who was openly hostile and verbally abusive to the woman.

There is sometimes a fine line between when it seems crucial to the treatment of a medical problem to come out and when it might be peripheral. For example, problems of contagious diseases put partners at risk and lesbians may need to request information about transmission. But what about conditions such as cancer that do not depend on a woman's sexual orientation? It may not be worthwhile for a woman to come out in these circumstances.

## Health Concerns

There are lesbians who believe that lesbians are healthier than heterosexual women and that they do not require routine medical care. I believe routine medical care is just as important for lesbian women as for heterosexual women, although it is not clear from the literature what the particular lesbian health needs and concerns are. The few articles written about physical health such as "Lesbian Healthcare" by Francine Homstein and "Self-Health for Lesbian Women" by the Emma Goldman Clinic for Women in Iowa, tend to focus on vaginal health and artificial insemination.

There is speculation in the medical and lay literature about other health issues affecting lesbians. Questions are beginning to be posed about hypertension, menopause, emotional health, substance abuse, motherhood choices, and breast and vaginal health. It is difficult to define areas of concern for a broad range of women who come from diverse social, racial and ethnic backgrounds. There is a danger that lesbians may be even more likely to be stereotyped on the basis of sexual preference.

Within the last year several groups in the United States undertook studies to define lesbian health issues. The National Lesbian/Gay Health Education Foundation in Washington received a grant from Ms. Foundation to carry out a national lesbian health needs survey. The Lyon Martin clinic in San Francisco began investigations into the incidence and nature of genital tract infections among lesbians. Both these studies will attempt to examine economic, cultural and racial factors. These studies conducted by gay and lesbian lay organizations may provide some very useful information.

Some lesbians have expressed to me a fear that the search for lesbian health issues may be used to stereotype lesbians. For example, a higher incidence of alcoholism among lesbians is reported in the medical literature. Statistics I have seen in *Lesbian Health Matters* and the *Sourcebook on Lesbian/Gay Health Care* estimate one in three lesbians is alcoholic. This information has been cited as evidence of the unhealthy lifestyle of lesbians and used to argue the negative repercussions of lesbianism. The bar culture is often identified as the problem. There is no recognition of the discrimination lesbians face and their need for a distinct culture, a culture that inevitably has both negative and positive aspects like any other culture. Alcoholism is a general problem in our society. It may or may not be any more prevalent among lesbians than within society as a whole. And if alcoholism is more prevalent among lesbians, we don't yet have a handle on why.

## Gynecological and Breast Health Concerns
Because so little is known about lesbian health issues, it is difficult to make suggestions about routine health care. Regular check-ups for breast and vaginal health are important for all women. Breast and vaginal self-help information is available from the Vancouver Women's Health Collective for lesbians who cannot afford medi-

cal coverage or who do not have access to supportive health care. I hope lesbian self-help groups and publicity about the value of regular health care will provide useful strategies for encouraging lesbians to seek information. The self-help approach, like the feminist health movement, stresses health, wellness and prevention.

Breast self-examination is crucial for all women. It is meant to familiarize women with their own breasts so that they will notice any changes. Lesbians without children may have a higher incidence of breast cancer because medical statistics indicate a higher risk for breast cancer among childless women. Fear of finding lumps and cultural stigmas against touching ourselves are two common obstacles keeping women from performing this exam. While health workers can perform the exam, a woman is more familiar with her own breasts; most women find lumps themselves. I suggest lesbians do this simple examination with a partner or close friend, or in the context of a self-help group.

A lesbian with breast cancer may suffer the same physical and psychological effects of mastectomy as heterosexual women, but she may additionally face the heterosexist assumptions of both hospitals and mastectomy recovery programs. Like many women, lesbians may face internal struggles about their appearance and wholeness following a mastectomy. However, these concerns are not discussed in a lesbian context.

Our society ignores the effects of mastectomy. From the moment a woman wakes up from her operation effort is made to pretend she is okay. In an attempt to be compassionate and reassuring, nurses often enquire about a woman's boyfriend or husband, in order to open a discussion to help her find ways to feel sure she is still feminine and appealing. Mastectomy recovery programs, frequently staffed by volunteers who have had mastectomies, tend to focus on the ease of regaining one's appearance by use of protheses and assuming a normal lifestyle; these volunteers likewise often ask questions about boyfriends and husbands.

Regular screening for abnormal cervical cells, done by Pap tests, may be something lesbians relegate to heterosexual women. Many women receive this test when they visit health workers for birth control check-ups. Warnings about the risks for abnormal smears in health literature and practice focus on heterosexual activity. However, two studies, "Failure to Identify Venereal Disease in a Lesbian Population" and "Factors Influencing Lesbian

Gynecological Care," suggest that the incidence of abnormal Pap smears among lesbians is comparable to that among heterosexual women. Nevertheless, these studies report lesbians only get Pap smears on an average of every 20 months rather than yearly.

Unlike breast self-exam, women need trained health workers to administer Pap tests. Self-help groups, lesbian clinics and access to sympathetic workers are ways I see to encourage lesbians to seek this test. Pap tests can be combined with cervical self-exam, either in a self-help group or in a worker's office. The condition of the cervix can be an indication of vaginal health.

According to the literature I have reviewed, lesbians actually get less vaginal infections than heterosexual women, though some problems such as Gardnerella, Chlamydia (both bacterial infections) and herpes seem to be increasing among lesbians. Medical guidelines for healthy sex rarely address lesbian sexuality. Organisms can be passed between women in a number of ways. Information about sexually transmitted diseases can be sought from women's health centres.

The percentage of hysterectomy among women over 60 years of age seems to be increasing in North America; estimates range from 25 percent in a Canadian publication, *A Friend Indeed,* to 50 percent in *Malepractice* by Robert Mendelsohn. A recent news report appearing in *The Vancouver Sun* cites total hysterectomy as the most common operation in the United States. There are numerous gynecological problems which are treated by hysterectomy including PID, fibroid tumours and endometriosis (a condition where the lining of the uterus grows outside the uterus).

I have met many lesbians under 30 years of age who have had hysterectomies for any of these conditions. Lesbians without children, an estimated 70 percent of lesbians according to a letter to the editor appearing in the December 1984 issue of *Ms.*, may have a higher incidence of endometriosis because of a higher risk reported for women without children. Susanne Morgan in *Coping With A Hysterectomy* speculates hysterectomy may hit particularly hard at lesbians; and women who do not want children may be offered the operation sooner than women who do want children. Lesbians who do not want children may accept the operation because they are not told of the possible side effects of the surgery, that the loss of the uterus and ovaries may affect their general state of health and sexuality. There are numerous studies which document hysterectomy overuse among poor women and women of colour, some of whom may be lesbian.

Lesbian health care and needs are being increasingly discussed and investigated. A growing number of medical studies are being published, and more and more literature about health care written by lesbians is becoming available. Some recent articles reported in *Lesbian Health Matters* address health care workers specifically in order to increase their understanding of lesbian health concerns. Other articles urge gay men and lesbians to come out. Advocacy work is also being done throughout North America to introduce lesbian health issues and sexuality into health care training programs. And I believe the International Lesbian/Gay Health Conference held in New York in the summer of 1984 provided the first forum for the discussion of lesbian health matters on a North American scale.

The increase in research, discussion and advocacy is intended to heighten the awareness of lesbian health issues both among lesbians and medical professionals and within the general population. Lesbians may then begin to feel more comfortable seeking health care, and the health care they receive may be improved. Lesbians within health care training programs may also begin to find it easier to come out to classmates and instructors.

I believe we will hear more about lesbian health care need and issues over the next few years. Think how reassuring it would be for lesbians if a book or pamphlet concerning lesbian health were available among all the other health literature lying around health care offices.

## Further Reading

Degen, K., and H.J. Waitkevicz. *British Journal of Sexual Medicine* (May 1982): 40-54.

Johnson, S., M.D., et al. "Factors Influencing Lesbian Gynecologic Care: A Preliminary Study." *American Journal of Obstetrics and Gynecology* (May 1981).

Robertson, P., M.D., and J. Schachter, M.D. "Failure to Identify Veneral disease in a Lesbian Population." *Sexually Transmitted Diseases* (April-June 1981).

**ROBIN BARNETT** is a member of the Vancouver Women's Health Collective. Her other writings include A Feminist Approach to Pap Tests and Understanding Vaginal Health. She attended the International Lesbian/Gay Health Conference held in New York in June, 1984.

*section two*

# The Medical System

Pat Armstrong's article offers an incisive description of the deteriorating working conditions confronting nurses. Armstrong identifies structural changes in hospitals such as increasing managerial control, increasing use of new technologies, reduction in primary care responsibilities, increasing use of part-time workers and cutbacks in capital and operational expenses, and problems inherent in those changes. Ultimately, Armstrong looks to the possibility of a meaningful collective response by nurses to deteriorating working conditions.

Bhooma Bhayana is interested in the interaction between the health care provider and the health care consumer when their cultural backgrounds are different, and, in particular, in the experience of immigrant women within the health care system. Bhayana identifies instances of potential "clashes" between caregivers and consumers based on differing systems of beliefs, and counsels the need for increased knowledge on the part of health care providers of the beliefs held by persons coming from other cultures.

Christina Lee outlines the experience of multiple disadvantage faced by refugee women in Canadian society based on gender, racial origin, educational background and, frequently, on their arrival in Canada as members of a "sponsored" class of immigrants, as defined by Immigration. Lee identifies the resultant stresses on physical and mental health borne by refugee women, as well as outlining limitations in the scope and effectiveness of current services for refugee women.

Janet Maher provides a description of certain broad developments within federal-provincial relations and the funding of health care.

Maher identifies concerns in relation to the coming into force of the Canada-U.S. Free Trade Agreement and the North American Free Trade Agreement, and anticipates a further undermining in the provision of health care services as the agreements are eventually applied to existing services.

# Where Have All the Nurses Gone?[*]

## Pat Armstrong

Across the country nurses are making the headlines: the recent strike by the Alberta nurses union, the severe nursing shortage in Ontario, and the continuing aftermath of the Grange Commission inquiry into the deaths at Toronto's Sick Children's Hospital. What is happening to nursing?

Recent media coverage focusing on the nursing shortage has blamed governments, hospitals and educational institutions for lack of planning. The argument goes like this. With the massive introduction of new technologies requiring special skills, more skilled nurses are needed. At the same time more nurses are needed to care for the growing numbers of elderly filling hospital and nursing home beds. The colleges and universities have failed to prepare a sufficient number of nurses to meet the demand.

But nurses are finally making themselves heard. And theirs is a different story. It suggests a much more fundamental problem — one that is much less easily solved. For nurses, the problems stem from deteriorating working conditions: the emphasis on tasks, not on caring for people, the long shifts and most importantly the lack of power. Nurses are held accountable despite having little control over their patients' care or their own working conditions. The most blatant example of this combination of blame and lack of authority is the recent Grange Commission.

In this inquiry into the deaths at Sick Children's Hospital, nurses alone were interrogated about their performance. This happened in spite of repeated suggestions from nurses that low staff ratios and the limited time spent by high-risk children in intensive care were endangering lives. Nurses were prime sus-

---

[*] Reprinted from *Healthsharing* vol. 9 no. 3 (Summer 1988): 17-19, with permission of the author.

pects despite the fact that they were the first to draw attention to the alarming rise in deaths.

The subordinate position of nurses is not new. But the caring work of nursing is being transformed, making it increasingly difficult for even the most dedicated nurses to stay in the job full-time. In our study of a large metropolitan hospital in Quebec, we spoke with hospital workers about their work experience and examined the overall changes in hospital structure. This article presents some of our preliminary findings and explores the ways in which these changes affect nurses and the nursing profession.

Hospitals are cutting costs and increasing managerial control. Nurses' work has become both more intense and less satisfying. They are working harder for fewer rewards. According to one nurse in our study, "You don't have time to talk to patients. Your work is much more compartmentalized. You do this and then you do that and then you do that." "Work has triplicated," said another. The job is fragmented into a series of discrete tasks, the work involves "more doing things to people, not for people." There is little time for the caring work that nurses have learned to do. Under such conditions, it is not surprising that there is a shortage of people willing to take up or stay in these jobs. With short patient stays and heavy workloads for the caregivers, nurses and patients have no time to get to know each other. Patients leave long before they have made significant progress toward recovery. Consequently nurses not only work harder, but, as one nurse explained, nurses "no longer feel that they have helped patients get better and that was the satisfying part of the job, that made the rest worthwhile."

Both the intensification of the work and the alienation from the patients are reinforced by the increasing use of part-time workers, registry nurses (nurses who work for an employment agency), and "floaters." Nurses are allocated according to a formula based on time-motion studies of nurses' tasks. With this formula, administrators calculate the minimum number of nurses required in each area. Part-time, registry and "floating" nurses are used to fill in gaps, ensuring that there is no slack in the system. Gone are the days when nurses could relax their pace because fewer babies were born last night. Fewer babies means fewer nurses. The application of the formula and the manipulation of personnel have been made possible by the new microelectronic technology, which simplifies scheduling, payment and hiring.

When nurses work part-time or with a registry, they seldom follow their patients through their hospital stay, making it difficult to develop any rapport. Nurses request temporary assignments as a means of creating variety in their work or as a way of escaping close supervision. For many, it is a strategy for coping with their jobs at home. But these nurses are pressured to work very hard in shorter hours and often derive little satisfaction from the care of patients. In addition, workers who travel from ward to ward have few opportunities to develop relationships with other nurses. They often eat lunch and take coffee breaks alone and seldom gain the support and stimulation that long-term relationships on the job can provide.

The increasing use of part-time, registry and "floating" nurses also has consequences for the nurses who work regularly on a particular ward. Regular duty nurses spend more time training and introducing those temporarily assigned to the area, leaving all nurses with less time for patient care. Furthermore, it is difficult to develop team work and group morale when the work force is constantly changing. In this situation nurses share less and have fewer possibilities to get together to organize for change.

Cutbacks in capital and operation expenses mean that nurses spend more time soothing patients angry about waiting in halls, and more time searching for equipment and materials. Those we interviewed tell tales of trading sheets for hospital gowns, of running upstairs in search of extra syringes. Such shortages result in both more tension and less time for patient care.

Efforts to save money have also led to reductions in non-nursing personnel. Many of the nurses' aides and orderlies have been dismissed. There have been significant staff reductions in the laundries, kitchens and offices. It is nurses who have to take up slack, nurses who move the gurnies previously moved by orderlies and who change the beds previously changed by nurses' aides.

Not only has the workload increased, but the new technologies are transforming the nature of nursing work. Some of the new equipment requires new skills and knowledge, making the job more challenging. But much of the technology reduces the skill required which often means the work is less interesting and rewarding. For example, nurses no longer have to read thermometers. They simply have to record the digital readout. In some cases, the technology is simplified to such an extent that patients or patients' relatives can do the monitoring. Like self-service gas stations and banking machines, the equipment allows clients to do the work themselves. Even when particular skills are necessary to operate and monitor equipment, nurses frequently find the job less satisfying because they are "tending machines not patients." And some of these new machines can be used to monitor nurses' work speed and volume.

Patient care isn't the only aspect of nursing being affected by technology. The ways in which nurses document their care is being computerized. Computer terminals are being installed in nursing stations to record nurses' activities and patients' conditions. This produces more noncare work for nurses to do and greater possibility for error. Errors are particularly likely when a nurse is working on an unfamiliar terminal at the end of a 12-hour shift.

Cost cutting and new technologies have also contributed to the growing numbers and increasing powers of nonmedical administrators in the health care system. Consequently, health care workers find that they must respond to two bosses: doctors and managers. With lines of authority not always clear, nurses often find themselves caught in the middle.

These changes in the organization of nursing work have played a part in growing numbers of nurses suffering from what is diagnosed as burnout. Often defined as an individual problem that can be treated with therapy, diet and exercise, burnout frequently has more to do with the structure and process of work than to individual failures or habits. The increasing incidence of burnout is also related to the fact that most nurses are women. In the past, only single women without family responsibilities worked in nursing full-time. Most nurses were young and stayed in the job for a short period of time. Now more and more women with children and other domestic responsibilities remain in nursing. Many have agreed to take on the exhausting 12-hour shifts because these schedules allow them more days off to do their work at home.

Changes in nurses' training — changes which reflect management strategies, new technologies and nurses' demands — divide nurses from each other and increase tensions on the wards. Some nurses are trained entirely in hospitals, some in colleges, others in universities or management schools. With such varied background and different possibilities for promotion, team spirit is difficult to develop.

Nurses are responding individually to these transformations. They switch to part-time, registry or "floating" work, or they drop out of nursing for years, even for life. Many are retraining for other jobs. Nurses' collective response is, to some extent, limited by these individual solutions as well as by management strategies designed to hire more part-time workers and to move full-time nurses around. But nurses have made gains. They have won some significant improvements in pay, power and conditions of work in the post-war years. Current trends in the organization of work and the consequent shortage of workers may well strengthen nurses' opposition, leading to new directions in the organization of work. The recent strike by Alberta nurses clearly indicates nurses are prepared to put up a fight.

At the same time as new management strategies are creating the conditions for rebellion, they are also creating the possibility for significant improvements in work. The new technology has the potential to free nurses' time, allowing them to care for rather than to do things to patients. Primary nursing, which makes nurses responsible for the total care of patients, could expand the job in more satisfying ways, making it possible for nurses to employ their expertise and to develop a relationship with their patients. Whether this potential will ever be realized will depend, to a large extent, on nurses' collective response.

PAT ARMSTRONG is a teacher, writer and researcher currently teaching at York University. Her research focuses on women's labour in the home and in the workforce. She and her research partner Hugh Armstrong have just finished their study of working conditions and overall structure in a large metropolitan hospital in Quebec.

# Healthshock[*]

## Bhooma Bhayana

I am a family physician working with the London Intercommunity Health Centre in Ontario which was created in response to the need for culturally-sensitive health care and programming expressed by various ethnic communities and settlement services.

The centre works with newcomers to Canada, most of whom have left behind political turmoil or war and are mostly from developing nations. For this reason this article will explore "healthshock" as it applies to the immigrant experience In Canada and, in particular, my own experience with immigrants from the developing world as they try to access heath care services.

### Defining Healthshock

The *Fontana Dictionary of Modern Thought* defines culture shock as "the trauma or bewilderment and anxiety that is supposedly experienced, most often by those who, whether voluntarily or involuntarily find themselves isolated in an alien culture." The World Health Organization defines health as "the enabling process by which an individual is empowered to take control of ensuring his or her emotional,. physical and spiritual well being." Healthshock, then, is a term which describes the interaction that occurs between the health care provider and the health care consumer when each has different cultural backgrounds and experiences. Unlike culture shock the reaction is bilateral and has as great a potential to be positive as negative.

The first step in understanding healthshock is to recognize that we all have a culture. The health care provider has a culture, the consumer of health services and even health care systems, in both the "new" and "old" countries, have a culture. The second step lies in knowing there is also no "correct" culture, although

---

[*]   Reprinted from *Healthsharing* vol. 12 no. 3 (Fall 1991): 28-31, with
       permission of the author.

there are more dominant cultures, often due to imperialist history or timing.

## Defining Health

Being healthy does not only mean not being sick. It means being in control of the options you have to fulfil your aspirations. A sole support mother on social assistance, for example, may not be ill at any given point in time; she may have available to her free visits to the physician, the laboratory and the hospital and she may have free medication. However, on a fixed income, with little power over her future and that of her children, she is unable to achieve a sense of being in control of her options.

## Parameters of Healthshock

The parameters of healthshock are quite diverse. First, it rears its head in the meeting of health attitudes, beliefs and practices. Second, it affects the nature of the exchange between the health care provider and consumer. In fact, it impacts on whether or not that exchange is really an exchange at all! Third, healthshock is particularly apparent when it affects certain members of a society such as immigrant women and seniors.

## Health Beliefs

We are all indoctrinated with some system of health beliefs and attitudes. They can be as benign as the belief that going out in the rain may cause pneumonia or as politically charged as the belief that women should experience pain in labour. It does not matter whether or not they are erroneous. The fact that we believe them affects when we seek help, why we seek help, whether we are able to help ourselves and whether we eventually comply with the kind of help that is given.

We all have a belief about what defines good health. So our tolerance for poor health depends on that definition and our beliefs. In China and India, for example, there exists little tolerance for "abnormalities" or anomalies. Birth defects are less readily accepted in a newborn baby due to the high expectation of what is considered to be "normal." However, in the western developed world, our tolerance for such abnormalities or disabilities is greater because of the availability of technology to correct abnormalities and specialized treatment and care services for people with disabilities.

That is not to say that the threshold for marginalization is lower in the West. The western concept of the nuclear family has a lot to do with the tolerance of the young and healthy and the isolation of the sick and elderly. The point at which the elderly are institutionalized has a lot to do with our cultural beliefs about their place within the home. Home visiting nurses caring for a dying elderly immigrant whose needs they believe would be better served in an institution can feel frustrated because, despite their pleas, the family refuses to institutionalize. This is an example of healthshock.

Many beliefs have a function in a particular time and place and can become antiquated and nonfunctional elsewhere. For example, many women believe that it is imperative to bleed profusely postpartum. Not bleeding is considered unhealthy. Before the routine use of synthetic syntocinon (a hormone that contracts the uterus after birth preventing hemorrhaging), bleeding was seen as a healthy sign that membranes were being cleaned out of the uterus. A woman who delivered her first baby in a refugee camp on the Thai-Cambodian border delivered her second in London, Ontario. It took several visits during which she insisted something was wrong before we stumbled across her belief that she had not bled enough, to be at the core of her concern.

The belief that a balanced diet is a balance of yin and yang as in Taoist tradition or hot and cold as in Ayurvedic tradition, may make the Western belief in a balanced diet based on four food groups, as recommended in the Canada Food Guide, seem ill-conceived. I find this latter belief the most difficult to deal with and perhaps the only one I would call erroneous. The fact that we are encouraged to adapt Western beliefs around nutrition because they are considered to be more "advanced" is uncomfortable to accept, especially when we know that such adaptation leads to a higher incidence of heart disease in new immigrants even within the first generation of migration.

Beliefs about the course and purpose of life can impact on health practices as well. The quiet acceptance of one's fate, so pervasive in Eastern philosophy, is difficult to reconcile with a commitment to preventive methods. Heroic measures to salvage life are difficult to accept when there exists a deep-rooted belief in reincarnation for example.

Additionally, in Canada there are strong beliefs about the patient's "right to know" which argue that the individual should be allowed to grieve and settle her material, emotional and spiritual concerns if her condition is terminal. However, it is widely believed in Latin America and parts of Asia that to inform a family member that they have a terminal illness is to make them lose hope. The family conspires to keep the patient in the dark about his or her illness. This situation could prove to be challenging for the health care workers in Canada, caught between a sense of duty to an individual patient and a level of respect for the beliefs of the family members. On the other hand, the family may experience considerable stress in being in conflict with the health care professional, a situation that would have likely been avoided if they were still in their home country.

The clash of health belief systems becomes much more apparent in the area of mental health. I am told by people from rural areas of Northern Africa that, in their villages, people were not institutionalized for mental illness. Every village had its "town fool" who was cared for by all. That "town fool" might even be considered shamanistic. In the absence of urbanization, the stresses that associate schizophrenia with drug abuse or antisocial behaviour, do not exist. The presence of the extended family and inherent social support networks also make provisions for a quieter reprieve from existing stresses. There is certainly not the marginalization, isolation or identification of mental illness in the same way as in our health care system. In some countries, particularly those in Latin America, psychiatric facilities are often commissioned by the state, legitimizing abuse of human rights, with political prisoners incarcerated in psychiatric facilities for so-called "treatment." Urbanization, westernization, the removal of the inherent support systems, intergenerational stresses and the effect of migration itself, subject the family unit to a higher degree of danger in terms of health and mental health. This is particularly true for refugees leaving situations where they had been incarcerated or tortured. By the same token, beliefs or stigma about the mental health care system may make access difficult.

Furthermore, beliefs about the treatment of mental illness can be at odds. Today's western psychological approach to catharsis, be it in a supportive, insight-oriented or psychoanalytic vein is often at odds that the South East Asian belief in denying or attempting to channel feelings into other outlets. Beyond being simply a difference in methods of treatment, this also shows a strong sense of denial of mental illness or dysfunction.

Health practices also cause healthshock. The use of traditional health practices for a period of time before seeking medical attention can alienate the health care provider. Expressing such alienation can, in turn, disempower the patient. People generally need to be validated for what they do. However, the more foreign or unusual the practice, the more unlikely it is to receive validation. For example, feeding one's child honey and lemon for three days before seeing the doctor for a cold is more likely to be met with approval than the Cambodian practice of "coining," in which a coin is rubbed over the skin to produce marks in an attempt to alleviate pain and other symptoms.

But to suppress or eradicate health beliefs and practices would in some ways result in a form of cultural genocide. We have only to look as far as Canada's Native peoples and their need to revitalize Native healing to see this.

### Dynamics of the Exchange

There are different models of interaction between the health care provider and the consumer. They range from the view of the provider as a patriarch, technocrat or partner in achieving health goals. For many people who have been told what to do without informed consent or without partnership in the decision making process, there is a kind of learned helplessness. They have been used to being told that they are going to have surgery rather than being told the risks and benefits involved and being allowed to choose for themselves. For providers who like to be partners, healthshock is experienced in the frustration felt at hearing the statement, "Well you're the doctor, you decide."

In many refugee camps, the Intergovernmental Committee on Migration has developed a system of mandatory immunization whereby a family's food rations are tied to their compliance with immunization for the children. In Canada, though immunization is mandatory, save for a handful of religious dissenters, the same watchdog approach does not exist. Only a form needs be completed at school entry. On the one hand it is a wonderful libertarian approach to partnership, but on the other hand, as the recent rise in measles in North America attests, there is room for improvement.

I encountered an interesting case while visiting the All India Institute of Medical Sciences in 1984, which illustrates well the advantage of the patriarchal model. A woman from an outlying village went to a gynecology clinic complaining of infertility. She and her husband had tried for a year for her to become pregnant without success. Examination revealed that her vagina ended in a pouch and that she had no uterus and no ovaries. In fact two testicles could be felt in either groin. She was actually a male. In the context of the kind of exchanges the gynecologist was accustomed to, he made the unilateral ethical decision not to tell her and simply to decree irreversible infertility. I have often thought that if she had been given the full information of her condition, it might have resulted in some psychological trauma and subsequently more difficult choices.

## Immigrant Women

In Ontario, 25 percent of women are immigrant, refugee and racial minority women. This group accesses health care services far less than the other 75 percent. Recently the Women's Health Bureau of the Ministry of Health conducted community consultations in the six health regions of the province to identify the health care needs of immigrant women. The results may show what many of us already know. Linguistic barriers keep immigrant women in isolation and keep them dependent on their spouses, family members and friends to communicate for them. Furthermore, remaining dependent can make immigrant women feel powerless in a range of cases whether communicating with an immigration officer, dealing with their family physician or seeking help if they are in an abusive or violent family situation.

Given the many factors which confront immigrant women, it is not surprising that they experience healthshock more than other groups in our society. Providing health information and services in languages other than English is part of the solution in decreasing the effects of healthshock; having community and public health care providers who are culturally-sensitive and aware is another. However, health care providers must also validate immigrant women's experiences by becoming aware of the existence of healthshock and opening their minds to the beliefs of other cultures. In this way, we can begin to break down some of the barriers to access and equality that exist in our health care system between the health care worker and the consumer of those services.

**BHOOMA BHAYANA** is a family physician working with the London Intercommunity Health Centre which primarily provides services to immigrant women. A second-generation South Asian woman, Bhooma is a former board member of the Riverdale Immigrant Women's Centre and has also worked with the South Riverdale Community Health Centre.

# Not Quite a Refuge

## Refugee Women in Canada[*]

### Christina Lee

> Thousands of refugee cases reflect the pain and suffering of
> someone disappeared or a member of the family tortured or
> killed on the streets of our beautiful country. Now I ask myself
> when will it all be over, when will we be able to live in peace
> with some freedom.
>
> — Maria Rosa Ramirez
> from Toronto's New Experiences for
> Refugee Women, an agency assisting
> Latin American refugee women

The past decades have seen a dramatic restructuring of Canadian
society. Since the Second World War, almost half a million refugees have settled in this country. In the recent years, the majority
of refugees have come from Third World countries, mostly in
Southeast Asia, Latin America and Africa. Many new refugees
arrive in Canada with little or no ability in either French or
English.

Before arriving in Canada, a refugee may have spent a period
of anywhere from six months to two years in transit from country
to country. Particularly for those from Third World countries, this
flight to asylum has been preceded by months or years of war,
persecution, and torture in their country of origin.

The physical and psychological effects of a prolonged process
of terror, migration and resettlement are well documented. The
difficulties are especially pronounced for Third World women, for
whom the sense of cultural, socio-economic and sexual dislocation is most extreme. Despite the diversity of their cultural and
socio-economic backgrounds, refugee women tend to share a

---

[*] Reprinted from *Healthsharing* vol. 9 no. 3 (Summer 1988): 14-16, with
permission of the author.

common thread of experience — that of escaping from life-threatening circumstances, and being forcefully dislocated from family and homeland. Many are widows or single parents, others are unaccompanied minors. Before arriving in Canada, many women are subject to physical and sexual violence, family separation and death, or long stays in refugee camps with little protection. There is also the "double back" effect which occurs in many cultures when the violated women are considered worthless by their own families. In addition to the loss of homeland, the physical and psychological scars of torture, violence and deprivation may make it very difficult for refugee women to adapt to their new country.

The undeniable benefits of safe political asylum, better health care and education are often largely outweighed by difficulties created by lack of language skills, relevant work experience, and problems of educational accreditation. These sobering realities are often compounded by family responsibilities, social isolation and the loss of self-esteem.

It is in this context that the plight of refugee women in a predominantly white society must be understood. Three factors define their situation. They are disadvantaged because they are women, because they are often of a different racial origin (and therefore visibly different), and because most of them come from either uneducated or highly educated backgrounds, both of which pose many employment difficulties.

A further complication arises because many of these women arrive in Canada as "sponsored class" immigrants. This entry category enforces their dependence on their sponsors, who may be their spouses, for a period of up to 10 years. During this time they are not eligible for some of the major subsidized language training (for example, the federal government language training with six month allowances), legal aid, or social assistance.

All these conditions combine to cause physical and mental health difficulties for refugee women. Depression is high among refugee women. Other stress-related problems include anxiety, psychosomatic disorders, insomnia and menstrual irregularities. These symptoms often tend to go unnoticed because of the deeply rooted reluctance to let outsiders know about personal problems. Some develop homesickness or guilt feelings at having survived and left their family behind; others resort to self-inflicted injuries or suicide. Some develop paranoia and great fears of authority as a result of escape from military governments or police states. Most women have a fear of the future, coupled with a general sense of hopelessness and helplessness. They feel that they have no control over their lives. Others are preoccupied with raising large families as a response to witnessing complete genocide.

The problems of adapting to a new society are increased by the extreme dislocation of traditional family roles. Domestic change may manifest itself in marital and other family conflicts, worry about the future, and underemployment. A recent Montreal study of Vietnamese refugees revealed sudden role reversals within families. Housewives and school children were forced to assume the role of primary economic providers, as their husbands and fathers were lamenting the loss of occupational status or properties in their homeland. Due to the time constraints of having to work several jobs outside the home, the women were progressively unable to fulfil their traditional duties of mothers and housewives. At the same time, the men were displaced from their traditional dominant role as the breadwinner of the family and were having difficulties finding jobs.

Other reports on refugees in the United States also indicate that while men tended to be most concerned with problems of finance, employment and learning the language, women were more concerned with such domestic problems as conflicts between spouses and children, and the often present threat of physical violence. The sharp contrast in women's roles between Western and non-Western cultures becomes a major stress when entry into the work force exposes the women to values that are diametrically opposed to that of their traditional cultures.

The problems of adjustment are further compounded when women move from the relative isolation of traditional home-based work to a highly socialized and industrial work force. As low-paid, nonunionized workers in such fields as the garment and service industries, they are subject to long hours, poor working conditions, and often to employers who display a flagrant disregard for occupational safety and employment standards. Illegal refugee women who fear being deported are placed in vulnerable and exploitative situations.

There are a number of barriers to refugee women seeking help from health care and social services. Many cultures attach a stigma to mental illness. Family pride and the fear of deportation prohibit the discussion of domestic and personal problems. Other barriers include a lack of familiarity with available services and the skills to access these services.

Currently, mental health needs of immigrants and refugees are served by community-based services in four relatively distinct service sectors. These include settlement agencies such as the Ontario Welcome House; multicultural or immigrant women's agencies, such as MOSAIC in Vancouver or the Calgary Immigrant Women's Centre; and ethnospecific mental health services (for example, Toronto's Hong Fook Mental Health Service for the Chinese and Southeast Asian refugees); as well as such mainstream institutions as Public Health Departments in Toronto, Vancouver and Edmonton. However, non-English-speaking refugee women seek help from community centres or immigrant women's agencies which are staffed by ethnic community workers or paraprofessionals who are sensitive to their needs.

But what happens when these women turn to health professionals for help? A 1979 study showed that if an immigrant woman approaches her doctor with complaints of nervousness, headaches and abdominal pain as a result of stress, the physician is likely to prescribe valium, sleeping pills or tranquilizers. Since most mainstream agencies or hospitals have no trained interpreters or bilingual/bicultural counsellors, the patient can generally expect to receive nothing more than medication or custodial care.

"If family violence occurs, women are further traumatized when they resort to emergency shelters," states Marilee Reimer, who researched immigrant women's use of these shelters. Since most shelters are developed for English-speaking clients, there are no trained multilingual staff. When immigrant and refugee women stay in a shelter, they are often forced into a dependent role, not being able to function or articulate their own needs. With the exception of Toronto's Shirley Samaroo Immigrant Women's Shelter, most regions of the country do not have suitable facilities with multilingual staff. In the case of sponsorship breakdown and wife assault, women are placed in extremely vulnerable situations legally and economically.

Most professionals view the mental health problems of refugee women — of all immigrant women, for that matter — in terms of adjustment difficulties created by the conflict between the women's cultural background and their new environment. Positive mental health is conceived primarily in terms of white, middle class values, such as individual fulfilment, competence and resistance to stress. This definition places the onus of blame on the individual's inability to cope with her new situation. Psychological problems of the refugee women are attributed to clash of cultures. The assumption is made that problems will be overcome once the woman and her family learn to adapt to the demands of (white, middle class) Canadian culture.

Refugee women who have been tortured have a past that is exceedingly vivid and painful. Often, professionals react to stories of torture with suspended disbelief or suspect exaggeration. Rather than discounting such important experiences, it is essential to validate them and to encourage refugee women to work at resolving their feelings. In addition to the lack of understanding of their past, most professionals tend to overlook the realities of the lives of refugee women, including language and employment barriers, and racial and sexual discrimination.

Many counselors are unable to counsel effectively because they don't understand their clients' backgrounds. There is also a shortage of professional translators. Often, interpreters are recruited from the ranks of clerical and cleaning staff. Women's husbands or children are sometimes assigned the responsibility for translating personal and family problems. It is unrealistic to expect a young child to translate the complexities of family relations, and equally unrealistic to expect the husband to objectively translate marital conflicts.

Current mainstream services are not able to serve refugees adequately. Most services are plagued with little in-service training, which if appropriately provided, would help develop the cross cultural understanding and skills of people working with refugee women. On the other hand, services which are sensitive to these women's needs, ethnospecific and immigrant women's agencies, are constantly struggling with unstable and insufficient funding. Most agencies lack adequate staffing and resources. Ethnic counselors and paraprofessionals may have the cultural sensitivity, however, they are often placed in extremely responsible and stressful positions, having to cope with crisis situations with minimal supervision and training.

Only with a concerted effort and cooperation at all levels

## WHAT CAN WE DO TO ASSIST REFUGEE WOMEN?

> Existing services must be changed and expanded to meet the needs of refugees and to accommodate to the changing multicultural reality of Canadian society.

> This improvement of services must involve both the co-ordination and development of existing resources, and the development of new services where necessary.

> Refugee clients must have equal access to all services, including multilingual outreach and information on existing services.

> There should be development and distribution of culturally-sensitive health and mental health related materials, for example, brochures and audiovisual aids.

> Present services should incorporate bilingual/bicultural professionals and the use of volunteer resources within the respective communities.

> It is important to develop culturally sensitive mental health programs for refugee women, taking into account their experiences, the need for child care, transportation and flexible hours of access.

> Alternative support structures should be developed to help compensate for the loss of the extended family. These could take the form of self-help support groups or peer counseling services. Such groups provide an opportunity for women to share common experiences and lessen their sense of social isolation, while encouraging them to make positive changes in their lives.

> It is crucial that refugee women themselves participate in the planning and development of programs, so that the mental health services offered truly reflect *their* needs and priorities.

(individual, community and institutional) can the needs of refugee women be appropriately addressed. As Sharon Rusu (from the United Nations High Commission for Refugees, Ottawa Branch) emphasizes, the needs of refugee women should be considered "as distinct from men, ... as workers and mothers, as heads of households and providers, and not exclusively as victims...; but as individuals with special roles, special strengths, and special responsibilities."

DR. CHRISTINA LEE, psychologist, is currently a Policy Analyst with the Ontario Women's Directorate. In addition she is a member of the Federal Task Force on the Mental Health of Immigrants and Refugees. The opinions expressed here are her own.

# Health Care in Crisis[*]

## Janet Maher

Is universal medicare in danger in Canada, as suggested by many of our politicians and news media? How will the North American Free Trade Agreement affect medicare in Canada, if at all?

The short answer is that the funding of health care in Canada has really been at risk ever since the passage of the Federal Hospital and Medical Insurance Acts in the early 1960s, which marked the beginning of public health insurance, or Medicare in Canada. The Acts worked by providing federal funds for provinces to pay for physician and hospital services. The North American Free Trade Agreement (NAFTA for short), threatens not only Medicare, but all the social programs Canadians have fought for years to receive and maintain.

### Medicare and Its Original Promise

Medicare, the sacred trust of Canadians, is in fact a very limited program, and has been eroded significantly over the past decade — so much so that it is unlikely to survive the current round of deficit reduction and all too likely to undergo further attacks from NAFTA.

The original vision of Medicare had two components. The first addressed the elimination of barriers to access — through a public insurance system — to all services considered medically necessary. It was anticipated that the process of eliminating the barriers would be gradual, and would eventually extend from essentially acute care services (those given by physicians, primarily in hospitals) to services such as dental work, eye care and nutritional counseling — first for children and seniors, and then for the rest of the population.

The second component involved the implementation of a

* Reprinted from *Healthsharing* vol. 14 no. 2 (Summer/Fall 1993): 10-13, 36, with permission of the author.

comprehensive public and preventive health care strategy. This includes programs like seat belts and child restraint seats in cars; effective anti-smoking, anti-drug and anti-alcohol campaigns; prenatal nutrition; population programs; and better occupational health and safety. All these programs have been shown to have a greater impact on improving the health status of Canadians and the citizens of other countries in the world.

The past three decades have witnessed some expansion in the range of services covered for some or all of the population, in one or more provinces. These include ambulance services, enhanced dental services for school children, and drug benefits for seniors and welfare recipients.

For preventive health care, however, progress has been extremely slow. While some small preventive and public health measures have been implemented in recent years (such as non-smoking areas in public places and helmet laws for motorcyclists) they are generally quite limited, not very seriously enforced, and have rarely been accompanied by the kind of public education which might lead to changes in behaviour. Although each provincial and territorial health budget reserves some funds for public and/or preventive initiatives, the amount generally accounts for a fraction of one percent of the total. In other words, what we spend health money on is illness care, not health care.

In the climate of economic growth and liberal social and political ideology of the 60s and 70s, governments were relatively content to spend on health infrastructure (modern hospitals, research facilities, labs and clinics) and health services. Until the late 70s few politicians or citizens were seriously concerned whether the responsibility for funding health care or other social programs was federal or provincial. Established Programs Financing, the original federal-provincial cost-sharing mechanism, ensured relatively open-ended funding to provinces. It was the Canada Health Act, passed after several years of funding erosions at the federal level, that attempted to ensure that provinces spent federal health care funds for health care alone. Passed in 1984, the Canada Health Act allowed the federal government to reduce transfer payments to any provinces that increased access barriers to a number of specified areas — generally acute care in hospitals.

The Canada Health Act is largely considered the bible on

Medicare in Canada, because it enshrines five principles for continued federal funding:

- *Universality* — Health care must be available to all residents of Canada, on uniform terms and conditions.
- *Accessibility* — Health care must be reasonably available to all residents of Canada close to where they live and work and without direct or indirect charges or other impediments.
- *Comprehensiveness* — Every province insures a full range of services for all residents as required.
- *Portability* — Coverage of health care services extends across Canada.
- *Public Administration* — Our health care system is administered and operated on a non-profit basis.

Although the Act was not perfect, it did lead fairly quickly to the elimination of balance billing or extra billing by physicians. Seniors' and social benefits recipients' access to drug benefit programs increased, and home care and long-term care services were extended, making community care cost-effective. But a working-poor adult with a bad toothache could expect little relief until an abscess or major dental crisis landed her in hospital. Incentives to corporations to be more respectful of the environment or occupational health and safety remained low. For many Canadians, especially Native people, people of colour, the poor and immigrants, the system has been less than universal and accessible. And a further decade of restraint budgets at the federal level have resulted in a chipping away at social programs which are even less able to meet the needs of Canadians already marginalized by the system, to say nothing of ensuring equity of access to all Canadians in 1993.

This erosion coincides with the aging of post-war baby boomers. By the year 2000 nearly a quarter of our population will be over the age of 60. While the majority can anticipate several good years after that age, advances in technology have raised our expectations of good health in our later years. If those expectations are to be fulfilled, we will need to have the resources for ensuring access *for all* to costly technology. The "cost-cutting" alternative will be increasing limitations on accessibility to those who are poorer, older, sicker or otherwise marginalized.

As federal politicians hasten to insist, direct federal health care spending has so far not been cut — only the rate of increase in spending has been reduced or frozen. To assist provinces in paring down their budgets, Federal Health and Welfare Minister Benoit Bouchard hosted a meeting of Federal-Provincial Ministers of Health, in June 1991. The provinces have responded in various ways, from de-insuring some services and procedures, placing caps on others, and introducing deductibles, co-payment fees, or user contributions.

Restructuring has already resulted in job loss, primarily of support workers: predominantly lower-paid female nursing assistants and ward aides. It has also meant a shift to more part-time and casual work in home care and attendant care services. Bed closures, particularly in smaller prairie and northern towns, threaten whole communities.

The new found interest of many provinces in community-based care options for seniors, people with disabilities and chronic psychiatric patients is ironic. Given the cost containment objectives of health administrators, many current and potential patients and their traditional caregivers, namely mothers, daughters and sisters, have reason for distrust. As acute and chronic care institutions reduce the number of beds or close down altogether, more and more of the burden will fall on women — many of whom are already caring for children to whom our child care system is woefully inadequate.

Furthermore, the declining role of the federal government in financing, regulating and supporting innovative new programs burdens poor and other marginal Canadians, and makes it easier for middle and higher income earners to lose interest in how universal health care is. Those with secure finances will be less and less likely to imagine themselves ever being recipients of government financed health care.

Universal family allowances have disappeared, to be replaced by a "targeted" children's benefit. Unemployment insurance coverage has been reduced and will be unavailable to the increasing numbers of contract workers. Not only has the federal government withdrawn funding for unemployment insurance, its own commitment to training now comes from unemployment insurance premiums paid by employers and employees — funds reserved for those eligible for or in receipt of unemployment insurance benefits.

Moreover, in spite of the rhetoric about the need for a more educated populace, cuts to student aid in the post-secondary sector have effectively shut the door to many promising young people. Those students who can come up with the money to support themselves are faced with overcrowded classrooms where it can be a challenge even to find a space to sit.

Two other disturbing developments deserve notice. The first is a substantial expansion of the use of private health care insurance to make up for service gaps. Particularly in the decade of AIDS, and other chronic conditions requiring costly intervention, there have been few incentives or sanctions for private insurers who disqualify potential users on the basis of certain risks or risk behaviours. At the same time, much of the middle class, or at least those still in relatively secure employment, are turning to private insurance as a back up to the deteriorating services, hoping that private insurance will cover them if they should need costly hospital technology.

The second distressing change has been the opening and expansion of a range of commercial services outside the publicly insured system. Some of these are licensed and regulated. Others include a growing number of unregulated and largely unevaluated counseling therapies related to such issues as eating behaviours or violence and incest survivor therapy, which are available only to those prepared to pay.

## So What About Free Trade?

The Canada-US Free Trade Agreement, implemented following the November 1988 federal election, was significantly more comprehensive than any previous trade arrangement. Although Medicare was formally exempt under the Agreement, Chapter 14 on Commercial Services outlined a number of exceptions to the exemption. These exceptions included a broad range of hospital and health care management services, like general rehabilitation and extended care hospitals; nursing homes; drug and alcohol treatment facilities; homes for physically and mentally disabled, and children in need of care and protection; ambulance services; home care; public health clinics; medical and radiology labs; and blood banks.

The basic provision of the 1989 Agreement allows US firms the same access to the commercialized or privatized market as

Canadian firms. While there has not been a great increase in commercialization since the agreement, the seeds have been sown for the takeover of hospital laundry and housekeeping, dietary, and security services by large US-based multinationals.

As Colleen Fuller of the B.C. Health Sciences Association noted in her presentation to the Commons hearings in the fall of 1992 on NAFTA, "private laboratories, walk-in medical clinics and various kinds of treatment facilities have sprung up like weeds in major cities across the country."

She goes on to suggest that the only reason US corporations have not moved in to the Canadian health system on a massive scale is that the Canada Health Act has acted as an effective barrier. However, as federal funding declines — at the current rate, Quebec will no longer receive federal cash transfers after 1996, Ontario will lose federal funds in 1998 and no province will be entitled by 2005 — the incentive to uphold the principles of Medicare will disappear.

Since the Free Trade Agreement came into effect, pharmaceuticals and medical devices industry have grown enormously. Encouraged by the first federal extension of drug patents and interest-free government loans and grants, a number of drug and biotechnology firms have put big money into new plant capacity in Canada.

### And What about NAFTA?

While we are led by supporters to believe that the North American Free Trade Agreement is simply an extension of the Canada-US Agreement to include Mexico, the reality is much more troublesome. Whereas the Canada-US Agreement addressed issues within the jurisdictions of the two national governments, NAFTA will eventually bind provincial and municipal levels of government to its rules.

NAFTA sets up a process to review public services that, because of existing laws, are excluded from the agreement. By the end of 1998, all exclusions in the areas of community, social and professional services, as well as health and education, will be examined to determine the extent to which they constitute indirect subsidies to Canadian traders. This whole examination will take place, not in our national, provincial or state legislatures, but by a closed tribunal with representatives appointed by the three governments. It is also worrisome to note that the deadline corresponds to a time when provinces will be struggling to cope with the final withdrawal of federal funds. The most likely result will be the further stripping of provincial health plans. The need for any review at all may well be pre-empted by the provinces themselves.

And if the Bill C-22 extension of drug patents from four to ten years were not enough to boost drug manufacturers profits, the Mulroney government's Bill C-91, which further extends patents for up to 20 years should have brand name manufacturers laughing all the way to the bank.

What the patent laws really do is give the brand name producer a full 20 years before the "recipe" for the drug becomes public property and can be used by a generic manufacturer even if it is only marginally different from another. It is hard to see how this will not mean astronomical drug prices — and the end of drug benefit plans delivered by most provinces.

Under the implementation procedure, all three federal governments must pass and proclaim the NAFTA legislation before it comes into effect on January 1, 1994. In Canada, the legislation has already passed both the House of Commons and the Senate. As of July 15, 1993, proclamation is still required for Canada to be bound by the terms of the Agreement. It is anticipated that passage in Mexico will not be a problem, but the situation in the United States is less and less certain. President Bill Clinton has indicated that accompanying its passage in the US Houses of Congress will be side agreements on labour and environmental standards. Even with those agreements, it is by no means clear that the deal will get congressional assent. In late June 1993, environmental activists secured a US court decision requiring an environmental impact assessment before the legislation passes the House of Representatives. If this court ruling stands, it is unlikely that the assessment will be completed within the required time frame.

## Can We Save Medicare?

Medicare, presumably the most sacred of the sacred trusts of social programs, has been eroded in such a piecemeal way that it is now difficult to restore as a national program. It has become even more challenging to move to the second phase of public and preventive strategies that hold so much promise for reducing our overall costs through maintaining a healthy population.

There is probably no question that women, as the lower income earners and those still socially responsible for the care of children and elders, have benefited from government policy initiatives like pay equity and affirmative action, and from transfer payments which make possible the expenditures on social programs. And so, it is no surprise that women have the largest stake in supporting Medicare and the allied range of social programs.

Although the situation looks bleak, we still have superior health care provision for virtually the whole Canadian population while spending less than 10 percent of our Gross Domestic Product (GDP). According to the General Accounting Office of the United States, it takes 14 percent of US GDP to provide very uneven levels of service to some 30 million Americans.

The reform of health care in Canada is long past due. But what we should be defending is not simply a system of illness care against "deficit fighters" and commercial interests. Community-based care need not be undertaken as a cost-containment measure, but as a legitimate option with adequate support systems and professional, well paid staff, in safe and comfortable working conditions. Investment in preventive and public health measures is every bit as important to the health status of Canadians as investment in new drugs and high-technology medical devices.

**JANET MAHER** has been active in the women's movement since 1968. Her interests are primarily in the areas of social policy, social planning and health care.

*section three*

# The Politics of
# Work and Health

A feminist perspective on health seeks to link work and health. Making such a link involves outlining ways in which Canadian capitalism has structured women's economic and social position. Moreover, this link forces us to acknowledge how race, class, disability, age and sexual orientation structure different women's experiences with health.

The articles in this section explore the relationship between work and health. Susan Wortman's "The Unhealthy Business of Making Clothes" documents how the organization of garment work impacts on workers' health. She points out that workplace health is affected by the design of machines, workspace and the work process. Thus workplace health issues include both issues of chemical and physical hazards as well as issues such as ventilation, heat, noise, the pace of work and job sex-typing. In "The All Pervasive Ache," Linda Lounsberry demonstrates that workplace health issues, such as the design of machines and the work process also characterize clerical and office workers. Lounsberry discusses the effect of fast-paced, repetitive clerical work on her health.

However, as the articles by Karen Weisberg, Joanne Doucette and Cathleen Kneen suggest, the impact of work on health goes beyond our workplaces. Karen Weisberg's "Board Games: Sexist Bias at the Workers' Compensation Board" raises the issue of how workplace injuries are dealt with in Canada, especially in relation to the work that women do. She analyzes the institutionalized sexism of the Workers' Compensation Board and its impact on the lives of women. Joanne Doucette's "Welfare: Far from Well" links poverty and health, and demonstrates that poor people have less access to the health care system while having higher health risks. In "Women and the Food System," Cathleen Kneen discusses how capitalism has transformed our control over the food system by industrializing not only the production and distribution of food, but also its consumption.

# The Unhealthy Business of Making Clothes[*]

## Susan Wortman

Imagine you work in a men's clothing factory. You sit all day bent over a sewing machine, putting collars on coats. You don't make the collars, or assemble the coats, just stitch the collars onto the coats at a rate of twenty per hour. You have to do at least that many, or you are let go, and you try to do more, because you are paid by the piece. You dread the rush season, because you start at 7:00 in the morning and you don't stop until 7:00 at night, but you pray that you aren't laid off when it is slow. The lighting is poor; you often leave work with a headache. The heat is oppressive. The girl across from you put a needle through her finger yesterday. The boss wanted her to go to the hospital alone. You can see how the older people are bent and stiff; you wonder if you will look like that in thirty years.

Many garment workers across Canada do not have to imagine this. It is their work, their life. There are 115,000 garment workers in Canada, concentrated in Montreal, Toronto and Winnipeg. Most of these workers are immigrant women. They work in an industry which has a history of intolerable working conditions, excessively long hours and extremely low wages.

Summer is the worst. We are making winter coats. They are heavy and hot and the dust from the coats flies around. There is just one fan for the whole factory (50 people). When we open the windows, the dust blows up from the coats. Or if there is no

* Reprinted from *Healthsharing* vol. 1 no. 1 (Winter 1979): 12-14, with permission of the author.

wind, no air blows in. We joke about getting air conditioning some day.

Women who work in hot, poorly ventilated shops sometimes faint from heat exhaustion. They suffer constantly from the effects of heat stress — headaches, fatigue, apathy, irritability. Some shops remain dark and dingy. However, even in those which are more brightly lit, lights may be poorly positioned, causing glare and shadows. Fatigue and eye strain results from trying to work in these conditions. Noise is a problem in many shops. While the levels are not high enough to cause hearing loss, the women working in a continually noisy environment get headaches, are fatigued and have other stress-related conditions.

There are also less well-recognized physical hazards. Some shop floors actually vibrate when all the machines are being used. This "whole body vibration" can cause nausea, disorientation, an inability to focus properly and chronic lower back pain. Women who operate button and button-holing machines experience local vibration of their fingers and hands which may result in wearing the smooth cartilage of the joints, contributing to osteoarthritis.

Noise and vibration can both be reduced by better designed and properly mounted machines.

Old, defective machines may present electrical hazards. One woman explained how she now sits on cushions to "protect" herself from shocks she received through her chair. Fire is an everpresent danger in an industry with combustible goods, fabric dust in the air and sparking from old electrical machinery.

### Unhealthy Design
The garment industry is rife with problems in the design of machines and tools, workspace and work process. (In the jargon of occupational health, these are referred to as "ergonomic" hazards.)

For example, the work of making a garment has been divided into jobs that require continual standing (pressers), or sitting (sewing machine operators). At certain times of the year, the pressure of production prohibits even a momentary rest to sit or walk around to ease weary or cramped muscles. Standing for hours at a stretch results in pooling of blood in the veins of the lower legs, leading to edema (swelling) of the feet and ankles.

Many women develop varicose veins. Many of the jobs that involve constant standing could be performed, at least in part, seated.

Any knowledge of comfortable and healthy seating design is sadly neglected in this industry. Women sit, all day, on hard, cheap chairs, piled with pillows to cushion and/or raise themselves to the proper workspace height. Adjustable chairs with adequate back support and cushioned surfaces are essential in any industry where workers are seated for most of the day.

Poor design is evident in foot-pedal sewing machine controls which are overly sensitive: "Practically a touch on the pedal makes the needle move very fast. This is how accidents happen. You have to be concentrating all the time." Operators have frequent hand and finger injuries. Puncture wounds from needles are not uncommon. These injuries are often belittled — the potential for serious infection ignored. Many cutting tools are designed such that the blade guards hamper the speed and ease of the task. Because of the pressure for rapid production the guards may be lifted, resulting in serious cuts.

Sewing shears are designed for the "average" male hand, and are therefore frequently too large for women. They must grip the shears tightly, causing the handles to cut into the flesh. This restricts circulation and causes numb or tingling fingers. Knee controls on sewing machines cause bruising of soft thigh tissue unless they are properly padded.

Innovative design has not been neglected everywhere in the garment industry. In the interests of increasing productivity, work processes have been restructured, often resulting in new ergonomic problems. The Ettron Line is an example. By this system, the partly finished garments are delivered automatically to the side of the sewing machine operator via overhead racks. She now must work constantly without her usual pauses to get or deliver garments, thereby depriving her of a stretch, a rest and a sense of accomplishment. In addition, she is isolated from her fellow workers by the rack of clothing surrounding her. She sees nothing, and hears only the repeated smack of each new article as it arrives at her side. Cramped muscles and fatigue are obviously not the only results of this new process. Isolation, speed-up and the elimination of visible goals are destructive to the emotional and psychological well-being of the garment worker.

## Manipulation and Dehumanization Equals Stress

Job sex-typing is evident in the garment industry. Cutters (using vibrating cutting tools) are almost invariably men, while choppers (using shears) are usually women. In most shops sewing machine operators and finishers are women. There is no physical rationale for this segregation. The "male" jobs are better paid than the "female" jobs.

The attitude that women are working just "for frills" or extras is also prevalent on the shop floor. In coat factories men as well as women operate sewing machines. Men are often given the easier, faster styles by the (male) foreman.

The women are aware of, and resent, this kind of discrimination. Stressful tensions, frustrations and suppressed anger can result in physical health problems such as ulcers, muscular tension, migraine headaches and high blood pressure. This situation also hinders all workers, male and female, from fighting together for better working conditions and pay.

In the modern garment industry, the creative job of making an article of clothing has been subdivided into many comparatively simple tasks. Because of this, the owner is able to hire people for very low wages, and underutilize their skills (and discourage acquisition of new ones). The worker has little control then, as she may be fired and easily replaced from the large pool of unemployed workers. In addition, because of this division of labour, the work is made repetitive and dull. The worker is seen as unskilled and ignorant. The paternalistic attitude evident in many shops is indicative of this concept of the worker. These attitudes promote feelings of inferiority and dissatisfaction in women, who in other aspects of their lives are seen as competent, worthy adults.

I like piece work because you can make more money [than on hourly wage].

Do you work faster on piece work?

Yes, I get more tired, but I make more money. The older people don't make so much money because they can't run so fast. But it is still better for them on piece work.

Piece work *means* rapid production. It comes under the guise of allowing the worker to go her own pace, but in practice, she will work as fast as she can, to earn as much money as possible. The hourly wages are kept low, so that the piece rate system is attractive. The physically exhausting pace promoted by the piece rate system results in chronic fatigue, high tension (nervous breakdowns are not uncommon) and, according to a British Columbia study, an increased rate of stomach ulcers.

The majority of the workers prefer piece work. The need and desire to earn a decent wage overrides comfort and health considerations. Most garment workers accept the ideology that the "good (fast) worker" is rewarded by the piece rate system. They believe that having the same hourly wage for all will lower their individual take-home pay. This keeps them from uniting to fight for a decent hourly wage and work pace.

## Chemical Hazards

The garment industry is not usually considered as having chemical hazards. Yet harmful dyes have always been used in clothing manufacture and a host of new chemicals has been introduced in recent years.

For example, beta-napthylamine and benzidine dyes, still widely used in the industry, are absorbed through the skin. They cause bladder cancers that do not appear for 10-15 years after exposure. Styrene and chloroprene are sprayed on edges of cloth to prevent ravelling. Both cause dermatitis (skin rash); chloroprene is a respiratory tract irritant and a suspected cancer causing agent. Benzene, known to cause leukemia (a blood cancer) can be found as a solvent or a contaminant in leather glue.

Some chemicals and fabrics produce allergic reactions in workers:

> One girl opposite me, she puts bandages on each finger every morning. I asked her, "Why do you do that?" and she showed me the skin rash all over her hands from the mohair.

> Can she ask for different material to work with?

> Yes, but she likes mohair best because it is so light (weight) and

fast. She can make more coats and more money. We all like mohair even if we are always itchy.

In addition to chemicals used in the work process, pesticides are frequently used to control rodents and insects. Among the many effects of the different classes of pesticides are nervous excitation, tremors, seizures, dizziness, vomiting and drowsiness. To minimize worker exposure to these chemicals spraying should be done on weekends, and the shop well aired.

In the past century in Canada, garment workers have led intermittent struggles for better working conditions. And yet, most workplaces remain unhealthy and unsafe. This is at least partly due to the structure of the industry itself. The 19th-century free enterprise model of small, family-run shops still characterizes garment manufacturing today. The high level of competition, both nationally and internationally, make it a cutthroat business.

In this context industry owners prosper by abusing the workers — by keeping wages low and minimizing expenditures in the factory.

The garment industry has traditionally employed immigrant women who are least able to fight for their rights. Their natural insecurity in a new country with a new language is played upon. They may be subtly or not so subtly intimidated. The fear and threat of deportation is ever-present.

Although 40 percent of the garment industry is unionized, the trade union organization parallels that of the industry itself: small craft unions competitive amongst themselves. The relatively weak unions that result are less capable of, or willing to, wage major struggles for pay and working conditions.

The workers, however, are not helpless in the face of this situation. One example of increasing awareness of health problems and activity towards improving conditions is a Toronto-based ad hoc committee. Their concern with health conditions in the garment industry has resulted in meetings with workers and a garment workers' health and safety newsletter. The committee has drawn people from different trade unions, though it operates without formal union support.

It is clear that much must be done to improve working conditions in the garment industry. It will be a difficult struggle for the right to an industry that is free from dehumanizing work practices and an unhealthy and unsafe work environment.

**Note**
Thanks to Nancy Price-Munn for her help with this article.

SUSAN WORTMAN is an occupational health researcher at the Humber College Centre for Labour Studies and is a member of Women Healthsharing.

# The All Pervasive Ache[*]

## Linda Lounsberry

For the past nine years I have sat glued to a video display terminal (VDT) at least seven hours a day. On the good days I enjoy what I do; on the bad days I notice most the dryness in my eyes, the ache along my spine, the deadness in my buttocks, the fatigue in my limbs, the never easing pressure in my brain and my hands to achieve more and more speed.

When I arrive at work, I pick up jobs and take the work into a cubicle seven feet by seven feet. There I spend the rest of the day sitting on a hard chair, eyes on paper, fingers on keyboard. The walls of the cubicle extend only part way to the ceiling, so I hear all the other machines in addition to the one on which I'm working. The cubicle itself is impersonal; the walls are covered with coding information and we're not allowed to put up our own decorations.

The most obvious problem of my occupation is my back. I don't remember what it was like when my back didn't hurt. Sitting in the same position for long stretches of time on a padless chair that gives no support, I know why I am in pain.

I researched chairs that give the kind of support I need. I gave my employer some brochures and prices; he gave me permission to get one — if I paid for it. The prices for these chairs start at $250.00 and I would have to share it with a worker on another shift.

I go to a chiropractor regularly so my back doesn't get much worse than it is already. I also try to work-out in the gym or swim every chance I can to counteract the effects of sitting still for such long periods of time. Even so, I am young enough that I am going to be at this job for quite a few years to come, and it worries me that my back might not hold out. After years of training I have a

* Reprinted from *Healthsharing* vol. 6 no. 3 (Summer 1985): 23, with permission of the author.

hard time imagining working at anything else, yet I need to support myself in some way.

My sore back isn't the only complaint I have about typesetting. I suffer from eyestrain, especially if I have worked overtime. I work a *lot* of overtime.

Most of what I do is very precise and close work with a lot of pressure and deadlines. Some of the print I have to work from is small enough to require a magnifying glass. Sometimes my eyes get so sore that the letters seem to jump up at me from the screen, and the room spins. Then I get a headache. This usually happens when I work more than seven hours without a break.

I have read articles written on safety and VDT operators, and I have to laugh! We should have a 10 minute break every hour, the articles say; I'm lucky to get a lunch-break. I try to sneak coffee breaks between jobs, but that can be tricky since we have to account for all of our time at work. Our unpaid half-hour lunch break comes right at the legal maximum time without a break, so there is no time allotted for coffee breaks.

My sore back and eye-strain are easy to identify as side effects of my job. Others are more difficult to identify. Working under such intense pressure is apt to cause side effects of sorts. Where I work, high productivity is demanded and mistakes are not tolerated. There are no excuses for anything. If I had *any* contact with a poorly completed job, if an error is my fault, I am in trouble; if it is not my fault, I am still in trouble. The fact that I have just worked 11 hours is never reason enough for making mistakes or for slowing down. "If you can't take the heat — get out of the kitchen," is a common reply to complaints when being tired and overworked have affected my or co-workers' productivity.

The strictness of working in a sweatshop has stifled my spirit considerably. The pressure never lets up and often with the pressure operators find management peering over their shoulders. I won't be fired over an error or two in a job, but the increased harassment and pressure on anyone who makes even infrequent mistakes takes its own toll. The emotional stress means I'm reluctant to stand up for myself. I attempt to meet expectations in speed and accuracy — no matter how unreasonable I think they are — in part because I don't want to make waves. I know I add to the unreasonableness of the job by staying quiet, but many times I would do almost anything just to be left alone with my work.

I always fear that the one day I allow myself to work when I am at low energy, and therefore make mistakes, will plague me for months. So on days when I wake up a bit tired, I load up on chocolate and coffee to give me enough "hype" to get through the day. Of course, I don't allow myself to do this for many days in a row, yet I still worry that my loading up on coffee is a problem. Even trying not to work mostly on artificial energy, I know that I and most other typesetters I know are among the heavy coffee drinkers. If I drink a lot of coffee, its very hard on my body; if I don't, it can increase stress with my boss — either way, side effects on the job.

It is next to impossible not to let the hype and pressure from work affect my personal life. I get off work on Friday evenings wanting to go home and relax and find that I am still "flying high" from work. It takes me at least two days of the weekend to unwind long enough to settle down to being myself and calm enough to relate to people at a human level. By then it is Sunday night and I start getting hyped up again. Needless to say, the three weeks holiday a year I get are very important for my sanity.

One would wonder why someone would continue working at a job that risks both her mental and physical health. I do it mainly for the money — although, as I said before, I do enjoy the work. What else could I do, without having finished university, where I can make good money, afford to travel, and have good job security. I find comfort in knowing that a steady income is there, and that if I decided to quit I could get another job in another typesetting sweatshop. Financial self-sufficiency is a priority to me and being a typesetter, although hurting my health some, allows me that.

I realize I will have to take a break from typesetting at some point to give my body a chance to rest, but hopefully I will have saved enough money to afford it comfortably.

**LINDA LOUNSBERRY** makes her living in Toronto working as a typesetter. She has also been a long-time volunteer with *Healthsharing*.

# Board Games

## Sexist Bias at the Workers' Compensation Board[*]

### Karen Weisberg

Loretta is a 63-year-old worker who now lives in a small Ontario town. She was employed for most of her adult life in the print-ing industry. In the 1970s Loretta developed chronic dermatitis on her hands as a result of exposure to chemicals in her work-place. She filed a claim with the Ontario Workers' Compensa-tion Board (WCB). The WCB initially agreed that her injury was work related and awarded her disability benefits. In 1982, her benefits were terminated. She appealed the decision but her appeal was denied at the lower levels of the appeal process. Finally in 1985 she appeared before the Appeal Board. This is an excerpt from the transcript of that hearing. Loretta was questioned by three male panel members.

Panel: Do you have any problem taking care of the house?

Loretta: I don't do dishes because I have a dishwasher, and I don't wash floors. I'm not to put my hands in water, so I don't.

Panel: Seems to me I've had help around the house that told me the same thing.

Panel Chairman: A typical cleaning lady reference.

Panel: Including a wife.

Loretta: I don't do windows either.

Panel: I don't think you're unique in that. Now, I have to ask you a question that you might think is ungallant, but how old are you?

(Not only do the Appeal Board panel members address her by

[*] Reprinted from *Healthsharing* vol. 9 no. 4 (Fall 1988): 25-8, with permission of the author.

her first name, but they also carefully question her on the nature of the work she has done for 26 years.)

Panel: Now, would you classify yourself as an unskilled plant worker?

Loretta: Well ...

Panel: You're not a carpenter, lathe operator, somebody that has long training and skill. You don't have any special skills at this time? You're not a bricklayer, you're not a carpenter ...

Loretta: I always worked in printing. I was a skilled machine operator. Is that what you mean?

Injured workers and their advocates frequently describe the experience of dealing with the massive bureaucracy of the WCB as "crazymaking." Most workers experience endless delays in the processing of their benefits, the fallout from inconsistent policies, and insensitive treatment. Women claimants experience additional hardships and indignities because they are women. The institutionalized sexism at the WCB has an impact on the lives of women in significant and subtle ways.

The workers' compensation system was originally established in Ontario in 1915. Based on employer contributions, it is designed to insure workers against "lost income" due to work-related injury or disease. Workers no longer have to prove in court that a work accident resulted from employer negligence. This no-fault system was a giant step forward for workers. However, there are many problems with the legislation, including definitions of who is covered under the Act and the types of injuries recognized as work-related. The devaluing of women's work render these problems particularly harsh for women. In addition, the establishment of a legal system which relies heavily (in practice) on the judgements of the medical establishment holds particular risks for women.

## Household Injuries
Industry propaganda frequently reminds us that the workplace is safer than the home. For most women, the home is our workplace, or at least one of them. The hazards of housework, including toxic fumes, injuries due to falls, and the stress due to the constant

demands of child care have been well documented. Although the economy is dependent on this invisible and largely unpaid work-force, women who work in the home are not protected under the Workers' Compensation Act (WCA). Most of us who work out-side the home still bear primary responsibility for housework and child care; we work a "double day." If we are injured on the "second shift," at home, and can't return to our paid employment, we are not eligible for compensation benefits. We must cope with the loss of income, rely on employer sick leave plans or apply for social assistance.

In fact, the possibility of "household" injury often becomes a major issue in determining a WCB claim. Adjudicators are careful to determine exactly where an injury occurred. If there is a suspicion that a woman injured herself while bending to do the laun-dry instead of at her place of paid employment, the adjudicators will rule that she not be compensated. This is clearly the "correct" decision according to the legislation; injuries incurred in the course of "housework" are not compensated. This is a powerful social statement on the value of housework and on society's view of "women's work."

The issue of housework surfaces in another form at the WCB. Janet was called to an appointment at the WCB in order to determine the extent of her disability. Her short medical assess-ment by a WCB doctor was followed by an interview with an adjudicator. In the course of her interview, she was asked if she was able to do "housework." She hesitated before answering. In fact, it was extremely difficult for her to carry out household work, but she had no choice. No one in her family helped out, and her home was a matter of pride for her, a reflection of herself. "Yes," she told the adjudicator, she did housework. The adjudi-cator noted this "inconsistency of complaint" and recommended that benefits be terminated since she was obviously not totally disabled.

Women are damned if they do and damned if they don't ... do the housework. In another case, Marlene had established a claim for psychological disability as the result of an injury and was being reassessed at the end of a two-year period. It was noted in her record that she reported being unable to do housework and that she spent part of the day "lying on the couch." The adjudi-cator noted that the worker sought increased help from her husband. This was interpreted as maintaining a "sick role" for the purposes of "secondary gain," not as a legitimate work-related psychological disability.

## Coverage Under the Act

> Leanna works by sewing at home. She has an industrial sewing machine set up in her basement. The contractor for whom she works brings her loads of pieces to sew. Some of the materials are very dusty and the lint from the cloth is everywhere in her house. The lighting is poor and after many hours her eyes are very sore. Sometimes she wishes she could go out to work but, at least, she says, this way she can care for her two preschoolers whose demands she must balance with the ever present pile of sewing to complete.

Laura Johnson in her book *Seam Allowance*[1] has documented the plight of homeworkers who are a particularly vulnerable part of the women's workforce. Immigrant women who sew garment pieces in their own homes for contractors form an invisible part of the garment industry. They often endure dangerous working conditions and long hours. Many try to combine child care responsibilities with homework. Dust, bad lighting and stress are serious problems for the workers. But, because they do the work in their own homes and on their own equipment, they are not protected under the Workers' Compensation Act.

Women who work in other people's homes have only recently been included under the Act. In 1985, major amendments to the WCA extended coverage to new categories of workers — the "cleaner," the "housekeeper," the "nanny." For the first time, women employed in traditional women's work were eligible for benefits (provided that they worked at least 24 hours per week at this paid work). This is an important reform but it remains to be seen how many domestic workers will actually file claims. Many domestic workers are immigrants, dependent on their employers for their immigration status as well as for a place to live. How many can risk conflict with their employer without the protection of a union or support organization?

## Stress and the WCB

Laura is a telephone operator with 12 years of service. Like her co-workers, she has experienced the sense of total lack of control over her work. Electronic monitoring, machine pacing and management style have been sources of acute stress. Several years ago, Laura began to suffer from a disabling psychological condition diagnosed as "clinical depression," causing her to miss several months of work. With the help of her union, she filed a claim for benefits at the WCB. The appeal was heard before the Workers' Appeal Tribunal in December 1986. By the fall of 1988, no decision had been reached.

Work-based stress tends to be stereotyped as the problem of the high-powered male executive, responsible for millions of dollars and hundreds of employees. The stress that accompanies traditional women's work — especially the "helping professions" or those performing highly routine, high-speed tasks — is largely ignored or trivialized. A disability such as that experienced by Laura, is often not even acknowledged to be stress-based. The WCB does not recognize stress claims per se. In order to establish a claim for psychological disability, a worker must prove that the disability resulted from an organic injury or relates to an organic injury. Thus, a major occupational injury resulting from the work that women do has not been compensated. Laura has challenged this interpretation of the WCA. She has argued that her injury is serious and work related and that she should be compensated.

### Sexist Bias
Sexism can preclude the recognition of a stress-based claim, even when the stress does result from an organic injury.

Rena was a food service worker who sustained a back injury. She was seeking to establish a psychological disability resulting from her organic injury. As part of her assessment she was sent to the WCB's Hospital and Rehabilitation Centre where she was assessed by a series of WCB doctors and consultants. The report of one of the WCB doctors described Rena as a "normally developed, generously nourished white female who looks her 39 years. She wears a perpetual frown and speaks with a long-suffering whine of perpetual misery." The conclusion was that her psychological problems were unrelated to the work incident.

Sexual harassment is also a source of stress which has not been recognized by the WCB. In a precedent-setting case in 1985, the Quebec WCB recognized sexual harassment as a work-related injury. The Quebec board held that sexual harassment had resulted in an occupational injury to the worker, including extreme stress, depression and physical symptoms caused by sexual harassment. In an Ontario case, Bonnie Robichaud, a Department of National Defence worker, filed a lost-time accident claim of stress resulting from sexual harassment she had endured at work. The decision in this case is pending.

### Women and the Psychiatric Assessment

Workers have access to their own WCB files. However, it can be a very disturbing experience for a worker to read her medical and WCB reports. She may feel that she has had a conversation with a very sympathetic adjudicator, only to find in his report references to her evident "overreaction," "hysterical nature" and "exaggeration of injury." Many women who are attempting to establish psychological claims meet face to face with the basic misogyny of the medical and psychiatric professions.

The WCB perpetuates the exclusive use of medical-psychiatric systems for women in need of psychological support. WCB benefit coverage, like OHIP (Ontario Health Insurance Plan), does not include women-centred services or feminist counseling programs. Women who want or need psychological help have no option but to use what the WCB makes available.

### Who's Minding the Kids?

Luisa spent two hours on the phone trying to find someone who could explain why her benefits were being cut. Finally the anonymous voice at the WCB told her to just come down to the Board and see someone. They'll answer all your questions. Without her full benefits, Luisa could no longer afford her babysitter. So with a baby and a three-year-old in tow, she set out for the WCB office. She went to the designated area and

waited in the small seating space. Injured workers moved un-
easily in the uncomfortable chairs; others paced the floor.
Luisa's children grew restless and began to whine. The baby
was tired and Luisa's shoulder injury made it exhausting to hold
him. She was tense. She didn't want the children disturbing
injured workers or the WCB staff. Finally someone called her
name. Then there was a further wait to find someone to speak
to her in her own language. By then Luisa's anger at the unex-
plained loss of her full benefits and the tension of trying to
control the children in a formal setting surfaced. The WCB
officer saw her as uncooperative and argumentative. He explained that her benefits had been cut because she no longer met
the criteria of a totally disabled claimant.

This was the beginning of an appeal process which would
take months to complete. Luisa left the office, overwhelmed by
what lay ahead in a panic about money and exhausted from the
ordeal with the children. At some point, Luisa, like other workers, will probably be ordered to the WCB Hospital and Rehabilitation Centre for assessment. This is mandatory; refusal results
in termination of benefits. Who would look after the children?
That was her problem.

In myriad ways, the institution has an affect on the real
day-to-day lives of women and children. Attending appointments
and often waiting hours at the WCB accompanied by young
children makes a stressful interview even more difficult. (In early
1988, the WCB reorganized services in the central offices, combin-
ing claims, pensions and rehabilitation into single units in a effort
to improve efficiency and case coordination. Hopefully this will
cut down on the excessive waiting time required of injured workers.) Hundreds of women share these experiences, yet no emergency child care funds exist; there is no supervised child care area
for use by clients.

## The Emotional Work

Ann stayed at home to take care of the children. From the day
her husband injured his right arm and shoulder at work, their
lives changed. First there was the immediate loss of income. It
took several tense weeks before details of the claim were sorted

out. They began to receive benefits. Her husband was in a great deal of pain. He didn't have to be hospitalized, but required a lot of help and encouragement. She wanted the children to understand and to be especially well behaved. As time went by, her husband grew more depressed and irritable. Money was short, and she had to stretch meals and children's clothing. Her husband's employer grew impatient. Since there is no law forbidding it, the employer decided to fire him. Ann's husband grew increasingly angry and withdrew from the family. The letters from the WCB began to suggest that there were problems with the claim. Within a short time, Ann had to get a job. While she was glad to contribute financially to the family, the changing dynamics in the family caused tremendous tensions. At times, she felt too worn out to continue.

Ann's story is a typical example of another side of women's experience with the WCB — the emotional work resulting from a spouse with a job-related injury.

When a worker is injured or suffers from an industrial disease, whole families are affected. The physical toll and suffering of a worker may go on for years, and medical treatment and hospitalization will ensue. Often the worker loses his or her job. Once a claim is filed, the worker faces long delays in receiving benefits, incomplete information and complicated appeals. This imposes great stress on a family already coping with serious health problems as a result of the injury and disability. Women do much of the emotional work, keeping their families together, supporting their spouses and making financial ends meet. But the partners of injured workers have no formal, recognized financial or social support.

Women whose spouses suffer from industrial disease may face years of watching the spouse's health deteriorate. They also face endless battles with the WCB to get recognition that the disease is job-related. Some summon the energy to research the link between industrial hazards and their spouse's health problems, while coping with the tragedy that has struck their families.

Survivors of workers who die as a result of a work-related injury or disease are officially recognized under the WCA. Since 1985, the financial situation of some survivors has improved. In order to qualify for survivors benefits, however, a worker must have died in a traumatic accident or have been considered 100 percent disabled by an injury or industrial disease. The WCB's assessment of a worker as 100 percent disabled is extremely rare. Though a family may have struggled for years on a severely limited income, in most cases they will not be entitled to ongoing benefits after the worker's death.

Further review would reveal many more dimensions of sexism in the policies of the WCB. The integration of medical and psychiatric structures with legal systems poses particular dangers for women. As feminists, it is important for us to articulate the larger theoretical issues in law, as well as the practical day-to-day ways in which these institutions affect our lives. Involvement with the WCB and its application of policies and procedures affects the quality of thousands of injured workers. Women as injured workers, as family members and survivors face tremendous difficulties.

Women who encounter the WCB have already been injured and disabled as a result of their employment. We must learn from their experiences and fight to prevent further injury from the legal and medical institutions which should serve them.

### Notes
The names of the claimants and their situations have been changed to avoid identification.

1. Laura C. Johnson with Robert E. Johnson, *The Seam Allowance* (Toronto: Women's Press, 1982).

**KAREN WEISBERG** once worked as a community legal worker at a legal clinic in Toronto that represented injured workers in their WCB claims.

# Welfare

## Far from Well[*]

### Joanne Doucette

Poverty is increasingly a woman's place. In the seventies, feminists said, "Every woman is only one man away from poverty." Now one-third of poor households are composed of single older women and families led by sole-support mothers fighting to survive on social assistance. Women with disabilities also compose a large proportion of those receiving social assistance. Minority women are much more likely to be poor and the greater number of oppressed minorities you belong to, the greater your chances are to be poor. University of Regina researchers calculated the odds and found that a Native disabled woman who drops out of school has a better chance of winning a lottery than she does of getting a job.

Since the 1970s, the number of poor people has increased dramatically in Canada. Inequality has increased. The bottom 20 percent of Canada's population gets 3.6 percent of all income; the top 20 percent gets 43.3 percent. The rich get richer, the poor get poorer. They get the Club Med; we get the rescue missions. A permanent underclass of single mothers, racial minorities, seniors, unemployed youths and disabled people is evolving.

Poor people have much higher health risks and reduced access to health care. According to the Ontario Advisory Council on the Status of Women in its brief to the Ontario government on sole-support mothers, "Poverty is the single most important factor in the perpetuation of ill health in our society."

There are three factors which contribute most to ill health for poor women — hunger and malnutrition, unhealthy environments, and stress — according to the National Anti-Poverty Organization (NAPO). Stress produces cardiovascular disease,

* Reprinted from *Healthsharing* vol. 9 no. 3 (Summer 1988): 11-13, with permission of the author.

infections and cancer, and drives us into addictive and unhealthy coping tactics like smoking, alcohol and drug abuse, and over eating. Deborah Sharpe of Low Income Families Together (LIFT), a Toronto based self-help group of low-income women, says: "Welfare mothers develop a weird kind of anorexia. Sometimes you can't eat because every time you sit down to a meal, it's like eating money."

People who live below the poverty line (euphemistically called the low-income cut-off level) spend 58.5 percent of their income on the bare necessities: food, shelter and clothing. If poor people get cancer, our survival rate is 10 to 15 percent lower than the affluent. We are more likely to get cancer because many poor women are forced to live near factories spewing industrial pollution, mercury, lead and other dangerous chemicals. We suffer from accidents and disease caused by the poor housing and wretched neighbourhoods, and from the overwhelming stress of fighting for day-to-day survival, all of which can contribute to a depressed immune system. We do not get enough protein or fresh fruits and vegetables. We live on cheap empty calories and suffer from malnutrition, obesity and anemia. Our children, starved in the womb, have low birth weights, increasing their odds of having physical and learning disabilities.

Hunger robs poor women of their ability to "interact with the environment so as to enhance their health," as NAPO puts it. Usually the housing we live in is poorly maintained by slum landlords, public or private, who do not maintain their premises or respond to our demands for improvements. Stairways are unsafe. Lighting is poor. For many, especially those of us in rooming houses, there are poor cooking and bathing facilities. It is hard to keep clean and eat properly in such circumstances.

We have reduced access to health care because of cost. User fees, incomplete coverage by drug plans or services and the indirect costs of getting health care (such as costs of transportation and child care) are effective barriers. For example in British Columbia, only one-half of the quarter-million people on welfare receive automatic medical coverage. In Saskatchewan, some recipients must pay the first $125 of drug costs a year. In many provinces, because reparative and preventive dental care is not covered, recipients must have their teeth pulled with destructive results for self-esteem and nutrition.

We have no access to alternative health care because it is not covered under health plans and most sliding scales start so high that they slide right by us. The attitudes of mainstream health care providers are effective barriers for poor women. "Doctors," according to Jane Bremner of Opportunity for Advancement, "often give totally unrealistic advice." For example, they will tell a sole-support mother with three children and a bad back to spend a week on bed rest or, if she is depressed, to take a week off and go on a holiday somewhere nice.

Too often efforts to help us or improve our health are moralistic or simplistic. They do not recognize the realities of poverty. Health promotion literature is written in jargon or at a literacy level of university. Programs are planned by people who have never been on social assistance and have little direct communication with us. They do not know our needs or believe us, or even ask us. Health promotion efforts aimed at us talk about better budget planning, better meal planning and more exercise. They do not look at our living conditions, the environments we endure, and our lack of choices. They are middle class solutions for poor women's lives. They don't work.

One disabled woman says, "It's a deadly curse." Her only escape from social assistance would be, in her opinion, to "marry a rich man."

The amounts paid by social assistance are simply inadequate to live on. You either pay your rent or you eat. You can't do both. Most often adequate food is given up for housing, perpetuating malnutrition and all the health problems it leads to. As well, recipients are often intimidated and unaware of their rights to health benefits and nutritional subsidies. Too often welfare workers refuse to supply basic information or do not have access to the information themselves. Often there is no printed matter to explain rights, benefits, etc.

Many social assistance recipients are talented survivors. No one knows budgeting better than a mother on social assistance. They get the best they can out of an intolerable situation. But woe betide you if you are shy, unable to speak English well, illiterate or so depressed you can not stand up for yourself.

The petty indignities of bureaucracy can drive one to despair almost as quickly as the gross injustices. Welfare workers often act as if the money was coming out of their own pockets and treat recipients in contemptuous and humiliating ways, concealing information and even lying. It is a common conviction of recipients that the system lies to them. Welfare workers can buy into the negative stereotypes and treat us like dirt. They can get burnt out and pass their resentment for their poor working conditions onto us. They can get burnt out by the sheer pressure of huge caseloads and inadequate resources and settle for a dehumanized approach to poor women. Victoria Hilderman, President of OPSEU Local 586, a union local for fieldworkers, says, "The case loads are so high that it is almost impossible to give high standards of service to our clients."

Yet many welfare workers are sympathetic to the needs of their clients. They know what is going on, but their hands are tied by regulations set from above which do not recognize the realities the worker sees every day. Worse, management watches caseworkers carefully to weed out the "shit disturbers" or those who too vocally point out the inadequacies of the system. The social welfare system, according to one former worker, "Is not a neutral place." She was working very closely with a poor woman's self-help group and found herself under police investigation. Management had tagged her as a subversive.

Those on social assistance often see social welfare workers as "soft cops" whose job is to regulate us not serve us or protect us from poverty. We think they are mostly there to look for "welfare cheaters." They walk into our homes without a moment's notice, looking to see if there's a man around. Yet if the workers are "policed," is it any small wonder that those at the very bottom live in fear?

Often government departments which are supposed to assist us do not communicate with each other, and recipients have to go through endless red tape to get what is needed immediately. One woman who uses an electric wheelchair woke up one morning with a dead battery. She spent three days trying to get her caseworker on the telephone. The line was always busy. It took her worker another month to process the red tape before the disabled woman could get a new wheelchair battery. For those four weeks, she sat in one spot looking out of her window, completely robbed of mobility and independence. Cruel and unusual punishment. But for what was she being punished? For being disabled? For being on social assistance? For being poor?

## WHAT CAN YOU DO?

While researching this article, Joanne Doucette spoke with Deborah Sharpe of Low Income Families Together.

Joanne: Is there anything readers could do to improve the situation for women on social assistance?

Deborah: Keep an eye on the rich. There are lots of studies done about poor people, but no one takes a long hard look at the rich — at who's got money, how they got it, what they are doing with it. Middle class women can do this better than welfare mothers. We need to know this information.

Support grassroots initiatives by poor women to organize themselves. Give money. Do child care so women can go to meetings. Provide attendant care for disabled women. Do the shitwork and the nitty gritty stuff like typing. Leave the glory to us, visiting the politicians, speaking publicly, dealing with the media. We can speak on our own behalf.

Assess your own lifestyles. How much of the world's resources are you using. The poverty of women on social assistance profits the middle class. Poverty is no accident. It is not something you "fall into." It is the result of our economic system.

Most women on welfare or social assistance are very well aware of the barriers within the system to our full social and economic equality and participation, but very tired of individually challenging the system. Things have not improved since the Royal Commission on the Status of Women in 1970 met with low-income women. Those women spoke of inadequate housing, poor nutrition, health problems, chronic illness, lack of education and training, the high cost of living, stress, lack of day care and decent jobs. Poor women's group organize, fight for equality and die slow or fast deaths. Outside the mainstream of feminism, without money or prestige, without operating funding or support, it is an uphill battle against hopelessness. We resign ourselves to perpetual, permanent poverty. In a competitive economy which values maleness, youth, physical perfection and white skin, someone is designed to be the losers and it's us — "poor sisters," sole-support mothers, disabled women, older women without men, Native women, immigrant women, women of colour and women in the north and rural areas.

Sometimes we feel that the affluent and powerful wish poor women to simply die quietly behind closed doors. But then who would clean their toilets?

## Note

This is written from the "we" point of view. It was the consensus among low-income women I talked to and the women that work closely with them that the "objective" narrative voice so often used by middle class writers helped to distance them from poor women. Usually middle class women speak of women's issues in such a way that "women" really means "women like us," that is, middle class women. The use of "we" is to challenge the use of language to obscure difference and, also, to recognize the input from women on social assistance, fieldworkers, and women working in health care.

JOANNE DOUCETTE is a feminist philosopher, writer, cartoonist, library board trustee, lecturer and social welfare recipient.

# Women and the Food System[*]

## Cathleen Kneen

Eating is an intimate affair. Even those of us who see health as a public issue tend to privatize questions of food. We worry about the effect of a certain food item or element on the health of the individual, forgetting the effects of the system in which that food item is produced, processed, distributed and prepared for eating.

In previous generations, and even at present in what we choose to call "less developed" countries, women have been central to the food system at every level. Even today, the majority of Third World farmers are women; indeed, women are virtually in charge of the domestic food economy. In addition to *producing* food by raising livestock and growing vegetables and grains, women are the food *processors*, grinding grain for daily consumption and preserving food for later use. Women control the *distribution* of food within the family, as well as the disposition of surplus. And of course, as everywhere, women are primarily responsible for food *preparation* and nutrition.

In Canada the role of women in farming isn't quite so clear. When my husband and I moved to the farm 15 years ago, I startled some of the neighbours by my insistence on calling myself a "farmer." The traditional role of the woman on the farm was certainly what I did: milking a cow, making butter and even sometimes cheese, raising a couple of pigs, a bunch of chickens, and a huge garden, selling off some of the surplus for cash, and pickling, drying, canning, freezing .... This is the work which in the Third World would be called farming. Here it's called being a "farm wife" (or even, a "farmer's wife") or at best, a "farm woman." A farmer is someone who rides around fields on a tractor.

To be more pointed: *we have stopped defining farming as the*

---

* Reprinted from *Healthsharing* vol. 8 no. 2 (Spring 1987): 10-13, with permission of the author.

*production of food*. I produced food for 15 years with the work of my own hands, and I was not considered a farmer. Farming is now *the production of a commodity for sale on the market*, subject to the same forces as any other commodity on the market.

This industrialization of agriculture is devastating at every level of the food system. Starting in the middle, with processing and distribution, industrialization has spread forward to the purchasing level, with the creation of superstores and franchise convenience stores, all controlled by a handful of corporations. It has spread back to primary production, transforming the face of agriculture by increasing the size of farms and radically decreasing the number of farmers. The capitalist belief that the profit motive will solve all problems has been at the base of federal agricultural policy since 1969 when the government's white paper laying down policy stated:

> ... there will be a substantial reduction in the number of commercial farms. Some will be family farms but all will be rationally managed, profit oriented businesses. Farm mergers and consolidation will result in much larger units, not primarily for production efficiency, but to structure units that are large enough to afford better management.

The governing principle which gives the system its logic and coherence is that food is merely a commodity, to be produced and traded for a profit. It is this principle that must be challenged if we want to effect meaningful change in any aspect of the food system.

If food is merely a commodity, social concerns are essentially irrelevant to a consideration of efficiency. At the level of production, then, industrialization involves replacing human labour with machines and chemicals. In many instances mechanization can be a genuine advance (for example, rock-picking machines). But as part of an industrialization process, mechanization can be the source of great hardship, both for those who remain on the land and for those who are displaced.

It goes like this. Because farmers are producing a commodity for sale, they have to produce enough to get back the amount of money they require — and except for those few areas where there are marketing boards, farmers have no control of the price. (Some of the reasons will appear when we look at distribution and processing.) They can't for example say, it cost six cents to produce this pound of potatoes, so we're charging six cents for it. If the contracted buyer will pay only three cents, the farmers' only recourse is to produce more in order to sell more and receive more money. Bigger and more complex machinery, bought on credit, can help increase the amount one can produce with limited land and human resources; but big machines are not efficient without a uniform crop to work. Chemicals of all kinds: pesticides to kill marauding insects, fungicides to ward off diseases, herbicides to reduce competing weeds, hormones to ensure that the whole crop matures at the same time ... these are an essential part of the modern farmer's struggle to continue to earn enough money from the crop to stay in business.

The link between the industrialization of primary production and distribution, or marketing, is clear. How has distribution itself industrialized? In the Third World village, when a woman has harvested her crop and fed her family, she takes the surplus to market to sell. Food is thus distributed through the community. Even here in North America, it was basically the advent of the refrigerated truck — a fairly recent development — that industrialized the distribution level of the food system. Food no longer needs to be consumed anywhere near where it is produced. The same procedure which was developed for bananas and coffee and sugar now brings tomatoes, grapes and beef across the globe. This means, of course, that food commodities produced here have to compete, in terms of price, with those produced in areas with vastly different climates, labour laws, and pay scales. The local market was once in the hands of local people, predominantly women. The industrialized system is now in the hands of large corporations (often multinational) whose bottom line does not include feeding the family of the food producers — or anyone else, for that matter — except as a side effect from the disposal of the commodity they are selling.

We begin to see how the system fits together when we consider the opportunities this vastly expanded distribution system offers for profiteering at the primary production level. Instead of dealing with small plots and variegated produce, this mode of distribution offers economies of scale for large plantations producing a uniform crop at set intervals, whether pineapples or beef, which can then be packed, palletized, containerized, and distributed worldwide. Similarly, in the industrial system, processing is removed from the site of production and of consumption. The simple techniques of canning, freezing and drying, which I practiced in my farmhouse kitchen, are speeded up and expanded to an assembly-line procedure to handle the large quantities of uniform products now available. High technology enters the picture with additives like BHT (butylated hydroxytoluene) which keeps the product from spoiling, thus increasing shelf-life and broadening potential distribution. Physics follows close on the heels of chemistry with irradiation of foods from spices to chicken, again, to reduce spoilage and increase shelf-life.

The last hold-out for local distribution was the dairy industry: milk sold for drinking has been produced close to where it is consumed because of the need for refrigeration. Local surpluses have traditionally been processed into cheese, or milk powder. Now we have UHT: ultra-high temperature treatment of milk which gives it a shelf-life, unrefrigerated, of six months.

As processing has become more sophisticated, the last level, food preparation, has also been undergoing changes which tend to remove it from the control of women towards an industrialized mode. The TV dinners which were the mark of the working woman in an earlier generation have now given way to such a staggering array of ready-to-eat foods that more and more of us rely on them. This is a result, not just of advertising, but of the whole industrialized system. We are being pushed out of situations where we could barter our work for the things we needed into the cash economy. As this happens, we depend increasingly on things we can buy to replace the things we no longer have time to make, since our time is taken up with "making a living."

According to those who now control the food system, nutrition doesn't suffer at all from this transfer of control. On the contrary, great care is taken to ensure that all *measurable* nutrients which are removed, are added to the packaged product. We have to take it on faith that they haven't missed anything important.

The final effect is that the whole food system, which was once in the hands of women, has been physically removed from our domain, along with the power and control of production, processing, distribution, and preparation.

Just how this happens will become clearer if we take a closer look at the primary production level. The industrial model of red meat production involves huge feedlots full of beef cattle being dosed with growth hormones and fed massive amounts of grains to fatten them for slaughter. But this a particular mode of beef production which arose only around 1960 or so as a response to a surplus of Western grain. Animals such as beef or sheep can also be raised basically on pasture, in an "extensive" as opposed to "intensive" feedlot system.

In an area like the part of Nova Scotia where we were, with abundant rainfall and relatively poor soils, this sort of grassland farming made a lot of sense. It has the advantage of using land which is unsuitable for row or root crops to produce grass which is inedible by humans but great fodder for ruminant animals such as cows or sheep. Manure from livestock is an important way of returning fertility to the soil, and improving the quality of marginal grazing lands.

But the fact of the matter is that we could not opt out of the industrial system if we wanted to make a living from farming, even on a modest scale. To be sure, we were careful to use drugs only as specific remedies for individual animals who were ill (intensive operations often feed antibiotics routinely as "disease prevention" in with the feed). We went so far as to build a new barn to keep the sheep in over winter so that we could retrieve the manure and cut down on chemical fertilizer (essential to keep up the fertility of thin stony soils like ours). Although one of our chief joys was the sight of the lambs playing in the pastures, we, too, ran a feedlot. The flock that lambed in April was only part of the flock. We also had sheep who lambed in February. Those lambs never did see grass. They stayed in the barn, eating the very best hay and whole grains, until they were ready for butcher.

Like every other farmer, we had problems of capitalization: we had to make maximum use of our barn space. We had to respond to demands of the market economy: in order to satisfy the chain stores who bought lamb from our farmers' co-op, we had to be able to provide top-quality (i.e. young) lamb year-round. And we had to make maximum use of our labour force:

since the daily care of the animals required that we be there on the farm all winter long anyway, we might as well be lambing.

Farmers are constantly being told to be more efficient, to improve their management, to maximize utilization of resources. But as we do so, we slip by degrees into the industrial system. The economic imperatives of our food system force certain practices on farmers so that they can survive as farmers. When the costs of production become too high, and the selling price of the commodity doesn't keep pace, the choice is to cut corners or go out of business, or both. In either case, it is always announced as the farmer's own fault.

If I learned one thing in the loneliness of an isolated farm in Nova Scotia, it was that the isolation is deceptive, fostering an individualist illusion that we are independent. The fact is that we were operating, not just on the world market for lamb, but also in terms of the world red meat market. In other words, the price we could get for our lamb was determined in large part not only by the price New Zealand farmers were forced to accept for their lambs, but also by the price Panama or Costa Rica were prepared to take for the beef produced on the lands "reclaimed" by destroying the rainforests. Indeed, we survive largely by virtue of persuading local consumers to pay a premium for fresh, local product; but the base line remains the world red meat market, controlled by the likes of Cargill, and the speculators on commodity futures.

If we give up, if we refuse to go on producing, year after year, for a price which rarely if ever reaches the cost of production — why then the corporations with which we deal will simply move operations abroad. Half a world away, we are effectively controlled, as producers, by the same forces that control the peasant farmers of the Third World. It is crystal clear that there is no real solution to our problems as producers that does not include them.

The same is true of consumers. Switching to tofu made from soybeans grown in Central America by a multinational corporation, on land which formerly grew sustenance crops for the peasants who now work as day-labourers for less than a living wage on that same land, using chemicals for pest and weed control which have been banned in North America as unsafe ... what kind of a healthy alternative is that?

Nevertheless, we must start somewhere if we want to change

the direction of our food system. The first step is to realize that "we are what we eat" in a deep sense: to begin at the personal level to make conscious and responsible decisions about what we eat. We need to develop what some have called "a taste for justice:" to eat foods which are grown locally, which are minimally processed, which are produced without systematic recourse to chemicals and which are co-operatively distributed. These actions, by themselves, will not alter the food system significantly: there are no individual solutions to the food system. They can, however, be the beginning of a process of empowerment.

Starting with the personal, we can move to such communal actions as working in a community garden or a food distribution co-op. We can make contacts with farm women (such as the National Farmers Union) and support them in their political actions to keep farmers on the land. We can organize the kind of global pressure that forced Nestle to back down on its promotion practices. We can lobby Parliament against legislation which increases corporate control of the food system, for example, the Plant Breeders Rights bill.

But whatever actions we undertake, the major task which confronts us is to *imagine* a different kind of food system. Rather than concentrating on what sort of food is healthy for the individual person, we must think about what kind of production system is healthy for the globe. Acting in the context of this vision of a different kind of food system, we will gain the freedom — and the power — to force change for some measure of justice in this one.

CATHLEEN KNEEN recently "retired" from a sheep farm in Nova Scotia and moved to Toronto, where she works with the Latin American Working Group. A long-time activist in the women's health movement, she was a founder of the Pictou County Women Centre in Nova Scotia. She continues her activity around issues of health and food through the newly-formed Nutrition Policy Institute and is co-publisher of *The Ram's Horn*.

# section four

# Options for
# Reproductive Health

Madeline Boscoe and Kathleen McDonnell, writing in the first issue of *Healthsharing*, evaluate changes which have taken place in the provision of care for women giving birth in hospitals in Canada. While they claim that such changes were made in response to consumer demands, Boscoe and McDonnell express concern that the home birth option may be undermined in the process of institutionalizing changes in the hospital, and that changes in the hospital context tend to be more formal than substantive. Their essay provides a clear articulation of the choice position with respect to birthing options.

Mary Neilans' article on midwifery was written subsequent to the coming into force of the legislation which provides for the regulation of midwifery by the government of Ontario, but before the actual establishment of the new regime. Neilans takes the position that history provides good reason for suspicion of the medical profession's unprecedented support for midwifery. Neilans expresses concern that midwives are being compelled to seek legitimation through the medical establishment, the very establishment which caused many women to turn to traditional midwifery in the first place.

Cecilia Benoit provides a rich description of the role of the midwife in Newfoundland and Labrador up to the early 1960s and her subsequent obsolescence caused by the takeover of modern medicine.

According to Benoit the midwife's approach toward health was vital to the whole community, not only in her assistance to birthing women, but also in her assistance to other members of the isolated society, "the young and old alike, of either sex."

Sheila Jennings Linehan opens her article by drawing attention to general concerns about the delivery of medical services to the First Nations of Canada. Linehan characterizes obstetrical practice as "the most aggressive 'advance' of medicine into the North," and in particular she looks at the practice of forcing Inuit women to leave their homes and families and give birth in the south. Linehan points to research which argues that Inuit women's loss of control over childbirth has become a metaphor for the Inuit people's loss of political control over their lives and their communities.

Bonnie Lafave counsels the need for women to be active in current discussions on the uses of human eggs, embryos and fetuses in biotechnology. Lafave expresses concern about how advances in biotechnology may have the effect of informing the abortion debate. Specifically, she discusses how the perceived separate status of the fetus and a concern with its independent health may conflict with the needs and wishes of the mother.

Katsi Cook questions our assumptions about the superior quality of breast milk and its importance to our babies. Cook describes the work of the First Environment Project, which was created out of a concern with the reproductive health effects of toxic contaminants carried by the St. Lawrence River.

Aruna Papp examines the use by the South Asian Community of a particular doctor's services to determine the sex of a fetus. Papp identifies some of the religious and cultural sources of the practise, but is unequivocal in her position that the doctor in question has targeted and exploited the South Asian community.

# Birthing Options*

## Madeline Boscoe
## Kathleen McDonnell

For most women, the experience of giving birth has been one of powerlessness, ignorance and alienation from our bodies and our surroundings. As women we've had to leave home and those close to us, giving birth in a sterile environment, surrounded by strangers. We have had to submit to a variety of drugs and medical procedures whose effects we understood little or not at all. Our babies have been brought to us according to the hospital's schedule rather than our own desires, and we have been actively or passively discouraged from breastfeeding by hospital staff.

All this is the result of the removal of birth from the home to the hospital, as well as the turn-of-the-century ban on the practice of midwifery. (See box.) Childbirth has been transformed from a natural process based in the community to a medical — even pathological — event. Doctors became the "heroes" of the birth process. Where once midwives "caught" babies, obstetricians now "deliver" them. In spite of some very real advances, the overall effect of medicalized childbirth in the twentieth century has been, in the words of one Ontario midwife, Willie Holmes, "to undermine women's confidence in their ability to give birth in a natural way."

In the sixties and early seventies opposition to the definition of pregnancy and birth as illness gained a wide public audience in North America. A consumer movement in childbirth grew out of the natural childbirth movement, the feminist health movement and mushrooming consumer activism. Some consumer groups offer classes and information in specific childbirth methods like Lamaze; others, like the International Childbirth Education Asso-

---

*   Reprinted from *Healthsharing vol. 1 no. 1 (Winter 1979): 8-10, with permission of the author.*

# MIDWIFERY IN CANADA

Midwifery is an ancient art, passed on through generations of women. Long before the healing arts became "professionalized," lay midwives practiced their skills within cohesive communities where they were known to their clients as relatives and neighbours.

Midwives have particular skills, knowledge and techniques that are oriented towards birth as a natural event, in which the woman and her baby are central actors. This body of knowledge and skills was discredited and buried away as a result of the medical campaign to suppress midwifery in the last century. Much of it is only now being rediscovered and revived by a new generation of birth attendants who see themselves as working within this long, time-honoured tradition.

Since the turn of the century, the practice of midwifery by anyone but licensed physicians has been illegal in Canada, except in remote areas without doctors' services. One way of looking at this exception is that midwives are permitted to deliver babies only where they pose no economic threat to the medical profession, and only in communities too poor or far away to interest doctors in setting up practices.

But pressure is beginning to build to change the legal status of midwifery in Canada. The New Family Centre proponents have precipitated a major discussion of the issue in British Columbia. Just this year, the B.C. College of Physicians and Surgeons ruled that midwifery is "part of the ordinary calling of nursing" and has approved the practice of midwifery by nurses in the proposed birth centre. Seizing on this important development, the Registered Nurses Association of British Columbia is actively lobbying for a much broader application of the College's decision, which would pave the way for the practice of nurse-midwifery throughout British Columbia, and perhaps in other provinces as well.

Recognition for the practice of midwifery by nurses or non-nurses takes time. In the meantime, a growing number of "lay" midwives are beginning to "go it alone" and attend births without medical assistance, though most have doctors they can call on in emergencies. These "lay midwives," as they are now being called, have been trained in countries such as Great Britain and the U.S., or in individually set up apprenticeship programmes.

At present these lay midwives are being tactically ignored, but they are worried about the possibility of future crackdowns, as happened in California in the mid-seventies. A few are ready to openly challenge the law in the tradition of people like Margaret Sanger and Henry Morgentaler, because they believe that only this kind of direct confrontation will bring about the changes needed.

Also they and other birth alternative activists fear that midwifery will be defined as a speciality of nursing. They are concerned that obstetrical care will not improve under the control of nurses. Nursing itself is still regulated to a large degree by the medical profession and the majority of nurses share the doctors' view of birth as requiring medical intervention. Midwifery may fit easily into the existing medical system only as long as midwives do not challenge the prevailing medical model of obstetrical care.

ciation (ICEA) also lobby for specific changes in hospital birthing practices: some organizations, such as Birthing Alternatives for a Better Experience (babe) based in Kitchener, are grass-roots political groupings. Individual physicians and midwives doing births at home are also part of this movement.

The consumer birth movement has made some headway in raising public awareness around the issues involved in birth, and is actually bringing about concrete changes and alternatives in the way we give birth. But how much have things really changed? How many parents are actually able to take advantage of the changes and alternatives in childbirth today? And to what extent have the various efforts at change really shifted the balance of decision-making power away from medical professionals and back to birthing women themselves?

Have things really gotten better in childbirth in Canada?

## In-Hospital Changes

Some hospitals, at least in large urban centres, are beginning to make concessions to growing consumer demands. New-fangled jargon such as "family-centred maternity care" and "home-like birth in-hospital" reflect an apparent liberalization of hospital attitudes. Parents are now labelled as "part of the health-care team."

A large number of urban hospitals now offer "rooming-in" for mothers and their babies, although fathers must still scrub and gown before entering the room, and the baby is removed for all other visitors. Fathers are also frequently allowed (if not exactly encouraged) to be present at the delivery — even occasionally, at Caesareans. For the most part, however, labour coaches, friends and other family are still locked out. In most hospitals women still labour and deliver in separate rooms, and give birth in the "lithotomy position" on an operating table. After the new baby has been examined, cleaned and suctioned, the parents may now hold it for a few precious minutes. Some hospitals run discussion groups for new mothers which aim at sharing birth experiences. A number of women, however, report that these groups end up being no different than traditional instructional sessions on baby care taught by nursing staff.

A few progressive hospitals such as McMaster in Hamilton, Foothills in Calgary and the new Grace in Vancouver now have or are building "birth suites," providing parents with a more home-like atmosphere, complete with music and private rooms. In these new units mothers have a little more control over who is present at the birth and how they give birth. For instance, a woman has a choice about her delivery position, can move around during the early stages of labour, and has some say about whether or not to have an epidural. However, even brass beds and hanging plants can acquire an institutional look. Parents having their babies in these new suites are still aware, at all times, that they are in a *hospital.*

## Birth Centres

Another promising alternative is the out-of-hospital birth centre. At this time Canadian birth centres, unfortunately, exist mostly on paper only. E. Clifford Tucker, a private obstetrician in Montreal, has set up the Carolyn Centre above his office as an alternative to time-consuming home births. A few groups across the country are studying the idea and are lobbying various levels of government for funds.

The most well-developed proposal is the New Family Centre (NFC) in Vancouver. Designed by a committee of consumers and faculty from the University of British Columbia School of Nursing, the NFC would be a comprehensive service, concerned not only with pregnancy and birth, but also with parenting, growth and development and whatever problems may arise for up to a year after the birth. Pre- and postnatal groups at the centre would be staffed largely by parents who had their babies there. All births would be attended by nurse-midwives rather than doctors. Nurse-midwives would also do most of the pre- and postnatal care. This, the single most contentious feature of the NFC from the point of view of the medical establishment, has already been approved in principle by the B.C. College of Physicians and Surgeons.

The NFC would be located in a remodelled house close to, but physically quite independent of, a tertiary care hospital. Emphasis will be on normal birth with a minimum of medication and intervention. Emergency equipment such as oxygen and resuscitation would be unobtrusively available. The staff will not be tempted to use sophisticated medical technology of dubious value (such as fetal monitoring) since none of these machines will be present. In case of emergency, the mother can be quickly transferred to the hospital, where the midwife will be able to stay with her throughout the delivery.

Even though liberalized obstetrical policies are not yet universal in Canadian hospitals, and alternatives like birth centres are still in the talking stage, the mood of some segments of the consumer movement is that a large part of the battle over birth practices has been won. "I firmly believe … that you can have the birth of your choice in any hospital across the land," Valmai Howe Elkins, author of *The Rights of the Pregnant Parent*, told this year's ICEA convention in Toronto.

## Backlash Against Home Birth

But have we come very far at all? While hospitals scurry to keep up with consumer demands, the medical campaign against home births is, if anything, stepping up. In fact, some doctors and medical organizations are supporting alternatives such as birthing suites and birth centres primarily as an attempt to cool out the consumer demand for home births. More and more we hear home birth being depicted as a form of "child abuse." One Toronto obstetrician has accused home birth parents of, "gambling with the … lives of their unborn children," in what he considers their selfish drive to achieve "emotional fulfilment."

Peer pressure on the few doctors who do perform home births is very strong. Numerous hospitals have threatened to suspend hospital privileges for doctors doing home births. At least one hospital, St. Paul's in Vancouver, did withdraw hospital admitting privileges several years ago for doctors who attended home births. Women choosing home births are put in a double bind. They can usually find a doctor to assist them, but cannot count on continued care from that doctor if they have to be transferred to hospital.

Doctors say they are opposed to home birth because the medical back-up does not exist to make it safe. Yet they do everything in their power to ensure that this continues to be the case. With the strength of the medical opposition to home birth, giving birth in the personalized setting of one's own home is at this time an option for only a small number of women who have extraordinary resources in terms of time, energy, money and plain gutsy aggressiveness.

## Getting Worse

In spite of a variety of advances, some aspects of hospital birth appear to be getting worse rather than better. Routine use of fetal monitoring is on the increase, in spite of the fact that its advantages have never been scientifically demonstrated. One-third of Toronto-area hospitals in a 1979 survey indicated a routine or near-routine use of fetal monitoring for normal births. In fact, some hospitals, such as Mount Sinai in Toronto, which overall have extremely liberal policies surrounding childbirth are among the most enthusiastic users of monitors. Caesarean delivery is also on the rise, now accounting for one-quarter of all births in a large urban centre like Toronto.

Despite the curtains on the windows and the "home-like" atmosphere for which hospitals now strive, the tendency of doctors is still to put more emphasis on technological intervention in the birthing process, rather than less. "We're going to combine warmth and a humanistic attitude with newer developments in electronics," an American obstetrician recently told feminist health writer Gena Corea for an article on the future of childbirth. The current trend towards regionalization of obstetrical facilities, already a reality in some parts of the U.S. and now taking root in Canada, is another reflection of this tendency.

A group of prominent teaching hospitals in Toronto, are now actively lobbying for a regionalization scheme which would involve a vast data bank on all pregnant women in the Metro Toronto region. Women would be screened by their doctors for risk factors and the information fed into the data bank, which would "assign" them to hospitals with appropriate levels of technology. Smaller community hospitals will get to do fewer and, ultimately, no births under this scheme. More and more, births would be shifted to large teaching hospitals with a bias towards technology and medical intervention. One member of the committee on regionalization, City of Toronto Maternal and Child Health Consultant Doreen Hamilton, has publicly expressed her view that it is a "costly and unproven system" which puts all emphasis on management of high-risk pregnancies rather than on prevention, where the emphasis belongs. Hamilton says the money spent on regionalization would be better spent on universal prenatal education, improved nutrition, primary care and better social services.

## More Changes Needed

The consumer movement cannot yet rest on its laurels. There is a very real possibility that all the liberalization will become window-dressing, which may make women feel more "at home" but won't give them any more real control over their births than they had before. Many of the groups working for change have up to now been reluctant to address this issue of control. They have tended to stress a nonconfrontational approach — parents should "work the system" to get what they want through "persuasion" and "communication," rather than challenging the system itself. The net effect of this attitude is to put all the onus for change on individual parents, says Montreal prenatal teacher Janet Torge. "If a couple doesn't get what they wanted, they end up feeling it's their fault — not the system. They just weren't diplomatic enough."

The real challenge for the childbirth movement is to work for a system in which there is a wide range of options — in-hospital, at birth centres and at home —

- *all* of which are safe and fully supported by the medical system,
- *all* of which recognize a woman's right to maximum control over the conditions of her birth,
- *all* of which see medical professionals as resources to the parents rather than as the decision-makers.

Curtains in the birthing suite are, in the end, only the beginning.

**MADELINE BOSCOE** is a nurse who is planning to become a midwife and is a member of Women Healthsharing.

**KATHLEEN MCDONNELL** is a Toronto freelance writer and a member of Women Healthsharing.

# Midwifery

## From Recognition to Regulation
## The Perils of Government Intervention

### Mary Neilans

Anne Maranta, a practicing midwife in Kingston, always warns prospective clients that they are taking risks. But the risks she cites are legal not medical. She cautions, "Since there are no clear legal provisions for the practice of midwifery, we practice in an environment of unknown risk." That's because in Canada midwifery is only now beginning to be officially welcomed into the fold of the medical establishment.

In November of 1991, Ontario passed Bill 56, establishing midwifery as a recognized profession. The new legislation means midwifery services will be covered under provincial health insurance and midwives will have access to hospital facilities. A side effect of government recognition is public acceptance of the midwife's role in advising and supporting the expectant mother throughout her pregnancy and delivery.

Since Bill 56, Ontario's subsequent decisions on how to regulate midwives are bound to have a precedent-setting effect on other provinces considering such legislation. As such, it is important to examine how any changes will affect the current role of midwifery.

History gives us reason to suspect the medical profession's new-found support for midwifery. Since the turn of the century, the medical profession has waged a concerted campaign to convince women that hospitals are the safest place to give birth. Women eventually realized that access to medical intervention during childbirth is a mixed blessing. In the late 1970s, the demand for midwives increased largely due to a high medical

* Reprinted from *Healthsharing* vol. 13 no. 2 (Summer/Fall 1992): 27-29, with permission of the author.

intervention rate in the birthing process with uses of demerol, epidurals, episiotomies, forceps and Caesarean sections. Such intervention was more commonplace than many thought necessary. As well, typical hospital practices did not meet the needs of most women: babies kept in the nursery to be bottle-fed, husbands or partners not made to feel welcome, and families allowed to visit only if garbed in gloves, gowns and masks. As Anne Maranta wryly suggests, it was "not what you would call a family-centred birth experience." Women wanted more control over their child's birth. They wanted choices. And they wanted midwives.

The medical profession, however, was more than reluctant to acknowledge women's desires or meet their needs. In fact, in 1983, the College of Physicians and Surgeons of Ontario tossed statistics at women in an attempt to instill doubts about the safety of midwifery and home births. They referred to data from Great Britain which suggested that the perinatal mortality rate for home deliveries was more than 60 percent higher than the overall rate. A closer look revealed that these studies confused planned home births with the more general category of "out of hospital" births. Late miscarriages, premature births, taxi-cab deliveries and unexpected births not attended by qualified caregivers were lumped together with planned home births. Ironically, those same statistics demonstrated that births planned to occur at home with midwives in attendance were associated with lower rates of intervention and lower rates of complications than hospital births. In these cases, the perinatal mortality rate was extremely low, approximately two per 1000, compared to an overall rate of 14 per 1000.

Also in 1983, as a result of the need for greater public awareness on midwifery, a lobby group of health professionals and other supporters of midwifery formed the Midwifery Task Force of Ontario. The task force responds to any concerns about the qualifications of currently practicing midwives by stating that the "midwife has always been a skilled practitioner. Modern midwives are trained through apprenticeships as well as in direct-entry training programs and in universities around the world. The negative image of the midwife as an unskilled and careless birth attendant was largely the creation of the medical profession."

Yet it seems the new legislation in Ontario responds to the

myths rather than the facts. Newly-defined programs will replace traditional forms of training for midwives. The standardization of formal training for midwives would mean that all currently practising midwives would have to prove themselves, often going back to school for several years.

The approved schools, as well as meetings of any governing councils, would require attendance in large urban centres, most likely in Toronto. This would be difficult for many midwives, particularly those in rural areas. Yet, if the midwifery degree were not attained and other routes of entry are deemed unacceptable, the midwife would risk criminal charges by continuing to practice as usual.

Anne Maranta spells out the potential loss for women in rural communities, if their midwives are required to attend school in urban centres for formal training. "Historically, midwives in rural communities had little or no formal training, but they were very capable. They simply learned on the job out of necessity. And if they weren't around to help the woman, often no one was. Before medicare, rural families often couldn't afford to pay a doctor to come to them. And they couldn't afford to go to the city to give birth. After medicare, most of the doctors wanted to stay and practice in the city anyway, so the woman was still on her own, unless she had a midwife." If the rural midwife is threatened, the women who need midwives most may lose them.

Midwives who practice part-time, often while raising their own families, will also have to make some tough decisions. Potential problems surrounding funding may force licensed midwives to practice full-time or not at all. This will be a no-win situation for many midwives.

Are setting province-wide standards, evaluating all currently practising midwives, institutionalizing a formal education process, and enforcing a full-time commitment really necessary in order to recognize the role that midwives play?

Midwives are currently regulated by the Association of Ontario Midwives which provides professional standards for those practicing. These standards include guidelines for mandatory consultation and transfer of care, codes of conduct and ethics, and peer review protocols. It hardly seems fair that midwives are now forced to seek legitimization from the medical establishment — the same body that has sought for so long to discredit midwives.

Ironically, it is the medical profession and its impersonal and interventionist practices that have forced many women to turn to traditional midwifery.

The licensing of midwifery in Ontario should be viewed with caution. The mainstream medical profession is quite capable of undermining those that threaten its position. As one anonymous physician warned in *The Montreal Gazette*, "Midwifery is a turf battle, plain and simple."

Subtle changes in proposed policy demonstrate how midwives could end up losing their "turf." For example, in the *Guidelines to the Scope of Practice* produced by the Association of Ontario Midwives, certain medical conditions, such as pre-eclampsia (a toxemia of pregnancy characterized by increasing hypertension, headaches and swelling of the lower abdomen) or insulin diabetes, place pregnant women into a category of greater risk. Current guidelines state that if a woman falls into this category while under the care of a midwife, the midwife is instructed to consult with an obstetrician or specialist. She is then obliged to recommend to her client the advice given by the physician, which may involve transferring care to a specialist. Still, the final choice on what action to take remains with the pregnant woman herself.

The proposed guidelines brought forth by the new Interim Regulatory Council on Midwifery effectively eliminate that choice. If a woman were to fall into a high medical risk category, her primary care would be transferred automatically to a physician. No consultation or recommendations are required.

If the woman still desires to have a midwife as her primary caregiver, she is putting all three parties — herself, the midwife and the physician — at legal risk. In fact, it is up to the physician to give permission for any further involvement from the midwife. The physician can refuse the midwife's presence at the birth even if the mother desires it. Choice is therefore taken away from the expectant mother and given to her physician, often an obstetrician who the woman may not even know.

Since most women base their choice of a particular caregiver on trust, presumably they would follow the recommendations given by that caregiver, wanting to make the best choice for themselves and their child. But the proposed policy changes only reinforce the belief that the medical profession does not trust a pregnant woman to make the best decision.

In *The Trouble with Licensing Midwives*, Jutta Mason writes:

> Part of our struggle has been to recognize that our support as women and as mothers, not particulary as experts, can help women in pregnancy and labour. [When I had my child], I didn't evaluate midwifery services — I found Mary, the woman who was willing to sit with me during the birth, through the advice of a trusted friend. No carefully-laid plans, no self-direction or prior information could have orchestrated this gift of strength and union.

Women should ensure that the unique and valuable role of midwives does not get lost on its way from recognition to regulation.

**MARY NEILANS** is a feminist researcher and writer working in the area of women's health issues.

# Midwives and Healers

## The Newfoundland Experience[*]

### Cecilia Benoit

I was raised in the Stephenville area on the west coast of New-foundland. I am one of eleven children, ten of whom were born at home with the local midwife attending. I have vivid memories of our midwife making her rounds in the community. She was one of the village's most important and respected people.

At university I became involved in women's issues, but adopted a rather simplistic notion of women as perennial victims of a male-dominated society (if they were not involved in the women's movement). Armed with this theoretical approach and a tape recorder, I studied the role of mothering in a Newfoundland community and wrote an M.A. thesis which was on the whole bleak and lifeless. The women in my study were only partly real for I had left out the positive aspects of their lives.

I realize now that what was sadly lacking was a detailed picture of the history of Newfoundland women. But how was I to reveal what had so quickly become buried since industrialization? I went back again to the people and asked them about women in outpost Newfoundland. Over and over again they told me about the midwife and her special role in their lives.

The concept of "midwife" as it is usually used today — a woman who assists another woman in childbirth — severely limits our understanding of the community approach towards health which was characteristic of midwives and village women in Newfoundland and Labrador prior to the takeover of modern medicine. On the Island and along coastal Labrador, (and I suspect in other rural societies as well) the role of midwife was a many-faceted calling. These women were vital to the village

[*] Reprinted from *Healthsharing* vol. 5 no. 1 (Winter 1983): 22-26, with permission of author.

community, not only assistants to birthing women, but also because they were indispensable to the other members of their isolated society, the young and old alike, of either sex. In the words of one man, Phil, whose mother had been a midwife practicing in Conception Bay, "She was the midwife, an' she was the nurse ... . She made her own medicines. The government paid her nothin'. She was jus' there on call for any, any family who wanted 'er." According to Gertie Legge, from Heart's Delight, "She understood sickness and set bones and everything, even did animals."

In 1949 when Newfoundland united with Canada, there were about 1,500 rural communities or outports scattered in isolated places along the rugged coastline or on islands. Most of these communities had less than 300 residents. There were no modern facilities, such as telephones and electricity, and most roads at that time were not much more than cowpaths. Outport people, when they did travel outside their village, (for example, during the fishing season, to seek work in the lumber woods, or to purchase supplies and food staples such as flour, tea and molasses from the merchant store) used the sea as their highway.

The women rarely left their village and spent their lives working "at the fish" (curing cod fish for winter consumption), tending the gardens and farm animals, gathering berries and wild plants and, of course, caring for their families. In most villages there existed a sharp division of labour between the women and men. Even the men would readily admit that the women kept the household and village together.

Few villages had their own minister or priest nor was there usually a resident doctor or trained nurse. Prior to the establishment of the modern hospital system, doctors, trained nurses and emergency medical facilities were in extremely short supply. The modern facilities that did exist were almost exclusively located in the capital city of St. John's. In 1933, for example, there were only 83 doctors, of whom 33 were situated in St. John's. This meant that there was one doctor for approximately 5000 people. The nursing situation was equally precarious. In 1934, for example, only eight communities could afford a trained nurse.

The diet of the majority of the people was simple and limited, especially during the long winter months when staples were difficult to come by and fresh foods rare. Families were large (ten or more children was considered normal); houses were rarely insulated and inadequately heated, with drafts a perennial problem. However, as the people point out, no one starved. Villagers were expected to help each other out during times of hardship or family crisis. There existed a kind of informal barter economy in most villages which meant that no person was left destitute. Neither did anyone become wealthy. The greatest peril of most villages was the contagious diseases and fevers which were initially carried to their communities by foreign supply boats or man-of-war ships. During the first half of the twentieth century, Newfoundland and Labrador had the highest rate of tuberculosis on the North American continent.

In spite of this rather bleak picture, outport communities were not unprotected from illness. Each isolated community pooled its resources, developing a rational way of dealing with the health concerns of its residents. Healing knowledge, learned by a process of trial and error, was passed on through an oral tradition. Many techniques for curing illness were practiced: setting bones, mending wounds, employing poultices and plasters, using tonics and brews, practicing massage and so forth. Although some older men did practice as healers, few attended childbirth and few had the central role that the midwife had in most villages.

According to oral accounts, those women who became midwives/healers had certain character traits in common. Midwives were generally older women (40+). There were a number of reasons why this was so. During this period people associated old age with wisdom and respect. They believed that only after persons had lived through many trials and life crises, and had demonstrated their ability to meet these problems in a rational manner, could they be trusted with the job of village healer.

Midwives were almost always mothers and usually widowed. The villagers believed that only a woman who had experienced childbirth could know what another woman was going through when she was giving birth. In the older, widowed mother, they saw someone who was aware of the daily health concerns of the household. Moreover, she had experienced the death of her husband and thus had passed the test of endurance of one of life's greatest trials. Villagers no doubt felt a mixture of concern and respect for her, seeing the role of midwife as a way for her to make a living for herself and her children.

But to be a widowed mother was not enough. The midwife had also to express a strong desire to perform the duties of midwife/healer. She had to express an inner "calling" or deep "feeling" for her community role. In one sense this feeling was an extension of her mothering role. Yet it was more than this. Long before she set out on her own as an independent healer, the midwife had to demonstrate to the local people that she liked to care for them, that she was willing to go to them in times of sickness and that she desired to attend women in childbirth. The meagre monetary reward that the midwife might receive for her work was perhaps the last reason why she undertook her role as village healer. In fact few of these women received money for their work, accepting instead compensation in kind or sometimes just tending to the sick "out of the goodness of their heart." The midwife Aunt Ri from L'ance au Loup on the Labrador coast recalls, "I received one five dollars once, and that was for a month's work in Pinware. Usually it was only one dollar, sometimes nothing at all." (Aunt Ri attended people between Pinware in Labrador and Long Point in Quebec, a distance of 30-35 miles.)

The people were well aware that the midwife attended to their health care needs for other than monetary rewards. In fact, midwives were treated by everyone as their close kin, called "aunties" or "grannies."

One final characteristic which these women had in common was that they were uneducated. Like others in their communities, few midwives could read or write.

In contrast to the method of recruitment of health professionals in the modern era, via formal schooling and clinical training, these rural women learned their art of healing either by informal apprenticeship with an aging midwife or perhaps by going about with their mothers or female relatives who were experienced in the practice of midwifery and healing. One midwife, Aunt Mary-Ellen, who lost her husband at sea, described to me how she learned her art of healing from her mother:

I first learned to doctor the people by going about with my mother who was also a midwife. We would go out during hay-making time and pick seeds and dry them. I learned how to steep a caraway seed brew for a new child. Or if a youngster had "summer complaint" (diarrhea), we would use a brew of yellow root. Sour duck seeds made a healthy drink for anyone with fever. And I learned to give new mothers a nice drink of senna tea after the birth of their child.... My mother was still smart at the end, but getting blind when she gave up and I took her place in the village. People after that used to come to me with their problems and, of course, I always went to visit the sick, and when a woman was nearing her time, I'd be there at hand. The people I nursed were really close together; they trusted a woman like me over a stranger from some foreign part.

Sometimes a midwife would get her first opportunity to practice on her own when the older midwife was already engaged. Clara Tarrant, a midwife from St. Laurence, who practiced until the arrival of the hospital to her village in 1953, describes her experience:

I got into a situation when I just had to and there was nobody but myself. I had been at a birth and had seen deliveries and I had children. Seeing is believing, but feeling is the naked truth. So you knew what it was all about when you had some yourself.

Not all women, however, began their practice of village health-care by assisting a woman in labour. Flossie Noble, a midwife from Curling on the west coast of the Island, recalls how she first felt a calling for her future role during a time of family crisis:

When I was thirteen years old, my mother had pneumonia. She was unconscious and she used to go: "Aaah, aaah." She had such a fever; she was in [an] awful condition. I kept bathin' and bathin' her. With a little bit of boric acid in the water, bath after bath. She was burnt up with fever. But she got better ... . I went to Boston an' I had three months training of midwifery. Well, I got the details. I think I was born to be a nurse.

Regardless of their path to recruitment, each midwife had to meet the expectations of her community. Usually an informal process of selection took place over a number of years. Irene Bradley who practiced in the area of Eastport, Bonavista Bay, describes how she was chosen:

I always enjoyed public life and community work and at an early age I started visiting the sick and aged. My life ambition was always to be a nurse.... I learned some things about obstetrics from my mother who had also been a midwife. I delivered several babies in emergencies .... Then, knowing that, Dr. Smith (who travelled to numerous villages scattered along this stretch of the coastline) came to me to help him out. When I asked him how he came to pick me, he said that he had asked questions and that I had been recommended by several people. So that's how it all started.

These women did not hold a monopoly over the existing health knowledge nor did they consider themselves a class above the common folk. They were of the same social status as the rest of the villagers, and were always willing to share their limited expertise of curing practices with those whom they treated.

Because the midwives were mothers themselves, they had first-hand experience of the fears and pains as well as the special joys of being a woman. Like most other women in their community, they knew what it was like to be frequently pregnant and a mother of a large family. They believed that sympathetic understanding, encouraging words, a lot of touching, and gentle rubbing and stroking were the best tools for getting through life's natural hurdles. Hence they prodded their fellow-villagers to engage in self-care as much as possible, knowing well that, as one midwife put it, "an ounce of prevention is better than a pound of cure." Yet when the villagers really needed some extra help they knew that the midwife was close at hand.

The people remember these women with genuine warmth, often reminiscing how the local midwife could be seen coming down the outport road in her large white apron, with her black nursing bag under arm. Gertie Legge, from Heart's Delight, says "She was jist like an angel in 'er white smock." The contents of her black bag — a pair of scissors, cord ties, cotton wad, perhaps eye drops for baby, lotion, herbal mixtures, and, for Catholic midwives, a bottle of holy water to spread about the home in order to ward off any evil spirits lurking about.

Apart from her own family duties, and her treatment of the various illnesses of the villagers, the midwife was expected to be available whenever a birth was imminent. In some instances the midwife might visit the expectant mother in her own home beforehand in order to check for possible complications. Few women remember such formal visits, however. Instead they recall meeting the midwife in the village, perhaps at the church or merchant store or during a knitting or spinning frolic. Information concerning pregnancy was often given by other women as well, perhaps when they were involved in their various productive activities — collecting berries, gardening, hay-making, working at the fish, and so forth.

These midwives were well aware that the majority of women can give birth naturally, without complication for either mother or baby. In those cases, however, in which problems were anticipated (such as breech birth), most midwives did their utmost to see that the expectant mother received special medical attention. There are numerous accounts of midwives accompanying a sick expectant woman for many miles over rough terrain or stormy seas, to a hospital or nursing station where a doctor or trained nurse could be sought out.

If all appeared well, the midwife would caution the expectant mother on how to prepare for the birth itself. Prior to the beginning of the "lying in" period (usually a period of ten or eleven days, from the onset of labour to "up-sitting-day"), a special birthing room had to be prepared, away from the main routes of the household traffic, and warm and dry in winter. Birthing sheets, layers of paper covered by a clean white sheet, were made to collect any blood and the afterbirth, and to provide protection for the mattress. A clean sheet had to be secured to catch the baby at delivery time. Baby clothes had to be made. Finally, a cradle had to be set up. James Carroll from Makinsons remembers that "Cradles were good and clean and every bit of the house was crystal clean waiting for the child."

If a new mother could not afford to pay for these various necessities, then either the midwife supplied them herself or, typically, the village women pooled their skills and material resources and came to the mother's rescue. Aunt Mary-Ellen recalls how the women's network operated in her community:

> Whenever one of my mothers was due, we all gave her clothes
> for the newborn that our little ones had grown out of. Often
> we'd also have a "bee" to make quilts and diapers and knitties

out of a piece of flannel or leftover things. Of course, it wasn't
fancy but it served the purpose well.

Midwives had to be prepared to attend a birth at any time,
day or night, and in all kinds of weather. They had to take
themselves to the birthplace which was often 20–30 miles away.

The midwife was an advisor to the labouring woman; she
counseled the expectant mother on when to anticipate pain and
on how to cope with it. According to Aunt Clara Tarrant, "They
had their minds made up to it, human nature being what it is. It
came naturally." During this emotional (and potentially dangerous) time of childbirth, the midwife brought compassionate understanding and reassurance to all involved. She would examine
the woman by palpating her abdomen with both hands. If the
labour was imminent, and if there were no problems, she would
encourage the woman to move about, perhaps to do a little light
housework together. Most women continued to move about during contractions and would sometimes lie down when they temporarily subsided. Gertie Legge explains: "You'd be all over the
place. You wouldn't be able to stay in bed sure. You'd have to
move about." The midwife encouraged the woman to adopt the
birthing position most comfortable to her, whether on her side,
on her back, supported against another woman or in a sitting or
crouching position. Aunt Elsie Piercey from Hopeall recalls how
she preferred not to give birth in bed at all: "I'd kneel on the floor
with my arms over the back of the chair."

The midwife had a spiritual role as well. After the birth she
was expected to offer words of thanks, such as "God bless the
baby." She then gave the infant to its mother for its first feeding.
Catholic midwives would often place a blue medal on the infant
in order to ward off the "evil eye." If the baby had a birthmark,
it was the midwife's duty to cross the mark three times with her
wedding ring to "bless it away." The midwife would then see that
the birthing sheets were disposed of. Aunt Clara Tarrant describes
this ritual, "It was a very private affair. The burning was seen to
by the midwife, that was all part of the performance. There was
never a speck of anything to be seen."

Of course, the midwife seldom coped with childbirth alone.
Almost always she was accompanied by a helper and she also
received help from the neighbouring women. As Aunt Mary-El-

len, who told me she assisted well over 500 deliveries, puts it, "There was always other women from around coming and looking out to things that needed to be done. No one starved, let me tell you, when a woman was lyin' in."

On the last day of the lying-in period, traditionally referred to as "up-sitting-day," the neighbouring women, accompanied by the midwife, would gather in the house of the new mother for a cup of tea and sometimes a piece of "Groaning Cake," often prepared by the woman's husband. This mini-celebration was seen as a token of appreciation given by the new mother to the women who had offered their assistance. If she could afford it, the mother would also give the midwife something special in payment for her services — perhaps a piece of cloth, some fish or, if available, a little money.

Finally, about a month or so after the baby's birth, or whenever a minister or priest would visit the village, a public celebration would take place in the form of a christening. Baptism was believed to further protect the child from the "evil eye" and its godparents were expected to guard the child in case of misfortune.

In the isolated areas of the Island and along the Labrador coast the midwife practiced her art of healing relatively unaffected by the outside world until the early 1960s. These women would no doubt have appreciated access to emergency medical services, which would have made it possible to combine their own caring skills and intimate knowledge of the local people with the positive benefits of modern medicine. But they found few doctors or trained nurses willing to adopt such a strategy. As Aunt Clara Tarrant puts it, "A doctor's work didn't seem to be in that then. Some of them ... didn't know too much about maternity either. Didn't want too much to do with it."

Ultimately, childbirth and most other life events (including aging and death) came under medical control. The scientific age arrived in most outports at roughly the same time as roads were built connecting communities to regional centres. Many outports were uprooted entirely and whole populations were forced to resettle in larger towns, serviced by modern hospitals and medical specialists. People, regardless of their status, gained access to the modern government health-care system and it was believed that every health problem would thereafter be cured. The once indispensable role of the midwife/healer was rendered obsolete. However, this "progress" also involved a significant loss. Irene Bradley, the midwife from Eastport, describes this loss:

> I really think that some ways were better. I don't think that women should be cut unless it is a must to save a life. I think that there's too much of that done and that people don't have the patience anymore. I always believed that lots of olive oil and the patience to let the mother do it slowly gave better deliveries. Nowadays the hospitals are in too big a hurry to get it all over with and the mothers are being torn up.

Or, as Aunt Mary-Ellen told me:

> Now the doctors are operating for this and that. Everyone seems to have their womb or some organ missing. I don't know, we were good for the people in many ways. I sometimes think that my homemade remedies and how I cared for the people were real good medicine.

## Note

This article owes a great deal to a number of people. I would like to thank the women of *Healthsharing* for their comments and assistance in writing this article. Special thanks to Phil Hiscock for access to material in the Folklore Archives at Memorial University, St. John's, to Sheila Wilson for interviews with people in Trinity Bay, and to Barbara Doran for her paper on midwifery. Hilda Chalk-Murray's *More Than 50%* gave me valuable information on aspects of birthing in outport Newfoundland. It was a good experience to knit our collective knowledge together to gain a deeper understanding of the history of women healers.

CECILIA BENOIT is presently working on her Ph.D. in Sociology at the University Of Toronto, and plans to do further research on women's health.

# Giving Birth the "White Man's Way"[*]

## Sheila Jennings Linehan

There is an ongoing discussion in the medical community on how to improve the delivery of medical services to the First Nations of Canada. Certainly Inuit communities want access to surgeons, ophthalmologists, pediatricians and general practitioners, for the times when they want or need medical care. Such communities actively solicit these services from physicians. However, the most aggressive "advance" of medicine into the North is clearly in the area of obstetrics. Most physicians have accepted the need for the "colonization" of childbirth in the North, and believe that Inuit women are in desperate need of "modern" medical management, and that they have been and continue to be grateful to be on the receiving end of it.

However, physicians are turning what the Inuit experience as a natural event into an event requiring medical intervention by forcing Inuit women to give birth in hospitals in the south. In doing this they are creating a market for their services at the risk of losing the Inuit's collective knowledge of birth.

Flying in specialists and setting up a referral centre is one thing. But flying out all pregnant women, on their own, against their will and the wishes of their families and communities in order to force them to have southern-style deliveries in a hospital, is quite another.

This compulsory hospitalization is not something that takes place only at a woman's due date; rather, the so called "evacuation" occurs for a time that ranges from two weeks to two months before the due date. When evacuated, Inuit girls and women are commonly billeted in boarding houses until delivery.

* Reprinted from *Healthsharing* vol. 13 no. 2 (Summer/Fall 1992): 11-15, with permission of the author.

Giving birth is a major life event that is definitely familial in nature. Forcing teenage girls, young mothers and mothers of large families to go it alone is cruel. Southerners would not tolerate this, why should northerners.

Years ago the Inuit resisted the effort to force women to deliver at nursing stations staffed by British-trained midwives instead of in their homes. Ironically, the government decided that while midwives were not acceptable for women in the rest of Canada, they could be tolerated for the purposes of preventing Inuit midwives (many of whom are men) from assisting Inuit women in the communities where they worked.

The legacy of quiet resistance by the Inuit to the medical co-optation of birth continues, manifesting itself in various forms. One form is when women delay reporting a pregnancy to create confusion about when they are due. Another is waiting to go to the evacuation centre until labour is so far advanced, it is impossible to get the woman onto a Medevac flight. These practices compromise the safety of the mother and child, but illustrate, at times the only way Inuit women can resist the practices being foisted on them.

In 1987, I read an article by Drs. Pierre Lessard and David Kinloch in the *Canadian Medical Association Journal*, entitled, "Northern Obstetrics: A 5-Year Review of Delivery among Inuit Women." I remember feeling that there was something unpleasant about the article, but I could not put my finger on what it was. Now I know. Like all the literature I had read on Native health care it did not consult Native people — it simply put forward the wants, needs and opinions of the physicians. It smacked of paternalism.

After reading another article earlier this year in the *Medical Post* on the Stanton Yellowknife Hospital finding a new purpose as a referral centre, I sought literature on maternity care written by Native Canadians. I contacted the Ottawa offices of the Native Women's Association and the Pauktuutit (The Inuit Women's Association).

The Native Women's Association directed me to a book called *Gossip: A Spoken History of Women in the North*. It is a collection of works by Native and non-Native women involved in the North, and if there is any doubt that Inuit women are discontented with what the Inuit call "giving birth the white man's way," a quick reading of the book dispels it.

Says Marie Kilunik, an Inuk woman: "In the old days I thought I was going through a rough time. That was before the white man came, but now it's worse for the young girls because of the white man's ways. I worry a lot that girls go south into hospitals to have their babies. I felt so homesick. I didn't know what to do when I was away from home for so long … . I was worried about my husband and kids. I think that women should have their babies in their homes, in their own beds."

Inuit Elders speak about their own experiences with birth in this book as well as their present concerns about the southern control of birth in the North. A major concern of the elders is the practice of their daughters and granddaughters being forced to lie on their backs with their legs up in stirrups (the lithotomy position). A further concern is their daughters' enforced isolation from family, friends and community. The elders also commented on the widespread use of drugs and anaesthesia during delivery in hospitals. Finally, the elders raised concerns that women return from "away" cut and stitched. They attest to a very low perineal tear rate from their midwife-assisted deliveries and do not understand why women fail to return home with an intact perineum.

I know two nurses and one physician involved in delivering Native women in the North. The nurses say Inuit women frequently balk at getting into the lithotomy position because they prefer to deliver squatting and refuse to hand over their infants to be cared for by complete strangers. *Gossip* quotes one Inuit woman as saying, "I'd always had my babies in the squatting position. But when I had my oldest son, they took me to Fort Simpson. I didn't like being on my back, I wanted to be in the squatting position, so I stayed in that position until just the last minute. They had to push me down on the bed to have my baby that way, even though I didn't want to have it that way."

Martha Greig is the National Health Coordinator with Pauktuutit. She is Inuk and since 1987, she has been involved in the organization's annual meetings where resolutions have been drawn up on the practice of evacuation. I spoke to Martha about birth in her community (both her grandmother and grandfather were practicing midwives). She told me "a pregnant woman is supposed to be in harmony. Pregnancy," she says "is not a sickness."

Greig emphasizes that Inuit women have a totally different perspective on pregnancy than the view held in the white man's world:

> In the 1940s, the Inuit lived at outpost camps and there were only Inuit midwife deliveries. In the late 1950s, the white man told the Inuit that they had to form into communities. The kids had to go to school and nursing stations were set up. In the mid-sixties some regional hospitals were set up, but occasional births still took place at home with the Inuit midwives delivering. In the early 1970s all women in their first or greater than fifth pregnancies were sent to regional hospitals, while all other births took place in the nursing stations. By the mid-1970s, all pregnant women were evacuated.
>
> Inuit women were moderately satisfied when the Department of Health and Welfare recruited British trained midwives who delivered in the communities. However, policy changed and suddenly new nursing graduates with little or no obstetrical experience were being sent up North. This was to promote Canadian nurses. All pregnant women started being evacuated. This practice is very hard for the woman's husband and other children; this was especially so in the winter because they could be gone for three or four months.
>
> Nowadays when a woman wants to remain in her community she must give birth in a health centre. This is hard because the woman is made to sign a waiver releasing the nurse from all liability for any faults on the part of the nurse or any problems if something goes wrong. This is risky. In view of this, some women choose evacuation instead and fly to a southern hospital even though they don't want to go.

Greig mentioned an alternative some Inuit women find palatable — a centre at Povungnituk in Northern Quebec where both local women and evacuees come to give birth. A team of three Inuit midwives works there year round. She said the aspect of having to live in a strange place and all the other attendant problems associated with evacuation still make Inuit women miserable, but the situation is tolerable since the women can give birth as they choose and can communicate in Inuktitut with their birth attendants.

She says the Native midwives at the centre do not work in shifts — Inuit women like to avoid the stress of changing birth attendants according to the clock. The Inuit midwife remains throughout labour, no matter how long and is dedicated to ensuring a drug-free labour and delivery.

The Inuit of Povungnituk, Greig explains, are conservative in the way they want to preserve Inuit culture. When the community heard of the intention of the government to build a hospital in the Hudson Bay area, they got together and formed a committee that put forward their proposals for maternity care. Although midwifery is not legally recognized in Quebec, they got what they wanted — a birth centre where husbands, partners or family members could stay with the pregnant women, where the women could bring in a labour coach, and where deliveries were conducted by Native midwives.

Although there are many Inuit women who would describe themselves as home birth advocates, Greig says "I prefer a centre such as the one at Povungnituk. I think it is good to have medical back-up if an emergency comes up. My ideal birth is a birth centre like Povungnituk where Native midwives work and have received further training from southern midwives. The way things are going with midwifery in the provinces, I am confident that Inuit midwifery will become re-established in the North in the near future. When that happens Inuit women will reap the benefits of both worlds."

There are several Canadian academics conducting research in this area. Dr. Patricia Kaufert with the Department of Community Health Sciences at the University of Manitoba, has been tracking the erosion of Inuit childbirth practices and traditions for some time. Kaufert says that the trend towards southern control over childbirth is perceived in the North not only as a hardship for Inuit women, but as a threat to long-term cultural identity and survival. It is experienced by the Inuit in a political context even more than a medical one. Many Inuit are concerned when their children are forcibly delivered outside the boundaries of the North West Territories. Inuit worry about their children's future rights to special status entitlements, which have been important in the past in economic benefit determinations. Nothing a south-erner can say can remove this concern.

One of Kaufert's studies examines the delivery of obstetrical care given to Inuit women in the Keewatin Region of the North West Territories. The epidemiological component of this study included an audit of the obstetrical records for all women in the area who gave birth from 1979 to 1985. After examining the data, researchers concluded that there had been a misuse of the rates, numbers and statistics by policy makers to justify extending medical control over Inuit childbirth.

Betty Anne Daviss-Putt has been a consultant to the Inuit Women's Association since 1985 and has been a practicing mid-wife for 15 years. In all that time she says she has not come across a single Inuit woman who prefers a hospital birth, and she also attests to a profound distaste of the medical approach amongst Inuit women.

In *Gossip*, she notes that the Northern Obstetrics Conference of 1987 in Churchill, Manitoba also exposed the faulty epidemiological rationale that is the basis for the belief that evacu-ations are the only safe alternative for Inuit women.

Kaufert's studies show increasing rates of Caesarean sections, inductions and forceps deliveries amongst the Inuit, at a time when many southern obstetricians are being chastised by the World Health Organization and Canadian health activists for overly interventionist and heavy-handed approaches.

Although physicians who have been involved in obstetrics in the North attest that Inuit women tolerate all the stages of labour well, reasons to "augment" are still being found. This should concern us all not just on humanitarian grounds but on fiscal ones also.

In one of Kaufert's studies, which took place over a seven-year span in the Keewatin region, not a single woman died in child-birth. Maternal mortality rates are often quoted to the Inuit in an effort to get them to see things the southern way. Kaufert points out that for Inuit women, maternal mortality rates are an issue only as an event which is feared, not as a reality. Stillbirths and neonatal deaths are the realities that the women face frequently. These serious problems point to the need for better prenatal care which could and should be delivered by Native midwives who speak Inuktitut. The need for medical advice for the neonate is self evident. This could be given by a nurse or a general practitioner. The infant mortality rate clusters around the first four weeks of life amongst the Inuit — a condition labelled "northern infant syndrome." Labour and delivery are manifestly not the problems. Importing specialists in the pathology of labour and delivery is unnecessary.

The excuse given for evacuation is that it is a sure fire method to save maternal and infant lives. But, evacuation is not always going to save a woman should an emergency Caesarean section be required. For example, women are evacuated to Churchill Falls regularly, yet C-sections are not available in Churchill Falls. The reasoning behind evacuation to this particular centre does not appear to be the availability of this service.

A second rationale could be the need for a blood transfusion in the rare event of a hemorrhage. But, as Betty Anne Daviss-Putt points out in *Gossip*, it would make more sense to cross-match the woman's blood ahead of time and forward it to a nursing station, than to evacuate the pregnant woman traumatically and at high cost.

Finally, Daviss-Putt notes that there is the assumption that the personnel waiting for the arrival of the evacuee in the hospital are better qualified than the personnel the woman just left. This, she says, is not always true.

There is also a strong sense of what Kaufert refers to as a "civilizing mission" among Canadian physicians who go to work up North. In the article, "Reconstruction of Inuit Birth," Kaufert and fellow researcher John O'Neil say: "... preoccupation with perinatal mortality rates transformed the death of a baby from a problem only for the individual women, her family and her community, into a concern for the Canadian government ...."

O'Neil and Kaufert further state that control over childbirth became essential to ensure constant proof of the advantage of power, and that when speaking with individual Inuit women, they found a recurrent theme: their loss of control over the place of birth, its timing and its process.

Both researchers feel this loss has now become a metaphor for the loss of political control by the Inuit people over their lives and their communities. They point to an ongoing campaign by the Inuit people to regain power over childbirth as having become as much an item on the Inuit political agenda as it is an issue for the individual Inuit woman.

Inuit people, specifically Inuit women, were not asked if they wanted southern obstetrical practice before it was foisted upon them. The reason for this is obvious — if consulted, they would have wanted input into its implementation or resisted its implementation altogether...

*Gossip* points out that some researchers have concluded that midwives are the most suitable providers of obstetrical care in the North for both pre- and postnatal care in healthy women. The question is: Why the muted response to this finding within the medical community? Until real communication begins, control over birth will remain a profoundly political issue in Inuit culture.

## Note

For more information, the Inuit Broadcasting Corporation has made an excellent video entitled, "Ikajurti: Midwifery in the Canadian Arctic," produced by George Hargrave, Dorothy Kidd and Ruby Arngna'naaq. To order by mail call: (613) 238-3977; or contact Pauktuutit, 200 Elgin Street, Suite 804, Ottawa, ON., ($30.00 for individuals; $75.00 for institutions).

SHEILA JENNINGS LINEHAN is currently clerking in the area of Intellectual Property Law at a law firm in Ottawa. She will be called to the bar in February 1993. She is married and has two children: Rory, age two, and Chloe, age one. Rory was delivered by a midwife and Sheila says she and her husband hope to have one more child and to have a home delivery with a midwife.

# Who's in Control?

## Eggs, Embryos and Fetal Tissue[*]

### Bonnie Lafave

Currently in Canada, no laws exist to regulate the use of embryos and fetuses in research and experimental therapies. Yet human eggs, sperm, embryos and fetuses are increasingly used for medical and technological experimentation. Because eggs, embryos and fetuses come from women's bodies, it is essential that we participate in discussions about how these tissues are used in current biotechnology. We must also be active participants in decision-making about the direction biotechnology will take in the future.

Decisions about what kind of research is done, how it is done, and who is doing it, are too often made only by scientists, governments and big business. There has been little public discussion about egg harvesting, embryo freezing or the use of fetal tissue in transplantation.

Women require awareness and understanding of medical procedures, which, while often presented to us as benign therapies or liberating choices, may be insidiously threatening our control over our bodies.

Human gametes and embryos are in demand because of their value in research and product development. In research, they are used to refine methods of freezing eggs and embryos, and to develop tests which predict the normalcy of fertilized embryos. They are used for diagnosing chromosomal or genetic disorders and in cancer research. However, their best known uses are in the refinement of experimental reproductive technologies.

Fetal tissues are used by pharmaceutical companies in the manufacturing of vaccines for poliomyelitis and rubella. Fetal

---

[*] Reprinted from *Healthsharing* vol. 9 no. 4 (Fall 1988): 29-31, with permission of the author.

tissue also is desirable because of its ability to repair itself. It may prove to be of benefit as transplantation tissue for victims of Parkinson's disease, Alzheimer's disease, Huntington's chorea, spinal cord injuries, diabetes, leukemia, aplastic anemia and radiation sickness. Dr. Robert Gale of the University of Los Angeles (UCLA), used fetal cells to treat six of the victims of the Chernobyl nuclear accident in 1986. In January of 1988, Dr. Ignacio Madrazo of Mexico City, transplanted fetal brain cells into the brains of two individuals who were suffering from Parkinson's disease, and has since noted a reduction of clinical signs of the illness in both patients.

The cosmetic industry is involved in fetal research for product development. In a recent report to the Parliamentary Assembly of the Council of Europe, Mr. Haase, a member of Parliament for the Federal Republic of Germany, cited several examples of corporate purchase of fetuses. In 1981, for example, French customs seized a consignment of fetuses from Romania being shipped to a cosmetics firm. Similarly, California police discovered in 1982 more than 500 fetuses preserved in formaldehyde, "allegedly intended for a clinic specializing in cosmetic surgery." We routinely use cosmetic products made from various parts of various animals as well as from human placenta. How long will it be before it becomes routine to use products made with human fetal tissue?

"Little embryo research is being done in Canada at present," says Connie Clement, family planning coordinator for the Toronto Department of Public Health. "But as of 1988, funding for such experimentation is available from the National Research Council following the release of Guidelines on Research Involving Human Subjects."

Some doctors performing abortions have been reported as donating fetal tissue for medical research without informing the women involved. It may be that most women who undergo abortions do not want to know or make choices about how their aborted fetuses are disposed of. Others may want to know what kinds of research are being done and may want to choose whether or not to give consent for their fetuses to be used. Even where the individual woman having an abortion or using the services of a fertility clinic is given the right to choose and to know how the fetus or embryos will be used, she could feel pressured to comply with the doctor's wishes since she is in a vulnerable position at that time. In any case, regardless of the question of individual rights or choices, the larger social and ethical questions involved concern all women.

There is a potential for misuse of new techniques used to obtain embryos. In particular, in vitro fertilization (IVF) is used more than other procedures to help women get pregnant because it produces a greater number of embryos than are implanted at one time. IVF is being used in Canada, the U.S., Great Britain, Australia, and other countries as a fertility therapy although it is still considered by many health professionals to be an experimental procedure with a very low success rate and a very high cost.

Women may be taking both physical and emotional risks because of researchers' desire to get embryos as drugs such as Clomiphene Citrate, more commonly known as Clomid, are used to make them hyper-ovulate. Clomid has a chemical profile similar to that of DES, a drug given to women in the 1940s and 1950s to prevent miscarriages. DES caused a previously rare and invasive form of vaginal cancer in a small number of the daughters born to women who used DES. The long-term effects of Clomid are not known, however animal studies are showing effects similar to those of DES.

Hyper-ovulation with Clomid produces up to 15 eggs per cycle although IVF only requires two to three eggs per cycle. The "spare" eggs, which have been fertilized to create embryos, can be destroyed but instead are frozen for later use or in experimentation. Infertility clinics across Canada are currently freezing embryos.

England's Patrick Steptoe, one of the founding "fathers" of IVF has said, "I would like to build up a panel of forty women ready to donate eggs." He once even offered free sterilization operations to any women who would donate eggs to his IVF patients, and incidently, to his research. Yet it is not only "services" that are being exchanged: money changes hands as well. Fertility and Genetics Research, Inc., a Chicago-based biotechnology company paid $100 per egg to donors in 1984. The money reimbursed the donor "mainly for the inconvenience of coming to the clinic," said Richard Seed, a live-stock breeder and coowner of the company.

According to Robyn Rowland, author of *Making Women Visible in the Embryo Experimentation Debate*, "Intimations are constantly given that IVF women are in fact in favour of embryo experimentation." Yet for many women, each embryo is perceived as an extension of her own body, her own being. It is not surprising then that women in IVF programs indicate that they are not totally convinced of the value of embryo research. The infertility group, Concern, in Perth, Western Australia found that the donation of embryos for experimentation was not acceptable to 35 percent of IVF couples responding to a survey, and a further 25 percent were undecided.

Here in Canada, it is illegal to buy or sell human tissue, according to the Human Tissue Gift Act. But it is not illegal to give or accept reimbursement for losses incurred by the donor, such as loss of wages. It may be that nobody buys eggs, but donors can be paid nonetheless. Clearly, lower-income women are most vulnerable when eggs, embryos or fetuses become commodities for sale or for donation. The desire for fetal tissue is as strong as that for embryos. There is already concern from researchers and the public that some women might get pregnant for the purpose of providing aborted fetuses to researchers in exchange for money. Arthur Caplan, specialist in medical ethics at the University of Minnesota says he "already knows of American women who are prepared to breed fetuses for spare parts."

The demand for fetal tissue is increasing, and according to the April 15, 1988 article in the *Montreal Gazette*, there is already evidence of an underground market. It was reported that a woman whose husband has Parkinson's disease attended a medical conference in Boston hoping to find help for her husband. She left her card on the bulletin board. She then received a phone call from a person who offered to arrange a fetal cell transplant at a private Mexican clinic.

How we view abortion may also have a direct bearing on how we view fetal and even embryo experimentation. Daniel Callahan in *How Technology is Reforming the Abortion Debate* notes, "the cumulative impact of a number of otherwise limited scientific developments could lead to a shift in public opinion, moral thinking and court decisions about abortion." These include the temporary separation of the egg, and subsequently the embryo from the mother, raising its status, even for a short time, to that of a separate entity; the increase in public awareness of and concern for fetal health, (to the extent that the fetus is now, on occasion, considered to be a patient, whose needs may supersede her mother's, as in the case of Baby R [see "Whose Womb Is It Anyway?" *Healthsharing* vol. 9 no. 2, Spring 1988]); and the increased "clinical efforts to improve the outcome for fetuses, premature infants, and otherwise distressed infants." In 1973, at the time of the Roe vs. Wade abortion decision, the age of viability was 28 weeks. At present, the age of viability has been lowered by the World Health Organization to 22 weeks.

We must continue to insist on our right to choose abortion. At the same time we are being threatened that if we elect to abort, we should be required to give up our right to determine what becomes of the fetus. Charles H. Baron, professor of law at Boston College Law School says, "Even if a woman has a right to be free of an unwanted pregnancy, she does not necessarily have the right to determine what shall be done to the fetus before, during or after its removal from her body."

Clearly, the use of eggs, embryos and fetal tissue gives us much to think about, even more to debate. We must continue to make ourselves aware of the advances being made in reproductive technology and biotechnology. Yet we must also be conscious of the potential for coercion and manipulation of women in the advancement of such research, technologies or products. Although women will disagree on the relative benefits of new technologies or research, our strongest defense is the collective opportunity for consent: if eggs, embryos, and fetuses from our bodies are used, then we must have the right of consent. As 52 percent of the Canadian population, and 100 percent of the bodies in this country producing eggs, embryos and fetuses, women are in a unique position of strength to make their voices heard on these issues of such ethical and moral importance.

**BONNIE LAFAVE** is a psychiatric nurse at The Clarke Institute of Psychiatry in Toronto.

# Mothers

## The First Environment[*]

### Katsi Cook

Native Elders know that the body of a pregnant woman changes to accommodate and nurture new life. For them, pregnancy is a re-enactment of the creation of the world. A child's birth changes both the family and the whole community.

In pregnancy, our bodies sustain life. At the breast of women, the generations are nourished. In this way, the elders believe the earth is our mother. In this way, we as women are earth. We are the first environment.

Our Native American traditions tell us that our unborn see through our eyes and hear through our ears. In the dream days just before their births, they learn from our thoughts and our emotions. And now, when they are born, they inherit a body burdened with toxic contaminants.

Where the St. Lawrence River meets the Canadian border at the 45th parallel, the Akwesasne community of 7,000 Mohawk people has drawn its subsistence from the local food chain for centuries. Generations have eaten fish from the river and birds from its banks.

But the beautiful St. Lawrence River carries with it chemical contaminants, dumped by industries all along the Great Lakes. Indian fishermen feel the effects of these toxins and have long-complained about the depletion of fish and other wildlife.

The First Environment Project, initiated by Mohawk women themselves in 1985, has also been concerned with the problem of toxic contamination of their water, air, soil and food chain by local industries.

Toxic chemicals like PCBs, DDT, mirex, and HCBs dumped by

---

[*] Reprinted from *Healthsharing* vol. 13 no. 4 (Winter/Spring 1994): 22-23, with permission of the author.

industries into the water and soil move up the food chain — through plants, fish, and wildlife — into our bodies. These contaminants resist being broken down by the body, and are stored in our fat cells where they collect and become more dangerous as time passes. The only known way to excrete large amounts of toxins is through pregnancy, when they cross the placenta and contaminate the fetus and during lactation, when they move out of storage and flow into breastmilk. This means each succeeding generation inherits an increasing amount of toxins from their mothers.

The First Environment Project was created because Mohawk women were worried about the reproductive health effects of toxic contaminants, including high miscarriage rates and birth defects. Our aim is to give momentum to the search for answers about the effects of toxic exposure in our drinking water, and to learn its full impact on reproductive and family health. Since Akwesasne borders the U.S. and Canada, we have been appealing to governments in both countries to restrict dumping by local industries.

The project also conducts community-based research that focuses on the analysis of organochlorines in mothers milk, fetal cord blood, and maternal and infant urine. To date, over 100 Mohawk women have served as participants in the study, which is funded by the state of New York and State University of New York (SUNY), Albany. So far, the Canadian government has not provided any funding.

Principal investigator of the study, Ed Fitzgerald, is an epidemiologist with the N.Y. State's Department of Health and an assistant professor at the School of Public Health at SUNY, Albany. Brian Bush, another faculty member at the school, and analytical chemist for the mother's milk study, examines different forms of PCB compounds for the health department's Wadsworth labs.

The First Environment Project works in unison with the Akwesasne Task Force on the Environment, which is made up of tribal and Mohawk Council officials, members of the traditional Longhouse, and concerned community individuals. Its aim is to strengthen community efforts in response to environmental issues.

The project is working with the St. Regis Mohawk Tribe Environment Division in response to the August 1990, U.S. Environmental Protection Agency (EPA) guidance document designed for "typical" industrial sites. This document states that soil with 500 ppm (parts per million) of toxins is acceptable, despite N.Y. State's policy that 50 ppm is considered toxic waste. This is an indication of how good the industry lobbyists are in Washington.

One site of great concern is a landfill made by General Motors on the New York side of the reservation. Researchers say this dump is contributing to the high levels of toxicity found on Cornwall Island, Ontario. Chemicals of concern at the GM site include PCBs, such as phenols and volatile organic compounds. In 1983, the EPA placed the site on the U.S National Priorities List of the most hazardous waste sites in the United States. That same year, the company was fined $500,000 by the EPA for violations of federal environmental laws.

The U.S. Food and Drug Administration sets a limit of two ppm of PCBs in fish and a limit of three ppm of PCBs in poultry. Samples taken near the GM site included three ppm in a lake sturgeon, 318 ppm in a mallard duck and 11,000 ppm in a small rodent.

So far, the First Environment Project has created a Native American presence in the environmental movement and has trained women in health research. There is much more to be done. Canadian initiatives are needed, and adherence to stricter regulations on both sides of the border are imperative. But the environmental work being done at Akwesasne is a big jump ahead.

The next phase is to include men in the study, especially since they tend to eat more fish at Akwesasne. We are really only getting half the picture by concentrating on women and children alone. In order to see the full effects of toxic contamination we must examine the entire food chain.

The First Environment Project provides a good example of how a community can respond when there is an environmental need — something communities around the globe will have to face more and more.

KATSI COOK is a Mohawk midwife and childbirth educator. She is the Project Director of the First Environment Project.

# A Matter of Gender*

## Aruna Papp

Canadian society reacted with repugnance when newspaper stories about the East Indian community using Dr. Stephens' services to determine the sex of a fetus for the purpose of aborting fetuses. The reactions from the East Indian community were very diverse. Some screamed racism, some expressed disgust and some said that, while things like that may happen in India, they do not happen in Canada. I along with perhaps many of those who remained silent, know that aborting female fetuses is a common practice in South Asian communities. But we also know that it is common in many other cultures as well and we abhor Dr. Stephens targeting our community. Aborting female fetuses is not an inherent feature of South Asian culture, but rather a reflection of a deep-seated sexism which permeates all cultures.

While it is not surprising that many women use sex selection services, we must look at the underlying causes and find a way to challenge this practice.

In 1989, South Asian Family Support Services conducted research to study the issue of wife abuse in the South Asian community living in Scarborough, Ontario. Of the 100 women interviewed, 22 said that they had been unable to produce a son and this was the main cause of abuse in their marriage. The other 78 stated that until they had given birth to a son they had lived in constant fear and uncertainty. They knew that their marital status could become worse if they did not give birth to a son. Several of these women attended support groups for battered women and their fears were confirmed by those women who had been divorced because they had been unable to have a son. Seventeen of the 22 women without a son had been in the hospital receiving psychiatric care at one time or another. The women

---

*   Reprinted from *Healthsharing* vol. 12 no. 1 (Spring 1991): 12, with permission of the author.

blamed themselves for not being able to have an "heir." They felt that they had failed as daughters and as wives. It was very difficult for these women to share the blame with their husbands. They often made excuses such as, "What can a man do? He must have a son," or "One can expect a man to go mad once in a while, especially if he has to come home and look at daughters."

In the East Indian culture a female is socialized from the first moments of her life into a culturally defined sex role which teaches self-sacrifice, self-deprivation, renunciation, humility and death before complaining. This role of the ideal woman is defined through sacred scripture, believed to be divinely inspired and unalterable. This same scripture also states that the nature of a female is wicked and deceptive; being a girl is a penalty for sin committed in the previous incarnation. A woman's only way to salvation is to bear a son so that her husband can receive incarnation, a good form of life in the next world.

These cultural values are secured by a variety of means; gender inequality from birth, educational deprivation and dividing women from one another. For example, special songs of respect are sung for women who are mothers of male offspring and when a woman marries, she receives the blessing "pray you have a dozen sons."

Why did South Asian women become the biggest clients of Dr. Stephens? The abused women in my support group said that they are not only the victims of their religion and culture, but of the racist and misogynist Canadian society they live in. It is difficult for South Asian women in such situations to visit friends who have sons; they are always in fear of any conversation turning to the subject of children and ultimately, to having sons. They feel ashamed for having failed as a wife. Some women stated that they live in constant dread that their daughters might be harmed or that the daughters will do something that will shame the family. This would reflect upon the mother and intensify the abuse.

In cases where police or other social service agencies have become involved, often the abuse has escalated. When the agency was able to assist the woman to leave and go to a shelter, the anxiety about the future, the concern that no South Asian man will marry a divorced woman's daughter, the lack of financial and emotional support from relatives, and the lack of social support systems usually forced a return to the family. Their state of mind is unimaginable. These women feel they have not only failed as women by not producing a son, but they have also destroyed their marriage.

Until South Asians come to terms with the fact that women in our community and in Canadian society as a whole, do not have the same rights and equality as men and until the community decides that women have the right to live with dignity, Dr. Stephens and his cronies will continue to exploit us. South Asian women are taking steps towards change. We're making our contribution to putting Dr. Stephens out of business.

ARUNA PAPP has worked with South Asian battered women for the past 15 years and is founder and executive director of South Asian Family Support Services.

## section five

# The Ongoing Fight for Reproductive Choice

From its inception, *Healthsharing* had an ongoing interest in reproductive health and the fight for reproductive freedom. The magazine featured numerous articles and updates on birth control methods and the politics surrounding the abortion issue. The articles in this section examine the legal and medical context for reproductive decisions and feminist campaigns for reproductive freedom.

"Legal Assault" brings together two major reproductive rights campaigns on a key common concern: the increasing medical and legal surveillance of women's reproduction which increasingly defined the fetus as a patient separate from the woman. Defining the fetus in this way allows doctors to appoint themselves the guardian of fetal interest and to intervene to protect those interests even against the woman's wishes. "Whose Womb is it Anyway?" shows how this intervention has worked in practice to control and confine women.

"No New Law!" gives and overview of the long but victorious struggle in Canada to remove abortion from the criminal code and increase access to save legal abortion for women. "Women Lose Freedom of Choice" shows the fragility of women's right to choose legal abortion.

"The Birth Control Gap" was the earliest of all the articles written in this section. It is a detailed examination of the problems women face making our contraceptive choices. It argues that higher safety standards, and methods that women can control will never be fulfilled until there is a fundamental change in women's role in society and until attitudes towards sex and sexuality are transformed.

# The Birth Control Gap[*]

## Dianne Kinnon

Contemporary women are now entering the second generation of modern, technological contraception. Since the Pill and the IUD (intrauterine device) ushered in a new era of contraceptive options, we have been introduced to contraceptive foam, suppositories and sponges, sympto-thermal birth control and now, awaiting us on the horizon, are hormonal rings, injections and implants. Only the condom, diaphragm, cervical cap and the rhythm method remain in popular use from before this technological revolution in birth control. And while these tried-and-true methods are far from having gone the way of the dinosaur, they are no longer treated as serious options by large numbers of women. Younger women, particularly, share an almost universal distaste at the very thought of using barrier methods. They are also put off by the idea of the IUD, and, while they may exhibit an interest in the science of sympto-thermal fertility awareness, they can't imagine using it for birth control themselves.

As most birth control counselors will testify, the Pill has first billing among teenaged women long before they walk in the front door of the clinic. The vast majority begin their thirty year odyssey of controlling their reproduction by using it.

On what basis are women making contraceptive decisions, and why? Is it just a matter of choosing "the best method for you, one that fits your lifestyle," a favourite phrase of clinicians and birth control counselors? Have we won the contraceptive battle, because we now have the choices our grandmothers couldn't imagine? Or are these "choices" something of an illusion? How far have we really come in our struggle to control our fertility?

The medical reality is that contraceptive methods as a whole are shamefully inadequate. Many pose real health hazards to

* Reprinted from *Healthsharing* vol. 6 no. 2 (Spring 1985): 15-17, with permission of the author.

women who use them, and none is totally effective. Contraceptive "choice" is really a matter of selecting the least unattractive option, and usually means changing methods several times throughout the reproductive years. Moreover, women have not really won control of our choices in birth control. Contraceptive research is still in the hands of male doctors, by and large, and reflects their biases and assumptions of what kind of contraception is best.

Perhaps an even more important aspect of reproductive choice is *how* we use the existing technology. Our ideas about our bodies, and the choices we make in our relationships have profound effects on the birth control we use. The result for women is often that we cheat ourselves in order to please our partners or fulfil some unrealistic sexual expectation of our men.

Use of barrier methods such as condoms, the diaphragm and foam is a good example. Any contraceptive that must be used just before or at the time of sexual intercourse is considered undesirable by many couples. Barrier methods, most say, interfere with the sex act and make sexual encounters less spontaneous and therefore less pleasurable. This attitude is rooted partly in the expectations of the sex act. Sex has been given an exalted position in our relationships, and we are willing to go to great lengths to achieve what we see as better, even perfect, sex.

Some women in new relationships don't like to bother their partners with birth control and some men do not consider it their responsibility to inquire or offer assistance. Virtually everyone who uses barrier methods has taken chances with them — not using condoms "just this once" to preserve an intimate moment, going ahead with sex even if the diaphragm has been left at home. Even in the most liberated of relationships, many women still put a high priority on the romance of a relationship, and often this means taking responsibility for using a non-intrusive birth control method.

Natural family planning, or sympto-thermal birth control, which can be a highly effective and medically safe method, is used by few couples because of the high degree of commitment and cooperation necessary. Some men flatly refuse to even consider it because it involves a week of planned abstention from intercourse (not necessarily from other forms of love-making) each month. In fact, though many of us are not conscious of it, the sex act sill largely revolves around male pleasure. For example, though barriers are not used because they supposedly detract from lovemaking, barrier methods do not affect female sexual response, and some actually enhance it. The extra lubrication of contraceptive foam is very helpful for a dry or semi-aroused vagina. Condoms may enhance a woman's pleasure by slowing down her partner's orgasm until she is fully aroused and also capable of orgasm. Use of a diaphragm or cervical cap has no effect on physical sexual response of men or women — neither can feel it — and their intrusion into the pre-coital encounter probably affects women less than men, since women seem more able to sustain a level of arousal. So often our rejection of barrier methods is a protection of our traditional expectations of male pleasure.

Is spontaneity in sex more important to men or women? Certainly *planning* is of more crucial benefit to women, if unwanted pregnancy is to be avoided. Whether through preference or necessity, women have been the holders of the key and, more often than we know or want to admit, the planners of supposedly spontaneous sex! We should ask ourselves to what lengths we will go to maintain this illusion of spontaneity. On a very crude level, some men believe their women should always be sexually available, and there are some women who want to stay readily available, in order to hold on to their boyfriends. But is natural sex so important a value to men and women that it should be the deciding factor in birth control?

Women's difficulty in consciously planning pleasurable sex is tied to another deciding factor in contraceptive choice. The double-bind thinking that punishes strong, self-positive sexual women and rewards shamed, passive women is still with us. A dominant message in pornography, advertising and party jokes still equates women's sexuality with promiscuity and evil, while male sexuality is filled with images of power and dominance. The old ideas of the dirtiness of sex and our bodies "down there" die slowly. An amazing number of women, young and old, have difficulty thinking about, looking at or touching their own genitals. For example, though many women have an academic interest in fertility awareness, the thought of actually examining their own vaginal mucus is abhorrent. Many women cannot use the diaphragm, cervical cap or sponges for the same reason. Some women are also turned off by the idea of an IUD in their uterus; others can accept it because a doctor is inserting it.

The reality for many women is that their sexual encounters are still filled with such embarrassment and ill-ease that a frank discussion of sexual pleasure, much less contraception, is still not possible. For teenaged women, the problem is even more acute. Most cannot countenance the idea of going to a family doctor to be fitted for a diaphragm to be carried around in their purse, because this assertive action belies everything they have learned about what makes a woman sexually desirable.

Male attitudes toward contraception are also an important factor. The idea that virility is tied to fertility is an important factor in many men's rejection of vasectomy as contraception. Condoms, too, have an age-old reputation for being less masculine.

The issue of safety of various birth control methods has affected patterns of contraceptive use. There has been a significant rise in the use of barrier methods over the last five years, as more and more women become concerned about the safety of the Pill and the IUD. Many of these women have in fact almost used up their "Pill years" (10-15 years of use before the age of 35) before switching to other methods. The Pill is still the overwhelming choice among young (15-25 year old) contraceptive users. Much of the conflicting opinion about certain health risks of the Pill is no longer in doubt. We don't just suspect that the Pill carries a higher risk of heart attack, stroke, breast cancer and cervical cancer; the research is conclusive enough to be widely accepted even in the medical community, which historically has been strongly pro-Pill. Yet millions of women undertake these risks in order to prevent conception.

Recorded side effects of the oral contraceptive number in the hundreds. Almost every woman experiences some common unintended effects: intermittent bleeding, headaches, depression, weight gain and increased vaginal infections. They are the price women pay for the effectiveness and ease of using the Pill. Young women are subjecting themselves to these so-called nuisance effects in the short run and are gambling on serious consequences in the long run. The payoff is another invisible means of contraception and a few extra percentage points of protection over most other methods.

IUDs appear to offer the perfect promise of invisible contraception. Once inserted, a woman's only responsibility, theoretically, is to periodically check the string to see that it is in place. In reality, many women endure very long, painful periods, recurrent infections and the threat of pelvic inflammatory disease. No wonder Germaine Greer and other women have begun to ask, "Is sex worth it?"

Despite all this the mystique of no-mess, no-fuss contraception dies hard, and women still gravitate to the Pill and the IUD despite the risks. An important reason is that many of them are not realistically informed about risks or about all options. You can't make a real choice when one option is heavily weighted by your doctor, the expert, and the other choices are discounted. Some doctors pooh-pooh other methods, or know nothing about them, such as sympto-thermal methods or cervical caps. Medical advertising is also heavily pro-Pill. Oral contraceptives are marketed as the modern woman's answer to contraception. Advertising of the Pill and the IUD encourages removal of contraception from the sexual act and from "down there," and plays on our ambivalence toward our own sexuality.

Why do women choose methods that privatize and separate contraception from sex, giving them more individual control in preventing unwanted pregnancy but also leaving them with the total burden? Because, in today's world, this is preferable to having to convince their lovers to get involved. Most of us do not yet have the kind of relationships with men that allow us to make contraceptive decisions on grounds of mutual choice and preference. As long as we are economically and emotionally dependent on men, we will continue to compromise our contraceptive decisions instead of striving for mutual respect, equal relationships and pride in our sexual selves.

A better contraceptive world is not hard to imagine. But it will not depend entirely or even mainly on the development of new technologies. More crucial is a change in sexual attitudes on the part of both men and women, as well as a change in women's role in society. Both are essential to real reproductive freedom for all women. When women reject squeamishness about "down there" and teach their daughters pride in their bodies, ideas about sexuality will begin to change radically.

Imagine, for instance, a world where sexual activity is not focused on vaginal penetration. Sex in this new society wouldn't mean intercourse as it does now, but a wide spectrum of sexual activities leading to mutual orgasms. This change would be an improvement in women's sex lives. The majority of female orgasms come not from vaginal penetration but from other kinds of stimulation, so variety in sexual expression would make sex better for many women. Freedom from intercourse would open up whole new vistas of sexual pleasuring, or as one visionary man put it, teaming to "make love with my whole body." Natural family planning would not be the burden that some find it now since a week of protected intercourse or no intercourse at all would not be unusual. Condoms and foam would be less of a hassle, since they would only need to be used occasionally.

Outercourse, or non-penetration sex, is on its way in. It will not happen until we teach young people and adults that self-masturbation, mutual masturbation, oral sex, etc. are good expressions of sexuality. For men, it would mean a major, but positive change in orientation. Perhaps a freedom from the need for penetration by men is necessary for the acceptance of the condom, for instance. Once men can let go of the idea that their sexual identity centres on the tips of their penises, encasing them may be possible. When heterosexual men start to accept condoms as being in their own best interest, we truly have some hope for use of the only present male contraceptive; more importantly, we will have brought about a change in attitude.

We must continue to press for more research, higher safety standards and more effective birth control. The priority must be less intrusive, less medically controlled contraception so that reproductive care is more self-directed and holistic. Access to all methods by all women who want them is a necessity, and abortion must continue to be available as a backup. The more difficult part of our struggle will be to exorcize the internal oppression that prevents us from making positive sexual decisions. Only then will women develop the power to challenge social expectations and the medical status quo.

DIANNE KINNON has been involved in women's health activities in a variety of capacities. Currently she offers workshops on both pornography and human sexuality. She recently resigned as the director of Planned Parenthood of Ottawa.

# Whose Womb Is It Anyway?[*]

## Maggie Thompson

On September 3, 1987 a British Columbia family court judge ruled that the apprehension of a Vancouver woman's unborn child and the subsequent coerced Caesarean section were entirely proper. The Baby R case, as it has become known, is a precedent setting one. For the first time the B.C. Family and Child Services Act has been successfully used to seize a fetus and thereby force its mother into surgery she did not want. Further, the case relied on a prenatal apprehension as the basis for state custody of the child born. It is a dangerous precedent that will affect all pregnant women because the rights of the mother have been considered secondary to the rights of the fetus.

Events as described in the hearing clearly illustrate that the woman involved was treated as little more than a baby container. Along with other members of the Vancouver Women's Health Collective, Maggie Thompson attended the hearings.

On July 13, 1987 the New Westminster court room had a pretentious air about it. Fine oak panelling covered all four walls. Court officials were positioned on one side of a solid oak divider. Sheriffs watched over them. On the other side of the divider observers packed into long, uncomfortable wooden pews. The air was thick with anticipation. The case we had all been waiting for was about to begin.

### "All Rise!"
In strutted family court judge Brian Davis. He hurriedly seated

* Reprinted from *Healthsharing* vol. 9 no. 2 (Spring 1988): 14-17, with permission of the author.

himself on a high backed leather chair, examined the court room gallery over the upper rim of his half glasses and began to tap his pen impatiently. It seemed he was looking for someone. I immediately felt tense.

"Is Ms. R in the court room?" Davis asked. "Yes, your honour," responded legal-aid-appointed lawyer Jim Thompson. Thompson turned in the direction of Ms. R. nodding his head. Every gaze in the court room turned to her, a small 37-year-old woman we'll call Rose. The sudden rush of attention seemed to take Rose by surprise. Her eyes turned downwards, her long brown hair shielded her, deflecting glances.

From that moment on the looks, the whispers, the notes passed from person to person all said that people were already making their judgements. Rose was on trial.

Ministry of Social Services and Housing (MSSH) lawyer Tom Gove, a red-faced, stocky little man, announced he had 10 people waiting to give testimony. He estimated it would take him three days to complete his evidence. Rose's lawyer, Jim Thompson, said he had no witnesses to call and that he was unsure of whether to ask his client, Rose, to take the stand. Rose's prospects looked poor. The testimony that follows recounts the events on the day of Rose's son's birth.

At 3 p.m. on May 20, 1987 Rose entered a Vancouver maternity hospital, in labour. It was her fifth birth, the previous four resulted in healthy babies, all born vaginally. Her fetus was in a footling breech position (its feet rather than its head appearing first), the cervix already quite dilated. In the absence of her own doctor, attending physician Christos Zouves examined Rose and quickly concluded that "the baby would die or would be seriously or permanently injured" without a Caesarean section. Rose didn't agree with his assessment. She refused to give consent for the Caesarean.

Zouves then phoned the Ministry of Social Services and Housing in order to find a way to force Rose to have the Caesarean. He attempted to have her temporarily committed under the Canadian Mental Health Act, but a hospital psychiatrist and MSSH's emergency health team found that there were not sufficient grounds to take such extreme action. They assessed Rose to be competent and able to make her own decisions.

It then became apparent to Zouves that in order to proceed

with the Caesarean, apprehension of the fetus, declaring the child in need of protection, was his only option. He contacted a ministry social worker, Ivan Bulic, who had never met Rose, to ask how an apprehension could take place.

In virtually every instance, the State is only given the authority to seize or apprehend a child once it has evidence that the child has suffered abuse or neglect. Once apprehended, responsibility for the well-being of the child is transferred, temporarily or permanently, from the parent(s) to the State. The State then has the authority to decide what is in the best interests of the child.

In the testimony that continues, Zouves held that if the fetus was found to be in need of protection, then the ministry was responsible for the fetus, and he could perform a Caesarean section without Rose's consent. He went on to say that the fetus needed medical attention to survive, yet the only medical attention he mentioned was the Caesarean section.

For a moment I was stunned. Could this fetus be pregnant, I asked myself?

Continuing testimony, Bulic understood Zouves' plan and recognized its irregularity. He checked with the superintendent of Family and Child Services and was told to ask Zouves whether he was dealing with a child or a fetus. Zouves responded "In my opinion this is a child." Within an hour Bulic had made all the necessary arrangements. He'd had absolutely no contact with Rose. He didn't even leave his office. Everything was done over the phone.

While Zouves and Bulic were discussing their plans, hospital support staff tried to convince Rose to have the Caesarean section. After viewing ultrasound images, and hearing news that the apprehension had occurred, she succumbed to the pressure around her, saying "Go ahead, cut me open."

At 10:50 p.m. a healthy baby boy was pried out of her. He required no special postnatal medical attention, showed no signs of distress and was described by the doctor as "vigorous at birth."

The State-approved abuse of Rose which began in the hospital, continued over the five long days of the hearing in New Westminster. MSSH lawyer Tom Gove carefully planned an attack on Rose, her friends and lover. His case was nothing less than a character assassination designed to make Rose look so bad that the impropriety of events on May 20 would be overlooked.

Day after day, Gove prompted recollections and glib editorial comments from social workers and doctors. Testimony throughout was full of harsh, judgemental, uncorroborated comments about the most minute and insignificant details of Rose's life. Because the courts failed to distinguish between the apprehension of her fetus prior to birth and State intervention in the case of her children, we heard lots of testimony about alleged problems of a mother caring for her children. We heard that on one occasion the cereal Rose fed her first child was not appropriate, that her friends were not suitable, and that, while she displayed love and affection for her children, she could not provide for them. One social worker referred to her behaviour as schizoid. Another remarked that her breath smelled like she'd had two beers. Yet another claimed her friends used hard drugs.

The well-dressed, articulate social workers could remember the most microscopic details, yet they were forgetting one thing, for me a fundamental factor. Nowhere in the hours of testimony, or in Rose's lawyer's flimsy cross-examination, did it appear that her rights as a pregnant woman were being considered or defended. I sat there screaming inside myself "What about her right to protect herself from the wounds a Caesarean would inflict? What about her right to liberty and security of the person? What about her right to say no?" I was left with the obvious and terrifying conclusion that on May 20 Rose had no rights.

For five days Rose and her partner came and went from the New Westminster court room. Each day she made her way through the throngs of the hostile, the curious and the supportive, encountered in the hallways, in the courtroom, even in the bathroom. All the good intentions, the sympathetic glances, all the authority and rancour, the huddles of lawyers, social workers and advocates whispering about her and her chances. Outside, the swarms of cameramen readied themselves for the attack. Once out in the open they rammed their weapons where they could: her mouth, her crotch, anywhere, the closer the better.

By the last day of the hearing, tensions were high, the MSSH's case was reaching its crescendo. Rose tapped her fingers nervously. Glances darted all around the court room. The glances were briefer, sharper and more critical than before.

"This woman is not on trial," said Tom Gove in his summation. The court room broke into sarcastic, nervous laughter. Judge

Davis was offended. Unauthorized laughter in his court room was unacceptable. He gave a belligerent lecture about respect and boorish behaviour, and ordered the room to be cleared for a 30-minute break.

While the outcome of the trial seemed to be a foregone conclusion — considering the mood — Davis delayed his decision for six weeks. On September 3 he ruled that events on the evening of May 20 were entirely proper, and awarded permanent custody of Rose's baby boy to the Ministry of Social Services and Housing.

Davis's decision is clearly outlined in this quote:

> The evidence is that the birth was imminent and it in fact occurred within three hours of the superintendent making the apprehension. The purpose of the apprehension was to ensure proper medical attention for the baby. This is not a case of women's rights, Mrs. R. consented without coercion or threat to the operation .... This is simply a case to determine what is best for the safety and well-being of this child. It is clear that this child was in the process of being born and the intervention and redirection of its birth were required for its survival. It was at or near term. It required no life support: it was "vigorous" at birth and indeed he was born healthy ....
>
> Under those circumstances, namely where the baby is at or so near term and birth is imminent, the failure to provide necessary medical attention to prevent death or serious injury is sufficient to allow the superintendent to invoke the procedure of apprehension. I am satisfied that the apprehension was entirely proper.

Yet it was Rose who received the controversial medical attention, not her son. In essence, Davis contends that the medical rights of a pregnant woman are secondary to the rights of her unborn child or fetus. By implication Davis' ruling concludes that Zouves had the right to pressure Rose, cut her open and take her child.

I fiercely disagree. The right of anyone to refuse treatment was, I thought, firmly grounded in Canadian law. What still stands is the obligation of caregivers to seek free, full and informed consent for medical treatments they deem necessary. Rose was denied her right to refuse treatment. The so-called consent she gave was clearly forced, not free, full and informed.

I agree that during birth the needs of the mother and her fetus have to be carefully weighed. However, the needs of both are far better served when the woman's concerns are fully addressed, when she is fully informed and when she is treated with care and respect. Ultimately, I believe that the woman has the final say.

Indications are that we will encounter more instances of forced obstetrical interventions such as the one Rose experienced. We may see that women are presented with the threat of complying with medical intervention, rather than have the State apprehend before birth.

In Belleville, Ontario in March 1987, a woman who was eight months pregnant, and who seemed to be behaving erratically was committed to a hospital so that her unborn child could be monitored. In that case, presiding Judge Kirkland included in his decision a passage from a previous decision which read:

> a local psychiatrist was quoted recently as saying every child should have certain basic rights such as: the right to be wanted, the right to be born healthy, the right to live in a healthy environment, the right to such basic needs as food, housing and education and the right to continuous loving care.

This second hand opinion was used to justify the forceful detention of a woman so that tests assuring her baby's health could be done. The woman's rights were suspended so that the right of the fetus to be born healthy could be upheld.

This case and Rose's case together provide evidence of the increasing attack on women's reproductive rights and of the growing confidence of the State to launch these attacks.

A study quoted extensively in an article entitled "Court Ordered Obstetrical Interventions" by Veronica Kolder, Janet Gallagher and Michael Parsons, printed in the *New England Journal of Medicine* on May 7, 1987, reveals that like Judge Davis and Dr. Zouves, many physicians are prepared to disregard the rights of women during pregnancy and birth. In the study, the heads of fellowship programs in maternal-fetal medicine were asked to agree or disagree with a number of statements. Twenty-six of 57 (46 percent) thought that mothers who refused medical advice and thereby increased the risk of danger to the fetus should be detained in hospitals or other facilities so that compliance could be ensured. Fifteen of 58 (26 percent) advocated State surveillance of women in the third trimester of pregnancy who stay outside the hospital system. The U.S. survey reported court ordered Caesarean sections in eleven states, hospital detentions in two states and intrauterine transfusions in one state.

Yet doctors' opinions are not foolproof. The study states that "uncertainty is intrinsic to medical judgements. The prediction of harm to the fetus was inaccurate in six (out of 15) cases in which court orders were sought for Caesarean section."

Not surprisingly, the study reveals that it is women of colour, women on public assistance and unmarried women who make up the vast majority of those involved in unwanted obstetrical interventions.

Why do almost half the doctors in the survey dismiss a pregnant woman's decision to refuse medical treatment? I suspect that the primary reason doctors will attempt to overrule a woman's decision to refuse an obstetrical intervention is because they have bought the argument that fetuses should have rights and that those supposed rights should be protected. In other words the competition for rights is no longer between women and their authoritarian doctors. It is now that doctors are hiding behind defenseless little fetuses. The legal sands are shifting beneath our feet and women are being left beached.

Forefront in the legal fight for women's reproductive rights in Vancouver is the Women's Legal Education Action Fund (LEAF). In a fruitless effort to intervene in Rose's case, LEAF hoped to challenge the apprehension by arguing that charter provisions which "guarantee" Rose liberty and security of the person, freedom from arbitrary detention and the right to equal treatment with men had been violated. A report appearing in the *Globe and Mail* on June 10, 1987 stated, "Nancy Morrison, a former provincial court judge who is acting on behalf of the Women's Legal Education and Action Fund, said the apprehension order is invalid because a fetus is not a person under British Columbia statute or Canadian Common Law."

Kate Young, legal counsel for LEAF maintains that Rose's case is a clear example of discrimination against a pregnant woman. When we spoke she presented a useful analogy. "Lets imagine we have a child with kidney disease. His life is in jeopardy unless someone comes forward with a donated kidney. Would the coerced removal of the child's father's matching kidney be considered proper? Of course not."

LEAF plans to apply for intervenor status again when the Baby R case goes to a judicial review, probably some time in early 1988. Young contends it is a crucial case to fight because "if the British Columbian Family and Child Services Act is extended to include in its mandate the protection of fetuses, that would lead to extended violations against women."

Since Canadian law does not distinguish between a fetus 36 weeks old and a fetus six weeks old, this apprehension could be used to justify the apprehension of much younger fetuses. Apprehension of a fetus is simply a disguised way of apprehending a woman. When given responsibility for a fetus the State obviously has directly affected the autonomy and rights of the woman involved.

Few observers seem to recognize that doctors gain from court ordered obstetrical interventions. Without involving social workers and the courts as they have done, doctors would have to bear responsibility for their actions alone. In effect the courts are acting as a kind of liability screen for doctors. The court orders both reinforce the doctors' opinions and let them off the hook should something go wrong.

In an article entitled "Protecting the liberty of Pregnant Patients," George Annas says that physicians often disagree about the appropriateness of obstetrical interventions and they can be mistaken.

In Rose's case, on the word of one doctor, the Ministry of Social Services and Housing brought all the pressure it could bear to force her into a procedure she did not want. Her baby when born showed no signs of distress, scoring 9/10 on the apgar test, a postnatal grading scale.

The ultimate effect of this and other obstetrical interventions could be disastrous. The fear of having forced procedures, of being unwillingly confined, and of having fetuses apprehended, may be great enough to keep some women away from doctors and hospitals altogether. Apprehension before birth will likely give cause to women to stay away from prenatal care, not encourage it.

And as for Rose, her life goes on without the cameras. She has absolutely no access to her son who could be several years old before the appeal case is settled.

I'm left wondering what might happen if she gets pregnant again.

**Note**
Portions of this article appeared in *Kinesis* prior to publication in *Healthsharing*.

**MAGGIE THOMPSON** is a member of the Vancouver Women's Health Collective.

# No New Law!*

## Norah Hutchinson

The jubilant faces of Canadian women flashed on national television the night of January 28, 1988. Flushed, beaming faces, with traces of incredulity captured the essence of our feelings on a day few of us will ever forget. The Supreme Court of Canada had struck down section 251 of the Criminal Code (which prohibited abortions unless performed in a hospital after the approval of a therapeutic abortion committee). We could not hide our victorious emotions despite our caution to the media that the court's decision was *only* one step to making safe, easily accessible, medically insured abortion services available to women in this country.

After 16 months of deliberation, seven of the nine Supreme Court justices assigned to the "Morgentaler Appeal" rendered their judgement 5-2 in favour of striking section 251 from the Criminal Code of Canada. Pro-choice activists had worked extremely hard for years to have this section of the Criminal Code removed for reasons that Madame Justice Bertha Wilson articulated most eloquently in her judgement:

> The right to "liberty" contained in s.7 [section 7 of the Charter of Rights and Freedoms] guarantees to every individual a degree of personal autonomy over important decisions intimately affecting his or her private life. Liberty in a free and democratic society does not require the state to approve such decisions but it does require the state to respect them.

* Reprinted from *Healthsharing* vol. 10 no. 1 (Winter 1988): 27-31, with permission of the author.

She went on to state further:

> Section 251 of the Criminal Code takes a personal and private decision away from the woman and gives it to a committee which bases its decision on "criteria entirely unrelated to [the pregnant woman's] priorities and aspirations.
>
> Section 251 is more deeply flawed than just subjecting women to considerable emotional stress and unnecessary physical risk. It asserts that the woman's capacity to reproduce is to be subject, not to her own control, but to that of the state. This is a direct interference with the woman's physical "person."

It took 20 years for this disastrous section to be struck down and it took fewer than 24 hours before ominous rumblings were heard from MPs opposed to abortion, the various provincial governments with a strong anti-choice agenda (particularly British Columbia), and of course, the ever present "right to life" movement. As Henry Morgentaler declared that evening, "This battle is won but the struggle is far from finished."

## Recriminalization

The Conservative government's response to the decision was to attempt to recriminalize abortion. This past summer, the Mulroney Government presented the House of Commons with new criminal legislation on abortion, claiming a desire to "read the will of the House." The motion and all five amendments were rejected after several days of debate. The "will of the country" had been heard. However, it was an unsettling spectacle to watch one MP after another wax exhaustively about their personal thoughts on everything from fetal development, their religious beliefs, to their views on fatherhood, with the fundamental issue trivialized and manipulated.

If the government is sincerely interested in providing health care for Canadian women then it need not immerse itself in lengthy, needless debate. It should act swiftly and decisively, referring to the mountain of data in existence which documents the sorry state of abortion services in Canada. The government should dismiss the idea of new criminal legislation, understanding that there are already sections of the Criminal Code that deal with the regulation of abortion. (Sections 252, 45, 198, 202, and 245 require that reasonable standards of care be met in all treatment.) The federal government should also acknowledge that it is the provincial governments that set standards for medical practitioners and the provincial medical colleges that are responsible for ensuring that physicians practice medicine according to accepted protocol. (An example of this is the recent formulation of standards for the provision of abortion services in hospitals and in clinics by the Ontario College of Physicians and Surgeons.)

## Gestational Limitations

One of the issues that was raised in the debate in the House of Commons was whether there should be limitations put on how late in a pregnancy an abortion could legally be performed. Although Canada has never had gestational limitations on abortions, it is evident that women do not seek abortions after three months of pregnancy, except in extenuating circumstances. Approximately 87 percent of abortions are done in the first 13 weeks of pregnancy. This has been the case even with the delays inherent in the therapeutic abortion committee approval system. And only 0.3 percent of abortions are performed after 20 weeks of pregnancy. That many women have late abortions in Canada is a deceitful and disrespectful myth that the opponents of choice have tried (albeit, somewhat unsuccessfully) to perpetuate.

There have not been any reasonable or justifiable arguments posed by those that would legislate gestational limitations. The circumstances that compel women to have abortions after 13 weeks are as varied as the reasons for terminating a pregnancy at an earlier stage. To advocate that Canadians need protection from "potentially-criminal" women, not only distorts the concept of a fetus, but charges that women are incapable of making moral decisions and in fact are merely vessels in which to carry a fetus to term.

But instead of understanding the many reasons why women are compelled to have abortions after 13 weeks, the spectre of "fetal rights" is raised and promoted by anti-choice organizations. Talk of unscrupulous doctors surfacing to capitalize on "free access" is occasionally thrown into the argument. Both these arguments disregard women's physical autonomy and the rights we have as adult citizens to make choices and decisions about our personal lives in privacy and in accordance with our own beliefs.

In the second instance, unscrupulous doctors wishing to perform any medical procedures are dealt with by existing sections of the criminal code and by their professional bodies. Likewise for nurses and other health care providers.

We know that with increased access to abortion facilities the overwhelming majority of women will obtain an abortion in the earliest weeks of pregnancy. We also know from the American experience, from the clinic experience in Quebec and from the Morgentaler clinics, that the safe, supportive, confidential and respectful environment that clinics provide is far superior to hospital abortions. Clinics can also provide their services on a more cost effective basis than hospitals.

Shortly after the motion on abortion was defeated in the House of Commons, the Canadian Medical Association (CMA) finally adopted a more strongly worded policy on abortion and the provision of abortion services. The resolution acknowledges that abortion should be made available outside hospitals and that "counselling services, family planning services and contraceptive information must be readily available to all Canadians."

But the CMA makes no demand for all-inclusive medical insurance coverage for these services. While the CMA policy paper emphasizes what we in the pro-choice and women's movement have been saying for years, its glaring omission on that count lessens the effect substantially.

Theoretical support is simply not good enough. The excuse by some in the CMA, that medical doctors must steer clear of politics is ridiculous. We have ample evidence that many physicians have little concern about expressing their political opinions on other issues, especially when it directly affects them financially.

### Right-wing Response

The right-wing response to the Supreme Court ruling was swift and biting. British Columbia's Premier Vander Zalm, while unequivocally on the leading edge of right-wing politicians, had plenty of followers eager to jump on the bandwagon. Antagonistic voices, mouthing ignorant statements rolled in from all corners of the country. MPs like Jim Jepson, Gus Mitges, John Nunziata and Don Boudria joined in with provincial politicians like Vander Zalm and Grant Devine of Saskatchewan and various church clergy to denigrate women's experiences and call into question women's integrity. It seemed like open season on the women of Canada; an opportunity to "highlight" anti-woman positions on other issues.

The inflammatory language used to promote their position no longer shocks pro-choice activists, long familiar with the "right to life" agenda, but creates untold anguish among those women who have abortions and are more vulnerable to misinformation and ghoulish imagery. For example, on July 14, 1988, a $15,000 half-page advertisement in the national edition of *The Globe and Mail* featured a blow-up photograph of a 19-week-old fetus entitled "Baby Talk."

There was also Senator Stanley Haidasz's Bill S-16 to amend the Criminal Code which states: "Every pregnant female person who, with intent to cause the death of an unborn human being within her, uses any means to carry out that intent is guilty of an indictable offence and liable to imprisonment of two years."

In Calgary, a demonstration held outside City Hall protesting the public funding of the Calgary Birth Control Association (CBCA) was attended by at least eight members of the Ku Klux Klan, lending an ominous note to the struggling anti-choice movement.

Said Charles Smith, president of the Alberta Pro-Life Alliance, "other opinions that KKK members hold are irrelevant. If they want to unite with us on this issue, we welcome their support. We don't have to agree on everything … individual members of their group who do not condone the destruction of human life should come out in support." The obvious connection in mentality did not escape many people.

As the "right to life" movement has become more fanatical and more right-wing, their support has eroded. A prominent anti-abortion spokesperson in Vancouver has indicated publicly that they have lost support because of the increasingly right-wing approach, which has included opposition to all forms of birth control and sex education, as well as continued emphasis on harassing women on their way into abortion clinics. These positions, she said, have alienated previous as well as potential supporters. The fractious infighting within their ranks continues to divide and polarize their agenda. Witness the split of REAL Women earlier in the year and the attempt by a few to form small rightist political parties such as the Family Coalition Party in

Ontario. Several planks in this party's platform include a vitriolic anti-gay stance, support for capital punishment and opposition to day care funding.

While the anti-choice lobby has intensified, in conjunction with their steadfast tactics of picketing hospitals and clinics, widespread public education and high profile events organized by the pro-choice movement across the country continue to ensure that existing abortion services are maintained and expanded to meet women's needs.

### Access Hasn't Improved

Most centres in Canada are reporting that there has not been a substantial change in the numbers of women seeking abortions, nor in the method in which they are offered. In some areas of the country access to abortions has deteriorated and medical insurance funding is in doubt.

In response to the Supreme Court ruling in January 1988, British Columbia Health Minister Peter Dueck responded quickly to the Supreme Court ruling by ordering an immediate cessation of funding for all abortions through B.C.'s Medical Service Plan. What resulted was a state of unprecedented chaos in the province. While Dueck and Premier Vander Zalm waged an all out attack on women seeking abortions both in financial and emotional terms, confusion reigned within the hospital system. Hospital administrators, physicians and abortion referral agencies could not make sense of the daily pronouncements coming out of the B.C. legislature.

Mary Bloom, the executive director of the Arcadia Women's Health Clinics in Seattle, Washington, an abortion-providing clinic, noticed a 25 percent increase in the number of B.C. women seeking abortions within a six-week period. She realized that the increase was directly attributable to the confusion in B.C. Given that the cost for an abortion in a B.C. hospital now far exceeded the $275 it cost to have it done in Washington state, women with the financial resources found it easier to travel south of the border and have the procedure done quickly and quietly.

Barbara Hestrin, the education director of the Planned Parenthood Association of B.C. observed that the overturning of the abortion law produced some short-term and some long-term effects as far as Planned Parenthood is concerned. One short-term effect was that additional time was required to counsel women who were at that time attempting to resolve an unwanted pregnancy. These women, and often their partners, needed clarification regarding access to facilities, and (for a period of several weeks, in B.C.) details pertaining to the financial costs that would be involved in the termination. Additional counselling time was also required to deal with the emotional turmoil and fear that resulted from the invasion of political and very public action into the realm of personal decision-making, in an already stressful area.

There was an immense swell of support for choice in B.C. in response to the provincial governments attack on a woman's right to abortion. A demonstration held on the legislature grounds, attended by 3,000 and a petition with 20,000 signatures coupled with public forums and pro-choice editorials in B.C.'s major newspapers exposed the government to daily public derision and ridicule. Nationally, Vander Zalm and his cohorts were treated with scorn (occasionally with outright disbelief) not only by the general public, but by the major news outlets.

The culmination of weeks of pro-choice political pressure was an order by the B.C. Supreme Court, initiated by the B.C. Civil Liberties Association which forced the Vander Zalm government to reinstate funding.

In Quebec, the Board of Health is investigating abortion-providing clinics including the CLSCs for "possible overcharging." Odel Loulou of the Morgentaler Clinic, objected to "the breach of confidentiality" and said that "if the government doesn't want the clinics to 'overcharge' it should give adequate funding to provide for proper equipment and other things, not just for the abortion itself."

Members of the *Coalition Quebecoise pour la droit a l'avortement libre a gratuit,* the Quebec coalition for free abortions, have demanded that the government expand services, particularly in the more distant regions. As one coalition member said "the government looks for guilty parties to make the existing abortion services look bad instead of addressing the real problem of access and availability."

In Manitoba, the Conservative government refuses to provide insurance plan funding for abortions done at the Morgentaler Clinic in Winnipeg, or improve hospital access. The Morgentaler Clinic reopened in June, but clearly needs health care coverage and core funding if it is to provide comprehensive services.

P.E.I. remains the only province with no abortion access for women. The Liberal government refuses to ensure that existing hospitals do the procedure nor will it make any efforts to provide a free-standing clinic.

Ontario remains, relatively speaking, the second best province

---

## UNITED WE CAN WIN

*Nikki Colodny, the first woman medical doctor in English Canada to work in an "illegal" abortion clinic prior to January 28th, reflects back on her experiences:*

On the day I was arrested, September 17, 1986, the clarity of the contradiction between our rights as women and the state's attempts to limit our rights was illuminated like a flash of lightning. For several weeks the Ontario Coalition for Abortion Clinics (OCAC) had been hearing that the arrests were imminent. We even had a tip that it was to be the morning of the 17th. That day I went about my morning activities waiting for the doorbell to ring. When it didn't, I assumed our tip was wrong. I left the house with the rest of my household. We were all somewhat relieved.

Just as I was about to start the ignition of the car, two plain-clothed policemen walked over. One of them flashed his badge and said somewhat apologetically, "I think you know what this is all about."

Then came the lightening bolt. For an instant, the powerful struggle between the state and the women's movement was boldly illuminated. Our side was our world, where it is our birthright to control our bodies, our reproduction and our sexuality and where we struggle to organize to force reluctant governments to recognize those rights. On the other side was the power of the state which can be forced to certain concessions but is nonetheless opposed to the full emancipation of women.

OCAC organized the pro-choice response to the attack on abortion access posed by this arrest of Dr. Morgentaler, Dr. Scott and myself. The visible and overwhelming support for Toronto's free-standing abortion clinics forced the provincial government to stay the charges.

I had packed a small bag with my women's music tapes. But on the same day that I was arrested, I was released. The important lesson that "united we can win" has never been more real to me.

---

after Quebec, in providing abortions with the least obstruction and resistance. But the Liberal government falls very short of making abortion truly accessible to all women. As is the case in all other provinces, geography plays a major role in determining who gets an abortion, how quickly and at what financial cost.

Women from the Maritimes still travel to Montreal or Toronto and women from Saskatchewan and Alberta travel to Winnipeg. In B.C., those from the north and the interior come to Vancouver or cross the border into Washington state.

Activists across the country are rallying together with renewed strength to ensure that abortion is not recriminalized and that services are expanded and made more accessible. Carolyn Egan, a spokesperson for the Ontario Coalition for Abortion Clinics (OCAC) states, "We are watching very carefully what is developing and are emphasizing that a new law is not necessary. What we need is increased access to hospital abortions as well as a network of publicly funded clinics across the country providing comprehensive reproductive health care."

In May of 1988, the Pro-Choice Action Network was formed with the intention of providing a closer affiliation to pro-choice groups in all provinces. The first project of the Pro-Choice Action Network is to organize pro-choice demonstrations across Canada and Quebec for November 19, 1988, two days before the federal election to say "no" to any new abortion law.

It is important that federal politicians know that they cannot reintroduce legislation restricting the availability of abortion. The sentiments of Canadians are clear — over 75 percent support a woman's right to choose and respect her right to make this decision in privacy. It must be the federal government that guarantees (through the Canada Health Act) that abortion be declared an essential medical service.

Abortion, as one component of fundamental reproductive rights that women around the world have struggled for, is a catalyst for raising other women's issues. The fact that significant support for a woman's right to choose has come from women in the labour movement, in the health care field and from immigrant women's communities, emphasizes the importance of the abortion rights movement and the drive for control over all aspects of our health care.

**NORAH HUTCHINSON** is a member and spokesperson for Concerned Citizens for Choice on Abortion, a Vancouver-based organization and a board member of the Canadian Abortion Rights Action League.

# Legal Assault

## A Feminist Analysis of the Law Reform Commission's Report on Abortion Legislation[*]

### Vicki Van Wagner
### B. Lee

*Crimes Against the Fetus* is the provocative title of a February, 1989 working document on reforming the criminal law relating to "birth offenses." Published by the Law Reform Commission of Canada, it concludes that the existing law in relation to the fetus is needlessly complex, inconsistent, incomplete and outdated in light of the development of medical science and the Canadian Charter of Rights and Freedoms. Although strictly advisory, the Law Reform Commission is the federal body which analyzes criminal law and makes recommendations for its reform and rationalization.

*Crimes Against the Fetus* comes at a particularly important time in the debate over abortion, but it could also have a significant influence in ongoing debates about state and medical intervention in pregnancy and childbirth. The Commission rejects majority public opinion that abortion should be a woman's personal decision and recommends resurrecting criminal regulation. As evidenced by the title of the report, the Commission's overriding concern is the protection of the fetus. We believe it is vital to reverse this focus and ask what their reform proposals mean from the standpoint of women.

*Crimes Against the Fetus* acknowledges the irreconcilable differences of values and belief in contemporary society on the status of the fetus. Moreover, there is not even a basis of agreement on how the "problem of the fetus" could be discussed and settled. The Commission argues that in situations where differ-

* Reprinted from *Healthsharing* vol. 10 no. 4 (Fall 1989): 24-27, with permission of the authors.

ences of political and ethical opinion are so profound, criminal regulation is inappropriate. Up to this point, most feminists would not disagree.

Yet despite its own strong argument against using the coercive powers of the state in such sensitive areas, the Commission asserts that there are grounds for a criminal law to prevent "unjustified destruction of the unborn." Rather than explicitly stating its rationale for criminalizing abortion, it hides this important issue under an umbrella law to protect the fetus from unspecified kinds of harm. It also fails to clearly outline just what kind of serious harm it is concerned with and who decides what constitutes fetal destruction. While acknowledging the legal principle that the fetus is not a person, it compares fetal protection to protection of animals and the environment. This leaves out the central fact that the fetus is located in a woman's body.

The Law Reform Commission lands squarely in the middle of the most sustained conflict between the contemporary women's movement and the state — the long struggle to ensure that abortion is freely and equally available to all women who need it. The report comes at a particularly opportune time for the federal government as it continues to search for ways to justify a new criminal law on abortion. The Commission's recommendations are doubly important because they buttress the preferred policy option of the government, to restrict availability of abortion through gestational time limits.

The Commission's majority proposal is a two-stage model: abortion would be legal until the fetus becomes viable, which it defines as the 22nd week of gestation, but only when duly authorized by a physician that the woman's physical and psychological health is threatened. After that point abortion would only be allowed when serious physical injury or the mother's death may result or when the fetus is suffering from lethal defects; two physicians must authorize the termination. The Commission also offers an alternative minority recommendation with three stages: in the first 12 weeks abortion would be solely a matter for the woman and her doctor; in the second stage (weeks 13 to 22) abortion would only be allowed to protect the woman's physical or psychological health; in the third stage (after the 23rd week) abortion would be restricted to cases where there is risk of death or serious injury to the woman or where the fetus has lethal defects.

The Commission rejects the World Health Association's widely accepted definition of health and explicitly excludes social well-being. Incredibly, this makes the allowable grounds for abortion even more restrictive than under the old law overturned by the Supreme Court in the Morgentaler case. It is questionable whether the Commission's proposal would be constitutional. The Supreme Court threw out the old law because it violated women's ability to act on their own "priorities and aspirations." The Commission's recommendations would be just as bad, requiring women to satisfy criteria laid down by doctors.

Feminists challenge the concept of "medical necessity" that underlies such restrictive views of abortion. Is an abortion for a woman who decides she cannot raise a child decently because she doesn't have adequate housing and lives on minimum wage any less necessary? What gives medical experts the right to decide for such a woman whether or not carrying her pregnancy to term against her will will affect her health? How could it not?

The women's health movement has long argued for an expansive view of health which recognizes the wide range of social and economic factors that affect well-being. Being able to decide when and whether to have children — controlling one's body in this most fundamental way — is as essential to overall well-being as being free of disease. Free and equal access to abortion is a vital precondition of women's reproductive health, sexual freedom, moral integrity and full and equal participation in society

The restrictive concept of health proposed by *Crimes Against the Fetus* leaves doctors and hospitals as the "gatekeepers" of access to abortion. How could the Commission ignore the wealth of data presented to the Supreme Court on what happens when medical authorities have such power? Many hospitals across the country simply refuse to provide services at all. Others could adopt their own narrow views of what constitutes proper dangers to "physical and psychological health." What if some doctors are convinced, as the Commission is, that an unwanted pregnancy must "do more than create annoyance or inconvenience?" What if others decide, for example, that the young woman who has been denying to herself that she is pregnant, who has not known where to find counseling or who fears telling her parents has only herself to blame? The result will continue to be huge variations in the availability of abortion and pervasive inequality.

Why does the Commission feel abortion must be criminalized? Obviously it cannot be a pressing need to prevent late abortion: very few are performed past its cutoff point of the 22nd week. Does it believe that the absence of an abortion law since the Supreme court's ruling has had adverse social and moral consequences? It never says. Nor does the Commission provide a convincing justification of why abortion should be restricted after the point of fetal viability — a point around which there is considerable medical debate as well as political and ethical controversy.

The commission itself recognizes the limits of criminal law as a coercive instrument. It may simply prove ineffective, as Canadian experience shows so well. The Commission admits that criminalizing abortion "may represent too negative an approach."

In one of the only instances in which the actual constraints and conditions within which women make their reproductive decisions are recognized, it notes the lack of effective birth control services and counseling, especially for teenagers; limited support services for parents, especially single parents; and inadequate daycare. Given all this, how could the commission possibly conclude that criminal regulation of abortion is necessary? Because "criminal law, however, can still contribute symbolically by upholding respect for human life." Would not acting on the Commission's recommended "positive improved social programs of education and assistance" provide a more powerful indication of such respect?

Unfortunately the Commission avoids such a broad view: abortion must be regulated for ideological reasons — to define abortion as a moral problem of fundamental importance to society. Here again, the insidious underlying message of the Commission's concern with protecting the fetus is clear: women are seen to be too unreliable and fickle to be trusted with such an important responsibility — they cannot be trusted to make the "right" decision without official regulation. The Commission portentously notes that there must always be "some sufficient reason" for abortion. The ignorance and insult of such a statement is staggering. Can they really imagine that women would undergo a surgical procedure — let alone the bureaucratic hurdles they must overcome; the paternalism or hostility of so many health professionals; leaving their own community because of inadequate access as so many women are forced to do; and the still significant social disapproval for abortion — for "pure whim or caprice?"

Why such a punitive attitude to women having abortions? Underlying state restrictions on access to abortion is not the pious concern for the fetus voiced by the Commission, but the crude message that abortion can never be made "too easy;" that women must "pay the price" for sexual activity. Restrictions on abortion are a crucial part of the myriad of state policies and programs that regulate and control women's sexuality: inadequate resources for contraceptive services, sex education and counseling; prostitution, age of consent and pornography laws; taxation, social and welfare policies predicated on the nuclear family; denial of custody rights and family benefits to lesbians, etc.

We can acknowledge that the fetus is potential life worthy of serious consideration in the abortion decision, that fetuses at later stages of development are regarded differently by many people, and that there are many ethical dilemmas involved in the complex meaning of abortion. But we don't need to retreat into the abstract moralism of the Law Reform Commission or the criminal regulation it proposes. We believe that it is the woman herself who is best placed to weigh these complexities and all the other relevant facets of her life situation — not doctors, not judges, not politicians, but women themselves.

Women have been struggling not only to win the right to decide when and whether to have children, but also to control the process of birth itself. At first glance, it would appear that the commission takes a reasonable position here. It recognizes that its new law could place "intolerable restrictions" on pregnant women and exempts them from responsibility for all but purposeful actions which harm the fetus. It sees forced treatment of pregnant women as assault and court-ordered obstetrical interventions and apprehension of the fetus *in utero* as unacceptable. It is ironic that the Commission is opposed to forcing a pregnant woman to have surgery without her consent, but is perfectly willing to force women to continue unwanted pregnancies.

But the key themes of *Crimes Against the Fetus* contribute to a growing trend in modern obstetrics which sees the fetus as a separate patient, needing an advocate for its interests. By emphasizing that the fetus and woman are separate entities and by setting out a key role for the state in balancing fetal and maternal interest, the Commission is intervening, intended or not, in these ongoing conflicts and debates. The same ideological assumptions that the Commission uncritically propounds serve to legitimize increasing obstetrical intervention into pregnancy and birth.

Forced Caesarean section is the extreme result of this ideology which paints the physician as the appropriate guardian for the fetus. More routinely, many obstetrical procedures are used despite lack of evidence of benefit, justified by the claim that they are good for the baby. Although opposing the extreme of court-ordered intervention, the Commission's focus on protection of the fetus reinforces the common view that doctor, not woman, knows best.

While most women may not be directly coerced, the power and authority of medicine put immense pressure on women in pregnancy and labour who want what is best for their babies and trust in expert opinion. Women who question medical authority are not seen as having valid concerns about procedures that are often very poorly researched, but rather "in conflict" with their fetus. The Ontario Medical Association (OMA) has published a discussion paper for its members titled "When the Pregnant Patient Does Not Follow Your Professional Advice." It refers to the pregnant woman as the "environment" for the fetus. It defines women who wish to choose homebirth, have labour coaches accompany them in labour or vaginal birth after Caesarian section as non-compliant, despite extensive evidence of the benefits of these choices for women and babies. In a document condemning homebirth the OMA asks, "Who speaks for the newborn?" The implication is of course that it is doctors who must protect the fetus from women's bad decisions. The focus in *Crimes Against the Fetus* on the fetus as distinct and separate from the mother reinforces this point of view.

Women's demand for choice in pregnancy and childbirth is not a case of their seeking individual autonomy and liberty at the expense of the fetus growing inside their body They are concerned both with their own health and dignity and the well-being of their fetus. Pregnant women constantly balance their own concerns and their baby's health.

If the Commission is so concerned with crimes against the fetus, where is the discussion of thalidomide, DES, Depo Provero, and fertility drugs? Where is its indictment of the pharmaceutical industry for the harm it has caused? If the concern is for the health of the fetus during pregnancy, where is the discussion of the adverse effects of routine but untested medical procedures? If the concern is with the health of the newborn, where is the discussion of the effect of poverty, inadequate nutrition and limited prenatal education and, once born, the lack of daycare, affordable housing and all the other obstacles women face in raising children? Where is the Commission's condemnation of governments that knowingly neglect the social and economic support needed for all children to be raised in decent conditions?

The potential consequences of the Commission's proposals could be devastating. It calls for the criminal regulation of abortion without addressing how to ensure full and equal access and without addressing the consequences for those women unable to obtain essential services. Its proposals could justify increased surveillance and control of pregnancy and birth without addressing the pressing need for improved prenatal care, midwifery, birthing centres and a less interventionist model of obstetrical medicine.

The real message of the Law Reform Commission's narrow focus on fetal protection is that women cannot be trusted — that decisions about abortion and childbirth are too fundamental to be left to women. We reject the Commission's ideological agenda and would start from the opposite point of view — from the standpoint of women's conditions, needs and possibilities. We must establish the social conditions within which women will be able to freely make the best decisions about their reproductive lives.

What is really needed to ensure that every woman has access to the health care she needs for herself and for healthy babies? There must be no new abortion law, but there must be a commitment from governments to provide the resources to guarantee access for all. There must be community midwifery and birth centres, effective and accessible contraceptive and sexuality counseling, and all the other services and programs needed for women to be able to control their reproduction. The best way to provide all this is through a network of publicly funded community clinics working in whatever language women need, and providing the full range of reproductive care: from safe and effective contraception to abortion, from birthing and midwifery to well-woman and well-baby care, and from sexuality counseling to reproductive technology developed according to women's needs and priorities.

The guiding principles of such women's reproductive health centres would be comprehensive care, equal access, informed choice, responsiveness to community needs and, most fundamentally of all, providing care that empowers women. Let these be the goals of public policy and we will see a very different prescription than that offered in *Crimes Against the Fetus*.

**VICKI VAN WAGNER** has practiced as a midwife in Toronto for eight years and has been active in the struggle to win legal recognition for midwifery. She is also a member of the Ontario Coalition for Abortion Clinics and has spoken and written extensively on reproductive rights.

**B. LEE** has worked with the Ontario Coalition of Abortion Clinics in Toronto for six years. He is also a member of the Midwifery Task Force and AIDS Action Now!

# Women Lose Freedom of Choice[*]

## B. Lee

Amid noisy protests from pro-choice supporters, MPs voted on May 29, 1990 to turn the clock back on women's rights. The House of Commons passed Bill C-43, the act that puts abortion back in the Criminal Code, by a vote of 140-131. (The old law had been overturned by the Supreme Court in January 1988.) The new law if passed by the Senate, will make abortion illegal unless a doctor judges that the woman's mental, physical or psychological health is threatened.

When the legislation was first introduced, the Pro-Choice Action Network, a coalition of activist groups from across the country, predicted that it would have a chilling effect on women's health. Unfortunately, the disastrous effects of the bill are becoming clear even before the final Senate vote. On the weekend before the House of Commons vote, a man was charged with performing an abortion on a 16-year-old girl in Kitchener-Waterloo — was this the first result of the panic created by the bill? Regional public health officials expressed grave concern that "backstreet abortions" could increase as a result of the legislation. Dr. Janet Ames, Waterloo Region family planning physician, noted that the incident places "stunning" focus on concerns raised by opponents of the proposed new law. She was quoted as saying that "it takes us back to 1969 …. That's when about a third of the intensive care unit beds were filled with botched abortions."

An even greater tragedy followed. A 20-year-old Toronto woman died from a self-induced abortion, apparently with a coat hanger.

The effect of the proposed legislation on health care providers

* Reprinted from *Healthsharing* vol. 11 no. 3 (Summer 1990): 10-11, with permission of the author.

has already been felt. Fearing prosecution, doctors at the hospitals in Winnipeg and Halifax that provide almost all abortions in their provinces have declared that they would stop. Some began to cancel appointments. The main hospitals in Calgary and Edmonton are also planning to stop providing abortions. These hospitals provide services beyond their immediate areas and these cutbacks will be devastating for women from smaller communities or rural areas and from regions where access to abortion is nonexistent. In Ontario, Brantford General, which was the only hospital in the city performing abortions, announced doctors will no longer perform the procedure. The decision was made "out of concern that proposed federal legislation will leave doctors who perform abortions open to criminal charges."

Whatever the likelihood of doctors being convicted, their real fear is the adverse impact on their reputation and livelihood if they are investigated or charged. And, of course, anti-choice leaders have already promised to use the law to prevent women having abortions.

Even where doctors and hospitals don't stop providing abortions altogether, they may require women to have additional psychological assessments or sign waiver forms attesting to their state of health. Doctors will practice "defensive medicine" to avoid liability rather than to enhance and facilitate the well-being of their patients. Women face greater bureaucratic hassles and increased delay, which is in turn associated with a higher risk of complications.

Justice Minister Kim Campbell says that doctors need only practice according to accepted professional standards. Perhaps what she really means is the common practice of doctors telling women what is good for them. She clearly does not mean what should be standard practice for health care providers: providing information on available options and facilitating women making their own choices about the care they need. The idea of restricting abortion through arbitrary health criteria is outrageous and insulting. Being forced to carry an unwanted pregnancy to term is always a threat to a woman's well-being.

What this bill is really about is women's independence and well-being. Abortion is one of the most immediate — and therefore hotly contested — mechanisms of state regulation of women's reproduction and sexuality.

The fundamental political message of this legislation is that women will not be allowed to control their bodies and their lives. In the context of cut-backs to women's centres, publications, research and advocacy groups and attacks on the National Action Committee on the Status of Women, this government is saying, loud and clear, that it will not accept policies and programs that seek to empower women. And this is why we can't give up the struggle.

We must not be demoralized because the bill passed in the House of Commons. We did not lose the vote because of poor strategy or weak organizing. Thousands of people took to the streets to support choice on abortion. This popular support was never clearer than in the months before the vote: on May 12, 1990 there were demonstrations and actions of one kind or another in communities across the country and there were dozens of actions in the week before the vote. This bill certainly did not pass because of popular support.

We lost this vote simply because there is a majority of Tories in the House of Commons. There were nine more Tory MPs — and a few Liberals — who voted for their own narrow moralism or caved in to the pressure from the Conservative government to toe the line.

The task of the pro-choice movement is to build on this legacy of activism and the solid popular support for women's right to choose. We are still demanding that the law be withdrawn before more women are killed or maimed. If it does come into force, the new law will be challenged in court. We hope health care providers will follow the inspiration of the Quebec clinics that have declared that they will defy its provisions.

**B. LEE** has worked with the Ontario Coalition for Abortion Clinics in Toronto for six years. He is also a member of the Midwifery Task Force and AIDS Action Now!

# Aging through Menopause

*Healthsharing*, like other women's health publications, did not start talking about the process of aging until the mid-eighties when a generation of women's health activists began raising concerns related to their own experience of growing older. In 1986, the editor of *Healthsharing*'s first special issue on menopause observed that in the two years she had been in the collective, between 1982 and 1984, nobody was over 40 years old. In the nineties, menopause and women's aging process have received more mainstream attention due to the growth of the aging population and increasing pressure from women's health movements. Unfortunately, it is the medicalization of menopause through the focus on osteoporosis and hormone replacement therapy which has brought menopause into the public arena. *Healthsharing*'s treatment of this issue is illustrative of the magazine's predilection to come down the middle between medical dogma and alternative therapy orthodoxy.

"Take Control of Menopause" by Carolyn DeMarco defines menopause as a normal part of the aging process rather than as an illness. As a medical doctor herself, but one who has embraced a more holistic view of our bodies' aging process and a critique of the medical establishment, she advocates attention to diet and exercise as part of a healthy transition through menopause. Still, she acknowledges there are crisis situations which warrant medication. Most importantly, she confronts her own negative feelings about aging and locates the origins of these feelings in our society's systemic undervaluation of women.

Between *Healthsharing*'s first theme issue on menopause in 1986 and the second in 1990, the magazine, under pressure from women of colour, began to critically assess how it maintained racism by allowing a white, middle-class women's experience to define a non-existent universal female experience. The magazine introduced new content to the magazine and also more importantly new writers, board members, staff and illustrators. In "The Colours of Menopause" Margaret de Souza helps to delineate the diversity of Canadian women's experience of menopause.

# Take Control of Menopause
## Do the Right Thing, Eat the Right Thing[*]

### Carolyn DeMarco

Are women still dreading menopause? Or is it old age they are trying to avoid? And why in 1990, are women being heavily pressured into taking hormones not only to prevent osteoporosis but also to prevent heart disease?

In Prince Edward Island, where I recently gave a public talk on the topic, the conference organizer avoided mentioning the word menopause on the poster because she thought it might scare some women away. An earlier survey by the Women's Network in P.E.I. found that even members of women's groups were reticent to discuss how menopause had affected their lives.

How is this possible in this day and age? Haven't we overcome some of the previous taboos around menopause? I looked closely at my own attitudes toward menopause and how they have changed as I got older.

At age 25, I gave my first talk on menopause cheerily emphasizing the positive aspects of menopause and discussing the dangers of estrogen replacement.

At age 35, I organized a weekend workshop on menopause at my place. I was carried away by positive images of the old crone freed from all roles and responsibilities.

Now I have already seen in myself the signs of aging, the first wrinkles, the white hairs, a few more aches and pains, the two to three weeks of disabling premenstrual symptoms, subtle changes in menstrual flow and taking days to recover from a late night. In fact, is it premenstrual syndrome or is it early menopause? Or is this another example of how we are avoiding using the term menopause?

Recently, I met a friend who attended my menopause work-

* Reprinted from *Healthsharing* vol. 11 no. 4 (Winter 1990): 28-30, with permission of the author.

shop seven years ago. She experienced five years of severe and unrelenting premenstrual-like symptoms before her periods finally stopped altogether. Maybe this is one of the early menopausal signs which along with minor changes in a still regular menstrual flow are not yet described in the literature. All the hormonal cycles of our life probably overlap.

Now at age 42, I hardly feel anything positive about menopause. When a close friend the same age as me said she thought she noticed signs of early menopause — all of which I had been experiencing — I immediately advised her that she was too young to be concerned about menopause. This shocked me as I had a lot of positive programming toward menopause in the past — at least on an intellectual level.

There is truth in what Janine O'Leary Cobb says — that most women in our society cannot welcome menopause. "Not because a woman will necessarily feel unwell," she states, "but because it requires her to face her own aging. And aging is not a pleasant prospect for a woman in this society." That really hit home for me.

### Chilling Prospect

What do we as women have to look forward to about aging in our society? Dealing with teenagers, ailing parents, housework, partners retiring, death of close ones, separation and divorce, living alone, becoming dependent, becoming poorer and poorer, and having fewer job opportunities and choices. Worldwide, women are the poorest of the poor. In the United States, old women are the largest adult poverty group: 40.2 percent of elderly African American women are poor. Conditions inside nursing homes and old age homes where women predominate are often deplorable.

It is not only that aging for women in this society is a chilling prospect; women are also forced to suppress how they feel going through the immense changes that this period of life brings in order to function in a world defined by male values. Women are bombarded by ridiculous images of menopause.

The root cause of many of the problems of menopause and aging are the way women are treated in North American society — how our society, our religions and our medical institutions view women's bodies and how women's work is undervalued at home and in the workplace. Added to this of course is the role of drug companies, the multibillion dollar industries which seek to define menopause as a disease which only their drugs can remedy.

One of the big pushes by the drug companies is for the use of both calcium supplements and estrogen for the prevention of osteoporosis and heart disease. Osteoporosis is a serious condition each year causing 1.3 million fractures in the United States and 800,000 fractures in Canada. Up to 2.5 million Canadians may be at risk for fractures due to osteoporosis, according to one estimate. Studies into heart disease show that it is the main cause of death for women over 50. Researchers believe that the increased rate of heart disease in older women is linked to lower levels of estrogen. However, other causes such as smoking, diet, exercise and heredity are important risk factors that have not been researched among women.

## Preventing Osteoporosis
In my office, women going through menopause need answers to practical questions such as: How can I prevent osteoporosis? Will estrogen help? Should I take calcium? How much?

Recent articles on osteoporosis suggest that doctors prescribe estrogen to all women, starting within three years of menopause to be continued indefinitely. Women who have had hysterectomies face at least double the risk of osteoporosis. But, the use of estrogen does not increase bone mass, it merely halts further bone loss. Moreover, as soon as estrogen is stopped, the rate of bone loss is accelerated. However, I believe that osteoporosis can be prevented through diet and exercise.

Recent research into the trace mineral, boron, indicates that this element may play a key role in the prevention of osteoporosis. Meat, fish, milk products and highly processed foods have a low boron content. Boron rich foods include non citrus fruits, green vegetables and beans. In one study, the addition of boron supplements caused calcium retention as well as an increase in blood levels of estrogen and testosterone. Boron tablets can be taken at the dosage of three to five milligrams (mg) a day.

What is the optimal diet to prevent osteoporosis? John Robbins in his book, *Diet for a New America*, maintains that high protein diets inhibit the absorption of calcium. A study funded by the National Dairy Council in the U.S. had one group of women drink three eight ounce glasses of milk a day, in addition to their regular diet. The control group received no extra milk. Researchers found that the women who took the extra milk derived no benefit to their bone density from it.

High fat diets tend to counteract calcium absorption. Our need for high amounts of calcium is based on a "pathological dependency state, the result of our distorted diet," claims Dr. Gary Todd, author of *Nutrition, Health and Disease*. He goes on to say that calcium requirements increase in direct proportion to the amount of protein and fat in our diet.

Studies of different ethnic groups have shown that the higher the average intake of protein, the higher the rate of osteoporosis. What seems to be important is not the amount of calcium intake, but the amount that is absorbed.

For example, the Inuit consume a diet high in fat and protein based on fish and animal meat and take in more that 2000 mg of calcium every day. Yet, they appear to have the highest rate of osteoporosis in the world.

In contrast, the Bantu tribes of central Africa have low protein, high vegetable and grain diets and take in only 300 mg of calcium a day. Osteoporosis is unknown among the Bantu, even in old age.

Japanese women who have a low protein diet with only 300 mg of calcium have a lower rate of osteoporosis than their American counterparts who take in an average of 800 mg of calcium a day.

On average, female meat eaters have lost 35 percent of their bone mass by the age of 65. In contrast, female vegetarians have lost only 18 per cent of their bone mass by the same age.

If you are eating a low protein vegetable diet you will need a lot less calcium. I do recommend to my patients that they cut down on meat and dairy products.

A new drug for osteoporosis is now being tested — editronate cyclical therapy. In a paper published in the *New England Journal of Medicine*, researchers studied 429 postmenopausal women with osteoporosis. Results showed a significant increase in the bone mineral density of the spine within one year of treatment and a significant decrease in the rate of new vertebral fractures.

This drug is not yet available in Canada and long term effects are, of course, unknown. Personally I would not consider taking this drug unless you are in a crisis situation — losing a lot of bone and/or at high risk for fractures.

## How Much?
What do I recommend for calcium supplementation? If people cannot change their high protein diets, I recommend 1200 mg to 1500 mg of calcium a day combined with half that amount of magnesium. I prefer to use liquid calcium and magnesium as I think they are better absorbed and I advise women to take the supplements at bedtime. Other high quality calcium — magnesium supplements include Nu-life Framework, Karuna's Osteonex and Osteoguard, and calcium-magnesium boron effervescent powder.

I feel women on pure vegetarian diets (no meat or dairy) can probably take half the above amount of calcium and magnesium. In addition, I suggest both groups take SISU silica. This is an extract of horsetail which contains large amounts of the trace mineral silicon. The body naturally changes silica into calcium in a very efficient manner.

These supplements may be difficult to get outside large cities. Check with your local health food store first. Otherwise, all the above supplements can be ordered from Supplements Plus through their toll free number 1 (800) 387-4761.

Vegetarian dietary sources of calcium include deep green vegetables, tahini, dulse, kelp, lime processed tortillas, tofu made with calcium sulphate, mashed sunflower and sesame seeds.

## Preventing Heart Disease
If we cut down on our consumption of red meat and dairy, and move toward a low fat diet of fresh fruits and vegetables and whole grains, chicken and fish (deep ocean fish like cod, halibut and pollack, or freshwater fish from clean lakes are preferred), we will also be following current recommendations for the prevention of both heart disease and cancer.

Dr. Dean Ornish and his colleagues at the medical school in San Francisco have been conducting research on patients with severe coronary heart disease. Preliminary results so far indicate that severe heart disease can be reversed by comprehensively changing lifestyle without surgery or drugs. Lifestyle changes include moderate exercise and one hour a day of stress management techniques (including stretching, breathing, meditation, imagery and relaxation exercises derived from yoga). Participants also stopped smoking and went on a low fat vegetarian diet with no animal products whatsoever except for small amounts of nonfat milk or yogurt daily.

## A New Approach
This is the approach I use for any health problems relating to menopause:

- Tell yourself the truth about what you are experiencing, your hopes and fears about the whole process and the prospect of aging.
- Fight ageism in yourself, in women's groups, at work, everywhere. We have to establish our own standards, our own role models and our own language and images of aging.
- If you are having a health problem at menopause, use this problem as a message from your body to pay more attention to it.
- Seek out and create support for yourself. Solidify your network of family and friends.
- Make use of self-help groups or start your own. In many cases, these groups have been at the forefront of knowledge on many topics. They have accumulated more research than most doctors will ever find time to read. Often they investigate the natural alternatives as well as unusual or innovative treatments.
- Educate yourself. Read everything you can get your hands on, ask a lot of questions, find out, listen to tapes, go to courses, talk to as many women as you can, make use of local experts.
- Educate your doctor as well. Bring him or her appropriate reading materials, especially articles from the medical literature or pertinent textbooks.
- Play around with natural methods of healing until you find what works for you.

CAROLYN DEMARCO is a doctor who works as a holistic health consultant in Toronto and B.C. Her book *Take Charge of Your Body: A Women's Health Adviser* was published by Well Woman Press and released in 1989.

# The Colours of Menopause[*]

## Margaret de Souza

Two centuries ago many women died around the time of menopause. Today, improved nutrition and disease control mean that women live an average of about 30 years beyond the menopause. Women now usually experience menopause between the ages of 48 and 52, depending on heredity, racial background and hormonal balance.

In North America, books, articles and newsletters on menopause provide support and information for the health needs of the dominant white middle-class woman. Unfortunately, information and support is not geared for the Black, Asian, Latin American or Aboriginal woman in our multiracial/multicultural country. In working with women from different racial backgrounds I have observed their attitudes towards the "change of life" and how for some of them, their difficulties "adjusting" to the North American environment adds to the stress of their menopausal changes. There is a difference in the needs and expectations of non-white women going through menopause.

Understanding their attitude towards menopause will help in setting up better health care strategies which are different from those required by white, middle-class, and dominant culture women and which will combat the assumption that immigrant women and women of colour are not capable of understanding, choosing or acting in accordance with their own health needs.

I am the family life counselor at the Women's Health Centre at St. Joseph's Health Centre and have been involved with menopausal counseling for the past five years. The women I see at the centre are from many different backgrounds including Portuguese, Italian, South Asian, Polish, Chinese, Somalian, Latin American and Canadian.

[*]   Reprinted from *Healthsharing* vol. 11 no. 4 (Winter 1990): 14-17, with the permission of the author.

I would like to share stories of menopause from these women — stories of increasing power and status, a time of positive change and fear of aging. Their fears and strengths are largely determined by their cultural background, family and community experiences and the level of support they have as women.

Most medical literature defines menopause as a deficiency and decline — a living decay. It has been created by the medical profession as a disease needing treatment. Rarely, are women seen as a whole. A hot flash or a mood swing is viewed in isolation, ignoring other possible causes. Particularly for non-white women, how the social and political environment influences their lives must be understood and racist stereotypes dispelled.

There is also a myriad of physical and mental health problems caused by traumatic emigration experiences, cultural dislocation and loss of support systems. A 48-year-old woman from El Salvador told me how she came to Canada as a torture victim and refugee with her three children a year ago. Her husband was taken as a political prisoner. She has missed her ESL (English as a Second Language) classes because of severe palpitations and chest pains. She thinks she is dying so she wants to see a cardiologist. She has had bladder infections, hot flashes, sleeplessness and sweating for the past 10 months. She used her own cultural drinks because she has no time to see a family doctor.

In "western" culture our mental, physical and spiritual health is constantly under stress. In most non-western cultures there is no concept of stress because coping techniques are built into the culture. But it is difficult to transport them into another cultural environment; they cease to work and the dominant culture determines our health. A 49-year-old Chinese woman talks of her social life being disrupted with hot flashes and heavy periods. "I cannot concentrate, my joints ache, but my twin sister, who is a Tai Chi instructor back home, does not have any of these problems."

"Western" culture glorifies youth and menopause is viewed as a period of decline. In North America menopause is viewed as an aging disease needing medical intervention — either drugs, surgery or both. Some immigrants adopt this belief, but others will seek alternative health options or traditional medicine. A 50-year-old Sikh woman from India talks about how her mother dealt with menopause differently. "My mother never dyed her hair like I do. I have to take estrogen for my sweats. My mother used to complain of a "hot fever" coming on and off with sweating. When the sweating got worse, she went to the folk doctor."

At the beginning of the century, doctors in Canada hospitalized menopausal women for depression. Today, menopause continues to be treated with tranquilizers and hormones by physicians and psychiatrists. An Italian woman describes her experience. "When I had those panic attacks my hot flashes got worse. My husband told me that this was the beginning of a nervous breakdown. He took me to a psychiatrist and I was given tranquilizers."

In dominant Canadian culture there is an emphasis on the "nuclear family." Stress due to the triple burden of the roles of wife/mother/worker can negatively effect menopausal changes. "I could slaughter the kids!" says a 47-year-old Chinese woman. "I have a bad headache, hot flashes and these palpitations. I am leaving home! I am fed up of being a taxi driver and a housekeeper."

Some cultures that are influenced by "western culture" react to menopause with a sense of loss, a loss of their ability to bear children and their youthful image. A 48-year-old Polish woman describes her pain. "I am sad so sad — no more babies! These hot flashes remind me that I am getting old."

Many cultures view this midlife phase as a healthy balance because menopause liberates a woman from the fear of pregnancy, the nuisance of birth control and offers her more leisure time and privacy for love making. A 52-year-old Italian woman talked about how sex was better than before. "No birth control! No babies! We have a good sex life. We spend more time getting ready."

Some cultures have a positive view of menopause. The menopause stage gives women a rise in status of power, worth and privilege. Menopausal women are seen as confidants, advisors, decision-makers and leaders of extended family and community. The Chinese, Japanese, Somalians and South Asians celebrate menopause as a triumph. Women move from being powerless to being respected as wise and powerful. A Somalian woman described how her 54-year-old mother is a "wise woman," who takes the young girls to initiation huts. An Indian woman compares her menopause to that of her mother. "I am sitting at home with my hot flashes, joint pains and aches, but at my age my mother had no complaints. She became the village decision-maker and arranged prayer groups at the village temple."

Some religions and cultures view menstruation as "impure" and women are ostracized from their community, but these cultures view menopause with a positive goal. It is the end of their menstrual taboos and beginning of a new dimension. "I can now socialize with my husband and his friends," says an Afghani woman from India. "I am free, no taboo. I can visit my friends in my community."

Accessible and culturally relevant health care for menopausal women from non-white cultures is crucial. Management of menopause depends on the total culture. The menopause experience for these women could be either a positive change or a crisis. But Black, Asian, and Latin American women living in Canada experience linguistic and cultural barriers to health services. These women bring with them different cultural beliefs, traditions and practices which are not generally understood or respected by the medical system. This causes racist and inappropriate responses from health services.

An effective multiracial/multicultural perspective brings important insights to the area of menopausal health. Creative approaches are needed and could also help all menopausal women to deal positively with this life change. Healthy menopausal care can be achieved through a health care system which cooperates with community-based organizations to break down cultural barriers. Instead of menopausal women being the subjects of intervention by health care professionals, these women need the tools to advocate on their own behalf.

Women going through menopause can assume responsibility for our own health care by taking control. But only if we can make choices in our health care through education, information, self-help, support and interpretation. Black, Asian, Latin American and immigrant women need knowledge about reproductive health care and non-medical remedies such as diet, exercise and relaxation techniques in their mother tongue. This brings it closer to home and combats fear. Health information centres should be community-controlled by women with a strong consumer perspective. All health information and counseling should be available in easy to understand forms in different languages.

Food patterns and dietary habits of women from different

cultures must be respected. East and South Asians eat a lot of fish, sea weed, wholegrain and tofu — foods which are rich in calcium. These guard against loss of bone mass (osteoporosis) in later life. Herbal teas, herbs, licorice root, and Ginseng are used by European, Chinese, African and South Asian women for hot flashes, fatigue and heavy periods which are symptoms of menopause. This optimum diet often changes through the process of emigration. Skilful health professionals can help women to avoid this change and it would be useful for all women to adopt dietary practices that prevent negative menopausal symptoms — practices that are more reliable than medical remedies.

Utilization of community based organizations and hospital resources geared to their needs will give women from diverse cultures the confidence to make choices. We will be able to choose our own doctor or health care giver who may practice holistic or traditional medicine. We will be able to take control of our own health needs by asking questions, finding options or questioning medical treatment. We will also be able to explore and possibly use non-medical remedies. Tai Chi is popular among Chinese and Philippine women, giving them vigour, flexibility and inner harmony. Relaxation techniques like yoga and meditation are popular among South Asian women, helping them to calm the mind and eliminate stress. These exercises and relaxation techniques can be incorporated in community programs for immigrant women.

Some Chinese, Japanese, and African women treat joint pain, muscle spasms, and menstrual cramps with alternative methods like accupressure, shiatsu, acupuncture and massage. Sometimes these non-medical approaches are provided by the experienced wise women of their community. These wise women channel their energy through their bodies and hands to heal the ailments women experience at menopause. Women will eventually learn to combine alternative approaches with conventional remedies to their advantage.

"Self-help" is invaluable for any woman going through menopause. A self-help group can offer courage, strength and "body" information. This support can reduce the sense of isolation as we learn the social context of our common condition. "Sex talk," for example, is taboo in many cultures, so the physiological changes of menopause cause misconceptions and misunderstanding in both men and women. Women misinterpret lack of lubrication as a sexual malfunction and men sometimes think that a longer time for sexual arousal is a sign of disinterest. Women in post-child bearing years will benefit from the knowledge on sexuality and communication they receive through participation in a self-help group.

Multicultural menopausal women can be strengthened and empowered by allowing them easy access to all resources for multicultural health care. If immigrant women are dissatisfied with their health care they can make a choice, they can shop around, thus assuming responsibility for their own health care by being in control.

**MARGARET DE SOUZA** is a Ugandan-born Canadian of East Indian origin who works as the head nurse of the Family Life Program at St. Joseph's Health Centre.

# section seven

# Resisting Medical, Cultural and Social Violence

This section examines procedures, activities and conditions that are often understood as medical in nature. However, when viewed from the perspectives of women who recount their experiences in the following articles, it becomes clear that the medicalization/mutilation of women's bodies may function to repress or pathologize us, to make us unwell.

For many *Healthsharing* readers, Virginia Mak's article "A Tradition of Pain" on female genital mutilation and Hazelle Palmer's accompanying editorial will most clearly set forth the complex interrelationships between society, women's health and violence. But in understanding how this interrelationship works, in what for many readers is a culture not their own, it is perhaps easy to ignore the violent and repressive nature of medicine as it is practiced in Canada. "Body Image/Body Politics" by Donna Ciliska and Carla Rice effectively outlines the anxieties, both societal and internalized, which we attach to our bodies and the way we occupy our space in our wold. Zelda Abramson, Lorna Zaback and Colleen Ferguson write about medical procedures performed on women's sexual/reproductive bodies — breast reconstructions, hysterectomies and episiotomies — and relate these operations to social repression and sexual violence.

In one of the few *Healthsharing* articles which specifically addressed the health of young women, Patricia Gibson looks at the issue of violence in teenage women's sexual relationships and the challenge presented to older feminists who want to support these young women but find that their tried-and-true strategies do not always work for these young women.

# Under His Thumb

## Teenage Battering[*]

## Patricia Gibson

In the first week or two when we started going out he told me
his brother's house was weird. I said I wouldn't go to his
brother's place if it was weird. He started hitting me and saying
that his brother wasn't weird and not ever to talk about him that
way...

When I got my hair cut he would tell me how ugly it looked
or if I wasn't dressed properly. He'd cut me down when he
thought I was gaining weight. Finally I started wearing what he
wanted...

What a waste of my life. I wonder what other relationships
will be like for me. I'm scared that no one will be able to get
used to me and help me overcome some of my fears...

My plans for the future? I'm just starting to think about it.
It is hard making new friends. I can't trust people. I'm scared
they'll phone him or his family and tell them where I am.

Like many other young women in their teen years, Mary has
been the victim of extensive emotional and physical battering at
the hands of her boyfriend. The relationship began when she was
thirteen; at nineteen she is still trying to keep him away from
herself and her infant son.

Unlike a lot of other young women in abusive relationships,
Mary has laid several charges against her former boyfriend and
has been able to enter a second stage shelter providing longer
term housing for battered women. The shelter is only temporary.
Her former boyfriend threatens that she will never be safe from
him; and she now must deal with the isolation, loneliness and lack

---

[*] Reprinted from *Healthsharing* vol. 5 no. 3 (Summer 1984): 10-13, with
permission of the author.

of self-esteem resulting from her six-year experience in a battering relationship.

The problem of violence in dating relationships is well-known to most social workers, school counselors, and crisis workers dealing with teenage women on a one-to-one basis. Police encounter it regularly. In severe cases it may come to the attention of medical personnel. Young women themselves freely admit they are aware of it occurring in their schools, even among their friends. Rape crisis lines and women's transition houses are frequently contacted by young women who have been beaten or sexually assaulted by their boyfriends.

Despite extensive awareness about the problem of abuse in younger women's relationships, there is not a single shred of solid documentation available in Canada.

In the summer of 1983, Vancouver's Battered Women's Support Services (BASS) secured funding from the Secretary of State Women's Program to undertake a 12-week research project on the subject. The idea for the project came from women working at BASS who had received a number of calls from concerned parents, teachers and social workers encountering young women in violent relationships. The calls not only brought the extent of the problem to their full attention, but also made them realize they were without sufficient information, let alone analysis, regarding the nature of what has been termed "dating violence." Moreover, BASS staff understood they could not automatically transfer the theories and research regarding women who are living with their batterers to younger women.

Jean Bennett, Jeny Evans, and Miljenka Zadravek, the three women hired for the project, were able to gather preliminary information on teen battering. The information is valuable primarily for the light it sheds on the existence of the problem and the questions it raises for feminists working in the general area of violence against women.

Although the project workers had initially wanted to interview only younger women who had directly experienced a battering relationship, they were forced to start with those people actually working with teenagers. They began the project with a series of interviews with streetworkers, social workers, teachers, youth workers, and rape crisis and transition house workers. These "professionals" proved valuable not only for their insights into the abuse they witness, but they were essential in providing contacts with younger women in violent relationships.

Through these contacts, the project staff were able to talk extensively with three young women who were battered in their first dating relationships. The workers caution anyone interested in pursuing research on younger women in violent relationships to remember class and cultural differences. The project was only able to make contact with white women.

The project focused its research almost exclusively on young women who had not lived with their batterers. Mary, for example, was in a battering relationship for six years, but never lived with her boyfriend. According to the project's research, this is not uncommon.

The three young women talked at length about their experiences during the relationships, how they finally managed to leave their boyfriends, and what they thought could have helped them personally when they were in the situation. They were also asked for their views on violence against women generally.

Mary is only now beginning to understand what happened to her and she has a lot of questions.

"I never saw any battering relationships outside my own situation," she told the women on the project. "I thought it didn't happen very much. Now I see it all over. It's scary. What if the judge beats his wife? How will he react to my case if he does? What about the cops, the lawyers? Do some of them beat their wives or girlfriends?"

Each story is as unique as the individual herself, making generalizations or parallels almost impossible. However, all three women interviewed had considered their abuse a problem that was either solely her own, or at least solely her own fault. All three believed their boyfriends loved them and needed them; none of them had been able to keep up relationships with school friends or close girlfriends once the abuse began.

Linda, nineteen at the time of the interview, was fifteen when she left her middle-class home in suburban Vancouver to work the streets. She met her boyfriend in a local hotel and from time to time he assumed the role of her pimp.

"Between fifteen and eighteen he kept me isolated," she said in her interview. "He didn't start abusing me until six months after we got together, when he knew I had fallen in love with him."

But once it began, emotional and physical abuse became a regular occurrence. "He'd love to put fear into me," she said. "He'd tease me for three hours with his boots hanging over my face.... Once he threw me down a flight of stairs. Another time he killed my cat and dog." Like Mary, Linda is afraid her former boyfriend will find her no matter where she hides.

When asked what could have helped her when she was in the midst of the relationship, Linda was sure she wouldn't have talked with anyone. "It was already too late," were her words. "I needed it before. I already felt bad, like a piece of shit." Linda did say she thought greater resources would have helped, specifically suggesting a home where workers would be genuinely concerned about her welfare.

"I was always around people who were trying to toughen me up. No one realized how sensitive I was," she said. As to what she thinks will stop violence against women, Linda replied: "People have to stop victimizing the victims, and they have to stop who's the good woman and who's the bad woman stuff; who can be a feminist and who can't be. It's like I can't be a feminist because I shave my legs. That kind of stereotyping has to be stopped too."

The third woman, Susan, is now twenty-three and has experienced two battering relationships. At the time of last summer's interview she was working and planning to return to university in the fall. She sees her experiences in violent relationships primarily as self-abuse. She too was unable to talk with anyone about what was happening to her at the time.

"I really needed someone to talk to," she said. "It would have helped me to know other people were in the same position." She now believes she could fight back or walk out of a violent relationship if it were to happen again but wishes she had encountered resources after her first experience with a violent boyfriend. "If I had even been able to read something," she said, "I wouldn't have gotten into my second relationship."

According to the project workers, the most difficult thing for a young woman to recognize in a violent relationship is the steady stream of psychological abuse. From interviews with crisis workers as well as the younger women, they discovered a pattern of psychological abuse that results in the woman gradually losing control of the situation. Psychological abuse begins with being called fat or ugly or stupid. The boyfriend will end up deciding what his girlfriend should wear, who she should not spend time with, how she should conduct herself when they are out together. Without realizing it, the woman finds herself isolated from friends and soon sees herself through his eyes.

Isolation is a major factor making it difficult to reach young battered women. A person conducting research has almost no credibility with these women, explained Jean Bennett. Teenagers are particularly concerned about protecting themselves from inquiry and are reluctant to talk with anyone who could bring their problems to the attention of people in the justice system. People who work with teens were adamant that anyone wanting to talk with young women in an abusive situation cannot be judgmental or too eager to give advice.

From the interviews with the "professionals" and the younger women themselves, the project concluded that the inability to talk about abuse when it is happening is the major problem for a teenage woman.

"Who can a younger woman talk with who will believe or understand her," asked Jeny Evans in a recent interview. "She doesn't talk to her family or friends about something like this, much less strangers, and she is afraid if she does tell someone she will lose her control over the problem."

Evans says it is important for older feminists to realize that a young person has been silenced for most of the years of her life and has not learned how to discuss a problem she is having. "Basically she's been told to shut-up all her life or ridiculed for the things she does say. For a teenager there is no safe place where she can open up and talk about herself."

Zadravek, Evans and Bennett were all convinced at the conclusion of the project that, while battering situations for younger women have a great deal in common with what is known about battering in marital relationships, the context in which teenage violence takes place is quite different.

"But it is not a difference that sets them poles apart," says Bennett. "Both younger women and older women who are living with their batterers are part of a continuum of violence. Younger women lack a certain level of knowledge, whether it be about birth control, sexuality, the judicial system, or relationships, that older women have gained simply through the process of living. Older women in battering relationships suffer from a lack of power and control, but it is even more intense for younger women. Young people are not given accurate and useful information that enables them to have greater control over their lives. At the same time, these young women are trying to assert a place for themselves as adults and they feel that they get that from their boyfriends, especially when the rest of the adult world continues to view them as children.''

Susan went into a variety of group homes, but was unable to find someone who could talk to her on her level. ''They didn't understand that it's hard to come off the street where you've had a lot of freedoms and have acted like an adult in taking care of yourself and stuff and go into a situation where people want to treat you on a child level. They create a bunch of rules that don't work for kids who have had control over what they did. Kids develop instincts about who is trying to manipulate them and they manipulate right back.''

Women as young as twelve are known to have been beaten, raped or terrorized by their boyfriends. Many still live at home; some are working the streets; most are caught in a situation where they are being treated as children at home and in school, while they are beginning to see themselves as adults.

The pressure to have a boyfriend is extremely heavy within their own peer group. At the same time, the pressure not to have a boyfriend can be as extreme within the family. The ideal of romance and lasting love, with all the accompanying myths, is particularly strong at such a young age and the experience of dating or sexual involvement is almost non-existent. A teenager living on her own who decides she does want out of a violent relationship has nowhere to go and, because she's a juvenile, people who know about the situation are legally required to report her to the government (in B.C. the Ministry of Social Services).

A major trap for the teenage woman is the likelihood that her boyfriend may be the only emotional contact she has. This is not necessarily the case for a married woman who may at least have her children as an emotional comfort. Zadravek adds, ''These women really care about the guy they're with. If he's been a victim of abuse at home, she sees herself as vitally important to his welfare and doesn't want to walk out on him. In many ways, she sees herself making up for all the rough breaks he may have had down the line."

The women on the project talked about the escalation of violence toward women generally and the undercurrent of violence that exists in advertising directed towards teenagers, as well as rock videos and other forms of popular culture. There is more pornography directed at and accessible to young people than ever before. In the past few years there has been a steady stream of horror movies for young people that repeatedly victimize or terrorize the female characters. "Tough is pictured as acceptable, normal and ultimately attractive," says Bennett "while violence as real pain is left out of the picture."

And of course, the real economic effects of an ever-escalating depression mean there are far fewer opportunities in general for young people to go to college, receive some form of training, or secure a steady job. "The ideal of independence from the family (having a job and an apartment) still persists," says Bennett, "while in reality things are closing down."

In other words, the experience of abuse in teenage relationships cannot be understood without taking into account the whole range of dynamics involved in being young per se, and being young today in a world that is openly violent and riddled with severe economic disadvantage. Most young people have trouble seeing a future for themselves and as a result are all the more vulnerable to abuse.

On the surface one would think young women today would be less susceptible to traditional myths and stereotypes about females, the feminist option being at least one plus for teenagers growing up in the eighties. Not so, say the women from the project. The feminist role model for many young women is not an acceptable option.

"The feminist option is a lonely option, or at least it is seen that way," says Bennett. The women's movement has not been able to bridge the generation gap and, as a result, young women today are likely to be trapped in the same role patterns as the young women of a generation ago.

The women from the project believe this is a major challenge for the feminist movement, and one that should not be easily glossed over. Teenage women, they say, are caught in the cross-fire between two conflicting messages. On the one hand, mainstream socializing tools continue to present the image of beauty as the road to popularity. Teens are told they must be "feminine" or "pretty" if they're going to be popular, have boyfriends, and so on. On the other hand, feminists are saying they should be themselves, stand up for their rights, and demand respect from the men they are with. The force that wins out time and again is not the feminist one.

Often another roadblock for feminists trying to relate to young women is their general unwillingness to accept youth culture. "As we age," says Bennett, "we have less and less understanding of what young women's culture is all about. We have to develop a greater tolerance. We already assume, for example, that there is a different and legitimate cultural experience for women from other countries. It's the same thing with youth. "We can't put our own analysis onto another generation of women; we can't be patronizing; and we can't assume they are all the same."

Older feminists have to open themselves up to younger women, realizing we have things to learn from them and their experiences. "They know best what is happening to them," says Zadravek. "We can't set up a structure that tells younger women what their experiences are, or should be."

As to what needs to be done, the women say more information must be gathered regarding the dynamics of these relationships. "We are in essentially the same position we were ten years ago with wife-battering," says Bennett. "Various professions were aware of the problem, but nothing had been done to document it or analyze the dynamics of a battering relationship." The BASS project was very preliminary, they say, and much too short in its duration.

The younger women interviewed seem much more interested in the development of outreach materials and safe, one-to-one help, than support groups or any kind of consciousness-raising classes. Evans believes that well-publicized information about what to do in a battering situation would be particularly helpful. "Even if they don't act on it right away, at least they know some of the options that are there, and someday, when they're ready, they will use them."

One suggestion the women have for feminists working with

violence against women is to be sure the information contained in their materials includes younger women. And materials should be developed for, and made accessible to, younger women.

On a final note, the women on the project discussed their essential optimism about such a tragic and disturbing issue. "There's a tremendous potential for change here," says Zadravek. "There's an opportunity with teenagers to circumvent a pattern of abuse before it is set. There is a chance to teach women how not to lose control over their relationships with men before it actually happens."

They also believe a greater understanding of the dynamics involved in battering of younger women will ultimately shed greater light on the issue of battering as a whole. The role of economic dependence is one of those key issues which we may need to reexamine. According to the project workers, there is no evidence that teenage women in abusive relationships are economically dependent on their boyfriends. Many of these women still live at home and are primarily dependent on their parents' income; some have moved into their own places and have jobs; even those who are working the streets are functionally independent on a financial level. Yet most research on wife-battering assumes the woman's economic dependence on her husband to be a major, if not the primary component in maintaining the battering relationship.

"If economics is not the greatest factor in keeping a young woman in an abusive relationship, then some serious questions as to the weight we give the economic element in wife-battering must be raised," says Bennett. "On the surface it would seem more weight should be given to the psychological and sociological questions relating to wife-battering."

PATRICIA GIBSON is a freelance journalist living in Vancouver. She is also a member of the Kinesis editorial staff.

# Breast Reconstruction [*]

## Lorna Zaback

"Thanks to recent advances in Plastic surgery techniques," a pamphlet on breast reconstruction from the U.S. Department of Health tells us, "a mastectomy need not have the same physical and emotional consequences it had in the past."

Any woman who has had a mastectomy can consider breast reconstruction. Not only are more sophisticated surgical techniques yielding better results, but most medical insurance plans in Canada now cover the cost of the procedure. Breast reconstruction is the rebuilding of a breast contour after the breast has been surgically removed, most often to treat breast cancer.

The first silicon breast implant was designed in 1962. However, because of concerns that the implant might mask symptoms of the recurrence of breast cancer, these early implants were used almost exclusively in breast augmentation. In 1971, Reuven K. Snyderman of New York's Sloan Kettering Cancer Centre, paved the way for modern breast reconstruction by suggesting that silicon implants could be placed under the chest skin that was left after a mastectomy. He demonstrated that the skin was looser and more flexible than had previously been thought and that an implant would not interfere with its blood supply. Today, this procedure — the placing of an implant beneath the chest muscle and/or skin of a woman who has had a simple mastectomy — is common practice in reconstructive surgery. Breast implants consist of a pliable silicon bag filled with silicon gel, or a saline solution, or layers of both. There are variations in design — shape, size, thickness of the silicon bag — depending on which company produces them.

Some plastic surgeons prefer to gradually stretch the skin by using an inflatable silicon bag as a "tissue expander." The bag is

[*] Reprinted from *Healthsharing* vol. 8 no. 3 (Summer 1987): 16-19, with permission of the author.

first placed under the chest skin and/or muscle and filled with saline, little by little, over a period of weeks. When the reconstructed breast is about the same size as the remaining breast, the inflatable implant is removed and replaced with a more permanent one. Dr. Richard Warren, a Vancouver plastic surgeon, uses tissue expanders to give the reconstructed breast a softer look. "I inflate the tissue expander until it is slightly larger than the other breast. When I replace it with a smaller silicon implant, the breast settles a little and ends up looking less rounded; there's more of a natural contour."

Even the most skilfully reconstructed breast will never look or feel completely natural and will never exactly match a woman's remaining breast. Some plastic surgeons suggest having the remaining breast altered, either made larger or smaller, or lifted. This procedure often involves the use of a second implant, a rather extreme measure to achieve symmetry, especially given the fact that most women do not have breasts that match each other naturally.

A woman who chooses to have a nipple added to her reconstructed breast is usually encouraged to wait five to six months for the implant to settle so that the nipple can be placed as accurately as possible. Nipple reconstruction usually involves taking tissue from the woman's labia or from the nipple of her other breast and grafting it on to the reconstructed one.

Until recently, women who had undergone radical mastectomies (that is where the entire breast, the skin and underlying fat, the lymph nodes in the armpit and along the collarbone, and the major and minor pectoral muscles are removed) were considered poor candidates for breast reconstruction because they did not have enough muscle or skin remaining after the operation to stretch over an implant. In 1977 surgeons at Emory University in Atlanta, Georgia developed a procedure called the "latissimus dorsi flap rotation." The latissimus dorsi muscle from the back, along with some skin, is cut out and rotated through a tunnel high in the woman's armpit to the front of her body. This muscle tissue and skin is used to supplement what little remains after a radical mastectomy and enables the surgeon to cover an implant. Not only can the breast mound be rebuilt, but tissue transferred from the back can also be used to fill out the hollow areas beneath the collarbone left by removal of the major pectoral muscle and to recreate the front fold of the armpit.

Gaining popularity these days is a procedure that involves making a lateral incision across a woman's abdomen, removing tissue and skin from the area between the navel and the pubic hair line. The rectus abdominis muscle is then severed and everything is passed into the breast area through a tunnel under the upper abdominal skin. According to reconstructive surgeons, most women have enough flesh in the abdominal area (!) to eliminate the need for an implant with this procedure. Rectus abdominis transfer may appear attractive to women who have problems with or concerns about silicon implants and still want reconstructive surgery. However, the surgery is long and complicated requiring up to six hours under general anesthetic and tremendous skill on the part of the surgeon. There is usually a good deal of post-operative pain both in the breast and the abdominal area and a woman ends up with two fairly large scars.

There are risks and complications associated with all forms of breast reconstruction. Aside from complications that can result from any form of surgery — problems related to the anesthetic, moderate to severe pain, the development of infection in the area around an incision — there are other potential complications specific to breast reconstruction. Hematoma, a pocket of bloody fluid that results from hemorrhage around the implant (or at the donor site, if tissue is transferred) may need to be surgically drained.

Sloughing can occur. In rare cases, the skin of the chest wall literally peels away and the implant is rejected. According to Rose Kushner, who has written extensively about her experiences with breast cancer and subsequent reconstruction, "sloughing usually occurs if much underlying tissue was removed during the mastectomy itself. Plastic surgeons have devised techniques to avoid the problem by grafting healthy skin to the chest before the implant is inserted."

There is the possibility of tissue death, particularly in procedures where "flaps" (transferred tissue) are used. If the blood supply to the transferred tissue is impaired or is partially insufficient (having diabetes, smoking cigarettes or receiving radiation to the blood vessels in the flap can all decrease blood flow to the skin), skin death can result. Although reconstruction can usually be completed with the remaining portion, at least part of the flap can be lost as a source of tissue for reconstruction.

Other risks pertain to the implants themselves. Saline implants appeal to some women, first because they are made with a small valve through which the saline is injected to make the implant larger or smaller, depending on what is desired, and second because saline is known to be compatible with normal body fluids. This is important in the event that the implant leaks. And they do. According to Dr. Pierre Blais, of Medical Devices at the Health Protection Branch in Ottawa, virtually all saline implants eventually deflate, with the contents leaking out into adjoining tissue. The implant has then to be surgically replaced. So much for popularity.

Double lumen implants consist of an inner envelope filled with silicon gel surrounded by an outer envelope inflatable with saline. One supposed advantage of the double lumen design is that the outer saline-filled envelope, although it, too, will deflate in time, may act as a barrier to gel bleeding out from the silicon-filled inner bag.

Silicon implants, although they are the most popular, presumably because they don't deflate, *do* leak. Dr. Thomas L. Dao, chief of Breast Cancer Surgery and Research at Roswell Park Memorial Institute in Buffalo, was first to notice that a silicon implant, when placed on a piece of paper, will leave an oily residue after a day or two. Even though silicon is thought to be inert and nonreactive within the body (silicon implants have been used in breast reconstruction for 20 years), no actual studies looking into the long-term effects of leakage have been done.

One of the most common complications with gel-filled implants is capsular contracture. "The body naturally reacts to the silicon implant (to the bag as well as to its contents) the same as it would to any foreign substance," says Blais. "It surrounds the implant with a protective layer of fibrous tissue. In many cases, this fibrous capsule becomes so hard and thick that it squeezes or contracts the implant into a ball-like shape. The breast, consequently, takes on a hard, rounded, often misshapen appearance and can become very painful." This may occur, although to a lesser degree, with saline filled bags as well.

Individual women react differently to silicon. There is no way of telling to what extent capsular contracture will occur. Regular post-operative massage can help prevent the build up of the capsule. Placing the implant between or beneath layers of muscle seems to decrease the incidence of contracture. According to Dr. Warren, 20 to 35 percent of women with submuscular implants experience capsular contracture as opposed to 65 percent of those whose implants are placed under the skin or breast tissue alone. However, there is controversy about the submuscular procedure because, if complications do occur, the implant is much more difficult to get at when it is under the muscle.

Most women who experience capsular contracture do so within five years of reconstructive surgery. Their choices at that point are to do nothing or to have the surgeon squeeze the capsule of fibrous tissue, either manually or by machine, to try to break it up and allow the implant to resume its shape and position. There is, of course, a danger of rupturing the implant with this procedure. A third option is more surgery to remove the capsule and reposition the implant.

Silicon implants *do* rupture. Dr. James Mason, a dermatologist from Waco, Texas recommends "that women with implants who have had any hard blow to the breast seek immediate medical attention. Any fluid released from a ruptured implant can form a hard, unsightly, possibly inflamed mass requiring surgery. The fluid also has a tendency to travel around the body."

Implants can be defective. Product control in both Canada and the United States is poor. (See "One Woman's Story," following.) Defective implants can make their way into doctor's offices and, subsequently, into women's bodies where they can cause serious problems.

Why, given the risks and possible complications, do women want breast reconstruction? Surveys have been conducted, including one by Edward Clifford, a psychologist at Duke University. He found that most women had negative feelings about their bodies after mastectomy. They felt lopsided or unbalanced, they were self-conscious about their appearance. Some experienced strong negative feelings when they viewed themselves in a mirror or while bathing.

Most women I spoke with expressed extreme dissatisfaction with external prostheses (breast forms). One woman who had both her breasts removed in 1963 decided 20 years later to have them reconstructed. "It wasn't until 1982 or so that OHIP began to pay most of the cost. So I decided then to have it done. And despite the fact that my breasts aren't perfect — they aren't what I dreamed they would look like — I am *so* much more comfortable. Before [the reconstruction] I was in constant misery. The prosthesis kept shifting, once one floated away while I was swimming. They were hot and irritating. Now I don't even think about it."

Sally Thomas, a Los Angeles nursing professor, recently surveyed 102 women after mastectomy to find out why they had not chosen breast reconstruction. Most of their responses centred around fear that the implant would cause cancer or make any recurrence of cancer more difficult to detect. Some dreaded the possibility of more pain or repeated anesthetic while others didn't like the idea of having anything unnatural under their skin.

In our culture, messages that a woman isn't a whole person without both her breasts are extremely strong. Even women with small breasts or with breasts that don't conform to a specific shape are described in some medical literature as being abnormal. Dr. Hal Bingham, a professor at the University of Florida College of Medicine made this disturbing statement in a 1985 issue of *Midlife Wellness*:

> The *self*-image of an American woman is not complete without her breasts, particularly in our society where significant emphasis is placed on the female chest as portrayed on television, in magazines and in newspapers. We actually worship the female breast and when a woman has a breast removed, she loses one of her more important identifying features. This severely affects her body image [emphasis mine].

With attitudes like these surrounding us, it is not surprising women experience emotional pain and insecurity after mastectomy. Nor is it surprising that women who have their breasts reconstructed express feeling better about themselves afterward.

But poet Audre Lorde, in writing about her experiences with mastectomy in *The Cancer Journals*, says: "Society's emphasis on wearing a prosthesis or on breast reconstruction (in short, looking "normal") after a mastectomy prevents women from coming to terms with their own pain and loss and, in doing so, getting in touch with their own strength."

Women *do* need strength and support to get through breast cancer and mastectomy. For some women breast reconstruction can help in this process, for others it will only mean more physical and emotional stress. A woman considering reconstruction should thoroughly investigate the procedure and talk to other women about their experiences. She needs to weigh the desire to look more symmetrical and "normal" against the risks of under-going more surgery and possibly serious complications.

## ONE WOMAN'S STORY

In October 1983 Jane Stone (not her real name) had breast surgery involving the insertion of a silicon implant. Two days after surgery, a lump had begun to form in her right breast. Whenever she lay flat and lifted her right arm, she noticed an unsightly bulge where the implant was sitting. She found it uncomfortable, thought that the implant might be too low, but decided, for the time being, to live with it.

By March, 1984 her breast had become extremely uncomfortable and she returned to hospital where the plastic surgeon who had performed the original operation attempted to raise the implant. Recovered, or so she thought, Jane moved to Vancouver where she was enrolled in an industrial baking course. Six months later, she was having difficulty using her arm (a situation that interfered with her work). By now, there was a very large lump in her right breast.

She went to see a second plastic surgeon. He told her that the lump had nothing to do with the implant and asked her about breast cancer in her family. Now she was scared. He sent her to a general surgeon who told her the swelling probably *was* due to the implant either leaking or causing inflammation in her breast. She had three choices: have the implant replaced; try once more to have it repositioned, or have it removed completely. She decided to have it removed and returned to the plastic surgeon who had performed the original surgery.

After the operation, the surgeon phoned her mother with whom Jane was living to report: "Everything went fine," he said, "but it's the strangest thing. All we found in Jane's breast was free-floating silicon. The bag has completely disappeared."

Jane was shocked. She asked where the implant could have gone and was told that it must have been absorbed by her body. "But," the surgeon said, "these bags are made of material totally unabsorbable by the body." He searched her breast for the bag and couldn't find it.

Two weeks later, there was still a lump in Jane's right breast. The plastic surgeon sent her back to the general surgeon who said he'd heard of bags breaking. "When the silicon gel is exposed to tissue it causes lumps and pain such as you are experiencing." But he'd never heard of a bag disappearing completely.

The pain became more and more intense and began moving into her lymph area and down into the muscle of her right arm. By this time, Jane was employed as an industrial baker. But, unable to use her arm effectively, she was forced to leave her job. She went from doctor to doctor trying to find someone who could define the problem for her and tell her what to do.

It was at this point that Jane sought legal advice. Margaret Smyth, a Vancouver lawyer, agreed to take her case. Margaret's first step was to help find another team of surgeons that might give Jane some answers. Jane underwent further examination, mammography, etc., only to be told that the results were inconclusive: "The silicon particles are too minute to be identified as such. It's hard to tell whether what we're seeing is silicon or fibrocystic breast lumps. And then you have all this scar tissue from repeated surgery.

From there, she was referred to a neurologist because of the difficulty in using her arm. Tests were performed that confirmed nerve damage and some loss of function. Another surgeon thought he might be able to remove the major lump in her breast to give her some relief from the pain. However, when he opened her up, he found the tissue so congealed he could do nothing and reclosed the incision. Jane is now being offered a mastectomy.

They never found the bag. There is new mass developing in the area of her ribs. Doctors think that because the implant was originally inserted behind her pectoral muscle, it might have slipped into the rib area after it broke. The bag may have been cut during one of the attempts to position it correctly or it may have been defective in the first place.

Doing research for Jane's case, Margaret Smyth has come across numerous cases (mostly in the United States) in which women have successfully sued manufacturers for damages resulting from ruptured bags. There is a group of plastic surgeons in Toronto suing implant manufacturers for damages to their reputations and for the costs of repeated surgery to correct implant-related problems.

"Medical devices of this type have not been adequately tested or regulated," says Margaret. "In the States, independent testing is required. In Canada, most companies that currently make implants need only have registered their name and the name of their product with the Health Protection Branch. No testing whatsoever has been required before the product has gone on the market."

The American experience indicates that manufacturers know about implant defects and failure and continue to sell their products anyway. It's apparently cheaper to pay the odd damage claim than it is to improve the product.

"Judging from the number of lawsuits in progress, implant rupture is a real risk associated with this procedure. Responsibility lies with physicians to outline all the risks of a procedure for their patients. My client was apparently told she might experience some hardening in her breast, but that's all!"

Margaret would like to see more women coming forward. She suspects that the number of complaints is very small compared to the number of women who experience problems. "Undergoing breast surgery or breast reconstruction seems to be something women have mixed feelings about. They certainly get mixed messages about how appropriate it is from the rest of society. I think most women are too embarrassed to complain if anything goes wrong."

There have been enough complaints about breast implants recently to alert the Health Protection Branch in Ottawa. A Health and Welfare committee has been struck to study their safety and effectiveness. It will publish a report in the near future.

### Further Reading

Berger, Karen, and John Bostwick III. M.D. *A Woman's Decision: Breast Care, Treatment and Reconstruction*. New York: The C.V. Mosby Company, 1984.
Kushner, Rose. *Alternatives: New Developments in the War on Breast Cancer*. Cambridge: The Kensington Press, 1984.
Lorde, Audre. *The Cancer Journals*. Argyle, New York: Spinsters Ink, 1980.

**LORNA ZABACH** worked with the Vancouver Women's Health Collective for over five years. She lives in Vancouver.

# Body Image/Body Politics[*]

## Donna Ciliska
## Carla Rice

Three months ago, I felt so awful about how fat I looked! I was
desperate and determined to lose weight so I went out and
joined three weight loss programs at once, paying out over
$3,000 in the process. As usual, I lost weight for the first three
weeks or so, leveled off for a short time, became discouraged at
the lack of results, figured "Why am I killing myself sticking to
these diets?" and went on a binge. So here I am, weighing more
than I ever have!

— Beyond Dieting participant

You might think this quote is from a very "over"weight
woman. (The term "over"weight is used here acknowledging that
there is no good word to describe being fat. We have chosen to
use the term "over"weight when speaking about the medicalization of body fat to communicate that although a fat woman may
be considered at an unhealthy weight according to medical standards, she may be at a weight which is normal and healthy for her.
We also use "fat" — not in a negative sense — but to reclaim the
word and our right to be/have fat.) This woman was, in fact, 35
pounds heavier than the average weight for her height and age
by Canadian statistics. Moreover, her comments echo the concerns of any number of women of all shapes and sizes who have
struggled with weight and shape issues: whether a woman *is* fat
or is preoccupied about *having* body fat, she has been bombarded
with images of what successful women look like. She has been
filled with insecurity around her body and as a result is preoccupied with fears that it does not meet socially constructed ideals.

[*]   Reprinted from *Healthsharing* vol. 10 no. 3 (Summer 1989): 13-17, with
      permission of the authors.

The woman quoted is fairly typical of the nearly 150 participants in Beyond Dieting — a program in Toronto which offers large women an alternative to the usual weight loss fare. Most have gone, for lifetimes, the rounds of the various clinics, commercial centres and self-help books and articles. Most are like the woman above, in that they are uniformly successful at short-term weight loss and uniformly unsuccessful at maintaining the weight loss. Why is there a need for an alternative to dieting?

Both of us became interested in weight preoccupation and alternatives to dieting after struggling with weight and shape issues in our own lives. In her early 20s, Donna compared her body to fashion magazine dictates, concluded that it did not measure up and spent money and time on self-managed diets. Later she helped to develop and offer a weight-loss program which incorporated the most up-to-date ideas about diet, exercise and group support. It quickly became evident that the participants were sincerely following the program, would typically lose weight initially, reach a plateau, get frustrated with the lack of progress, binge and end up at a higher weight than when they started the program.

Carla felt the effects of weight prejudice as an "over"weight child and internalized the fat phobic attitudes that were constantly directed towards her. Through the process of confronting and resolving weight issues, we both began to perceive some of the psycho-social and political implications of weight preoccupation.

## The Cult of Thinness

The reality in the Western industrialized world is, and has been for most of the 20th century (certainly since Twiggy) that "thin is in." According to one North American study, the ideal (as measured by Miss America contestants and *Playboy* centrefolds) has become thinner and more "tubular" over the past 20 years — down to 76 percent of average weight, while the average weight for women has gone up about five pounds. Another study done by Susan and Wayne Wooley of Cincinnati for *Glamour* magazine, found that 75 percent of females rated themselves as "too fat" even though only 25 percent could be considered "over"weight. Canada's 1985 Health Promotion Survey, moreover, showed that 45 percent of Canadians of "normal" weight, and seven percent of those underweight still wanted to weigh less.

The wide gap between ideal and reality leads many women to feel that we have failed and that we lack the ability to "measure up." Moreover, most of us learn to internalize this social construction of the female body as our own and vigorously diet and exercise in an attempt to close the gap. Janet Polivy and Peter Herman at the University of Toronto have shown that dieting among women has become the norm — that it is actually more common for young women to be on a diet than not. Even more shocking is a study by a group in Ottawa which found that female children as young as five years of age expressed dissatisfaction with their bodies and fear of getting fat.

The cultural pressure for thinness and the related prejudice against fat contribute directly to low self-esteem among "over"weight women. Fat women are still the brunt of jokes by many professional comics and cartoonists. As early as six years old, children describe the "over"weight as "lazy," "stupid," "ugly," "cheats" and as "less likeable." Health professionals rate them as more disturbed and likely to have less favourable results from treatment than "normal" weight clients. As well, "over"weight obese have lower rates of acceptance to college, reduced likelihood of being hired for jobs and lower rates of pay. *Industry Week* magazine reported in 1974 that male executives lose an estimated $1000 in wages per pound "over"weight per year. This leaves us wondering how much more severe the punishment is for fat women who make it to that level!

Prejudice against fat is most often a gender specific form of discrimination. As the statistics have shown, it is primarily women who learn to equate thinness with personal worth and allow body shape to determine self-esteem. It is also primarily women who are most often harmed by fat phobic attitudes. In a culture where women are taught that our social value as women is equated with appearance, we learn that the only way we can legitimately access power as women is by achieving and maintaining the socially constructed ideal of beauty. In other words, we are told it is only when we can approximate the ideal (by becoming obsessed with our appearance and its consequent cycle of diet, over-exercise, binge/purge and starve), that we are entitled to like and feel good about ourselves and perceive ourselves as "successful" and "powerful" women.

## "Natural Weight"

As if the negative effects of living in a culture which idealizes super-thin and equates women's value with their physical form were not enough, the fat woman's body supports a physical conspiracy against weight loss. The body does not discern the cultural or internalized preference for the thin ideal. It has built-in survival mechanisms which interpret lower calorie input as famine. Many researchers are working on the theory that there is a "set-point" or biological control for amount of body fat in the body, around which the body allows only slight variation. The adaptive mechanism is such that if you try to create a deficit in the number of calories available to the body (such as by exercise and/or food restriction) the body becomes very "thrifty," shutting down the metabolic rate or the furnace which uses up calories. When that happens, any activity, including rest, uses fewer calories than if you were maintaining your usual calorie balance. Similarly, an effort to gain weight leads to an increase in metabolic rate so that there is a limit to the amount of weight gained and excess calories are burned off as heat. Simply put, calorie use is influenced by calories taken into the body.

In our culture, the condition of reducing calories to slow down weight gain or promote weight loss is not often viewed as a problem for women. However, the body's attempt to conserve calories is a problem for many weight preoccupied women. Weight loss attempts become a "no win" situation where, like the woman in the introductory quote, weight loss slows down after a period on the diet causing the dieter to become discouraged and break her diet plan — right at the point where her metabolism is at its lowest. She then eats more than she would normally to deal with her nutritional and emotional deprivation and weight gain takes place at a faster rate than if she had never dieted, usually resulting in a rebound gain higher than before the diet. The body is so adaptive that, unfortunately, it becomes better with practice — faster at slowing down the metabolic rate with each diet and faster at regaining weight after every diet is broken.

The theory of "set-point" is that each of us has a level of body fat, somewhat like height, which was probably determined by a combination of genetics and very early nutrition. Each of us has our own "natural" body weight which may be very different from what our culture tells us is the ideal. Thus, a woman may be at her set-point at 175 pounds, be very physically healthy and highly unsuccessful at maintaining a lower weight. Similarly, someone else may be underweight by the height and weight standards tables, but be at her body "natural" weight.

## Medicalization

"Over"weight is considered to be a major problem in most Western industrialized countries, where anywhere from 10-50 percent of the adult population is fat, depending on the measurement techniques and standards used. Medical conditions such as hypertension, diabetes, cancers and heart disease are commonly cited as related to "over"weight. Unfortunately many health professionals and the general public translate "related to" to mean "caused by," that is, they assume body fat causes medical problems. Thus, "over"weight, itself, has been labelled as both a physical and psychological disease. In reality there are many "over"weight women who are quite healthy. Some analyses of major population studies have concluded that having a moderate amount of body fat is even associated with some lessening of health risks.

Some of the confusion results from the fact that there are many factors which could lead or contribute to the development and maintenance of a high weight. Sclafani, an American researcher, has identified 50 known causes of obesity in animals. It is likely that most of these causes and probably others, contribute to fatness in humans. Therefore, it is reasonable to expect that some of these factors would be associated with health problems and some would not. Similarly, it appears that the location of body fat is more important than the amount of fat. "Pear" shapes (most women) are much less likely to have diabetes or heart disease than the "apple" shapes (most men).

Given the cultural expectation and the discrimination which exists against fat people, it is surprising that emotional problems are not more common in the "over"weight than in average weight individuals. As mentioned earlier, it is more common for those of us who are fat to dislike our bodies and express dissatisfaction with them. But so-called psychoses, neuroses and personality disorders are no more common among fat people.

Generally, in our society, health care professionals see "over"weight as a danger sign or in very moralistic terms, implying personality faults, weakness of will or laziness. The experience of most Beyond Dieting participants is that health care professionals often treat them as social deviants and attribute any complaints that they have to their weight, advising weight loss for anything from a vaginal infection to the common cold. Unfortunately, many well-meaning family and friends use the same rationale in attempting to help motivate fat women to lose weight. Out of ignorance, others encourage weight-loss programs for the "over"weight, assuming that all are able to lose weight and maintain the weight loss with a little work.

## Dangers of Dieting

Recently, researchers have begun to question negative effects of the diet craze and have looked critically at claims of effectiveness and lack of harm. It is hard to get information about commercial weight-loss programs but the best clinical programs all have positive results in producing weight loss. The catch is that they all produce similar dismal maintenance of weight loss with a rate of 65-95 percent regain at the end of one year. By far the majority of participants are heavier one year after beginning a weight-loss program than they were on entry.

Not only are diets ineffective in the long run, but it is now clear that they have their own set of hazards. In addition to inadequate nutrition and its consequences, dieting has been implicated in the development of weakness, depression, irritability, fatigue, social withdrawal, loss of sex drive, "semi-starvation neuroses," binge eating, bulimia, weight gain and "over"weight and sudden death from damage to the heart. Some of the association of body fat with diabetes and heart disease may be due to repeated dieting, not to the "over"weight itself, as a few studies have shown that harmful fats in the blood are elevated and glucose tolerance is impaired (a sign of diabetes) following a diet.

Susan and Wayne Wooley in Cincinnati have asked the question, "Should obesity be treated at all?" They feel that "over"weight should not be treated because: treatment is mostly unsuccessful, there is evidence for biological control over weight (set-point), a lack of clear evidence that obesity alone is a health risk factor, and that stringent cultural standards of thinness for women have been accompanied by a steadily increasing incidence of severe eating disorders.

The Wooleys suggest that what is really needed is to vigorously treat weight obsession and its associated problems: poor self and body image, excessive or inadequate exercise and disordered eating patterns, metabolic depression and inadequate nutrition caused by dieting. This has become the goal of the Beyond Dieting program.

"Over"weight women from the community are self-referred to the National Eating Disorder Information Centre, where the Beyond Dieting program is located. Even though "over"weight is not considered an eating disorder per se, the women who come often have eating problems as a result of years of dieting. They have unlearned how to respond to hunger and fullness signals, and often do not eat when they are hungry, restrict their food intake for a part of the day or week, then binge for a period of time. Therefore, in addition to educational issues, a primary focus of the time together is in defining what is normal eating, how to relearn hunger and fullness, and how to return to a pattern, amount and quality of food intake that will maximize health. This includes getting rid of the "forbidden food" list, which means learning to incorporate the foods that the women usually deprive themselves from eating in order to avoid binging on them when they cannot tolerate the feelings of deprivation any longer.

Another major focus of the group is to generate a feeling of competence and confidence in the body, that even if the participants cannot get to the place of liking their body at its natural weight, they can at least learn to trust that it functions well and appreciate that it allows them to do things they like to do. Many groups and individual exercises are devoted to this purpose, as well as to reducing the relative importance of body shape in determining self-esteem. As Geneen Roth states: "Thinner thighs are not my salvation," my boss, kids, strife in the Middle East will not be changed by reducing three inches from my thighs. Other parts of the program include body image exercises to reduce body dissatisfaction, assertiveness training to develop strategies to deal with discrimination or well-meaning friends who suggest another diet, as well as discussion of appropriate physical activity and strategies for incorporating it with relative ease into daily life-style.

A real challenge for the participants is to deal with the ambivalence produced by the information. The first reaction is, "What a relief! I have always knows that diets leave me heavier than when I started. Now I don't have to go through that deprivation anymore." Immediately following is the grief reaction over realizing that this information means they will never be thin. Much time is spent in the group and in the followup support group in dealing with grieving the loss of the dream of thinness.

The formal evaluation of the Beyond Dieting program has indicated that the participants have a significant increase in their self-esteem and a successful return to normal eating followed by dramatic reduction in binge eating. Women reported feeling that the quality of their lives is much improved. Loss of obsessiveness with food·allows them more time and energy for family, friends and hobbies. The feel that they no longer have their lives "on hold" no longer waiting until they lose 50 pounds in order to start an exercise program, go back to school, change jobs, think about their relationships, etc. One woman expressed great anger at herself, her family and society in general for allowing her to keep her life on hold for 55 years. She felt she was finally liberated to live without feeling restricted by her body shape.

### Fear of Fat

We do not live in a vacuum. The issues presented here are issues for all women. What is needed now is for a fundamental social and cultural shift to take place, for women and men to be able to accept variation in body shapes as we accept variation in height — as something largely beyond a woman's conscious control. Political action groups such as Hersize, a weight prejudice action group, are working to eliminate discrimination against fat women — discrimination that takes away our power and denies us basic rights.

In a world which accepted and celebrated variation in body shape and size, our buses, subways and theatres would be redesigned for comfort and ease. Fat people would find themselves judged on the basis of their abilities as opposed to their size when applying for jobs. Wages and promotions received would be based on job performance, not on hidden assumptions about body weight. Offices, stores and workplaces would be designed for access and comfort of everyone. Clothes would be designed in large sizes and available at all stores. Images of fat women would be present in the media, not as a symbol of the exotic or erotic, but as one of many images of strong, creative women.

Each one of us needs to begin accepting and learning to like our natural body size, both as a route to personal health and well-being and as an essential step towards empowerment for all women.

As one Beyond Dieting participant remarked: "I am so liberated! I threw out a whole box of diet books and my scales. My husband would prefer that I were thinner, but agrees that I am much easier to live with since giving up dieting. I am getting on with the important things in life."

## Further Reading
It is usually difficult to find these books, but any bookstore will order them for you.

Bennet, William, and Joel Gurin. *The Dieter's Dilemma*. New York: Basic Books, 1982.

Polivy, Janet, and Peter Herman. *Breaking the Diet Habit*. New York: Basic Books, 1983.

Schoenfiedir, Lisa, and Barb Wieser, eds. *Shadow on a Tightrope*. Iowa City: Aunt Lute Book Company, 1983.

Szekely, Eva. *Never Too Thin*. Toronto: Women's Press, 1988.

Roth, Geneen. *Breaking Free From Compulsive Eating*. New York: Signet, 1984.

DONNA CILISKA founded the Beyond Dieting program for the National Eating Disorder Information Centre, while a doctoral student at the University of Toronto. She is currently an Associate Professor at McMaster University, Faculty of Health Sciences, and a Clinical Nurse Consultant for the Hamilton-Wentworth Department of Health Services.

CARLA RICE is an activist and founding member of Hersize: A Weight Prejudice Action Group. She is also a freelance writer, educator and group facilitator, and is currently working on her Master's in Applied Psychology at the Ontario Institute for Studies in Education.

# Unimaginable? Not Really... [*]

## Hazelle Palmer

The first time I read Virginia Mak's article on female genital mutilation (FGM), my blood ran cold. I kept trying to picture going through the procedure myself; kept trying to imagine how young girls manage to survive such brutal mutilation.

Imagine having your genitalia removed entirely; worst, imagine being forced through this procedure as part of a cultural tradition which supposedly prepares you for marriage. Imagine having your body mutilated to make you more attractive to men.

For many of us living in North America, FGM may seem unimaginable. But if we look closely at the underlying cause for this procedure it may not seem so far-fetched. It is true that FGM is at the far end of a continuum which has young girls and women having their bodies redefined in order to be more attractive or pleasing to men. It is also true that, FGM is performed on girls so young they are unable to fight back or object to the mutilation on their bodies. But in North America, we are starving ourselves with unhealthy diets, having our faces stretched to erase the signs of aging and having breast implants surgically inserted to enhance our breast size, all to reach some unrealistic and unreasonable image of beauty; an image created by men.

This quest for "perfect" beauty is mutilation. We may not see it exactly that way and when we read about women undergoing such procedures, it may not have the same impact as FGM (and shouldn't). But anyone who has heard the stories of the women who have had breast implant surgery and are now experiencing problems, will know that the effects can be physically and emotionally damaging in their own way.

What joins the survivors of FGM with the experiences of North American women is that all of these traditions, and the

\* Reprinted from *Healthsharing* vol. 13 no. 4 (Winter/Spring 1993): 3, with permission of the author.

voluntary surgical or cosmetic adjustments are created around the wishes and fantasies of men.

As FGM gains worldwide attention, women and health activists are calling for an end to this procedure. We need to align our efforts with these groups to ensure that this goal is achieved.

Before, we dismiss FGM as being something that happens to "them" and not to "us," I beg you to re-examine the things we do here that also have us changing our bodies, voluntarily. And before we conclude that any form of mutilation in our environment is unimaginable....

**HAZELLE PALMER** is the managing editor of *Healthsharing.*

# Female Genital Mutilation

## A Tradition of Pain[*]

### Virginia Mak

At the age of four, Kowser Omer was prepared for marriage.

> A group of women came to my home. I was told to sit on the floor. One woman sat behind me to support me. She opened my legs and two women held them down. My mother supervised the procedure and told the woman with the razor blade to remove everything.
>
> She injected some fluid into me, which was supposed to be an anesthetic. Then she cut off my clitoris, my labia majora and part of my labia minora while I screamed in pain. Then she stitched my vulva closed, leaving an opening the size of a corn kernel for urine and menstrual blood.

A celebratory gathering followed the procedure. Women brought sweets to her home and Omer was given a piece of jewelry. This marked the beginning of her womanhood: she was now "prepared" for marriage. Omer, who was raised in Hargesia, northern Somalia, is just one of the millions of young girls who have undergone this procedure. It's called female genital mutilation (FGM) and it continues today.

Twenty-seven African countries; parts of Arabia, Yemen, Oman, the Arab Emirates; some Muslims in Indonesia, Malaysia, India, Pakistan; and newcomers to Australia, Europe and North America are believed to practice FGM. One hundred million women worldwide have been affected, and that figure increases by more than a million each year due to population growth.

Three types of FGM are practiced worldwide today. *Sunna* is the procedure where the prepuce (hood) or tip of clitoris is cut.

[*] Reprinted from *Healthsharing* vol. 13 no. 4 (Winter/Spring 1993): 10-13, with permission of the author.

*Excision* involves removing the entire clitoris and all or part of labia minora. *Infibulation* is the scraping away of the entire external genitalia — the clitoris, labia majora and labia minora. With the remaining tissue, the vulva is stitched closed, often with thorns, leaving a small opening. Infibulation is performed in Somalia to girls of every class. In Omer's case, her mother paid for the extra expense of anesthetics, stitches and antibiotics. Paid to perform this procedure are elderly women from an economically-disadvantaged clan called Meetgo. "My grandmother pressured my mother to have the procedure done to me since a young girl is not marriageable unless she has been infibulated," recounts Omer, who now works at the Birth Control Venereal Disease Information Centre as a Community Health Educator and Counselor in Toronto.

Omer says her own experience was under comparatively favourable conditions. For other girls, unsterilized knives and broken glass are sometimes used. Some have even been infibulated without washing. Up to eight women have been known to hold down a young girl during the procedure. Instead of stitches, thorns are often used to close the vulva. Cloth knots are tied at the end of the thorns to hold the stitching in place. Ash may then be used to close the wounds.

Despite the war and disruption in Somalia, women continue to infibulate their daughters, hoping to protect them from rape. The procedure is sometimes performed on the run — in refugee camps and often under unhygienic conditions.

Hawa Mohamed, who recently immigrated to Canada from Somalia, is the former director of the Human Education Department at the Ministry of Education in Somalia. She was responsible for sex education, including the topic of female genital mutilation. Much of her work involved speaking out against FGM. Recently, Mohamed spoke to the Toronto Women's Health Network about the history and beliefs that rationalize female genital mutilation.

> The origin of this practice is not clearly known. Many believe that it dates back to 500 BC. Mummies from ancient Egypt have been found with signs of mutilation. Some speculate the practice was used to distinguish aristocratic women from slaves. In the ninth and 12th century in Britain, it was used as a treatment on women with perceived psychiatric disorders.

Since Muslims, Christians and Jews in different countries practice FGM, it is based on culture rather than religion, although many people still see it as a religious requirement.

The first time FGM was discussed was at a seminar in Khartoum, Sudan in 1979. In 1984, the Inter African Committee (IAC) was formed by African women to prevent and eradicate these mutilations. The name "female circumcision" was officially changed to "genital mutilation" in 1990.

## Health Effects

Adverse health consequences range from injury of the urethra, bladder infections, hemorrhaging and trauma from the extreme pain, to long-term psychological scars. Young girls can die of bacterial infection, or simply bleed to death.

Omer recalls the aftermath of her own infibulation.

> My legs were tied together from my waist to my feet. I stayed bound like that for nearly three weeks so my vulva could heal shut. Urinating was excruciatingly painful. I had to be turned on my side so the urine could drip out of an opening.

During a girl's first period, blood clots block menstrual flow, causing infection. A keloid scar (a tough, raised scar) can form on the vulva, where cysts as large as a grapefruits are also not uncommon.

The vaginal opening of FGM women remains small until marriage. Omer describes what commonly occurs on the day before the wedding.

> Women from the groom's family visit and examine the bride. They check to ensure that infibulation has been done and that she is a virgin. The genital area should be smooth as the palm of one's hand. To make intercourse easier, the vulva may be cut open slightly. Otherwise, during the wedding night, the groom widens the opening with his penis which is painful for him as well as for the bride.

This "tailoring" of the vagina to the size of the husband's penis is meant to ensure monogamy on the part of the wife. Having too large an opening is grounds for divorce in Somalia.

On the wedding night, a cloth is placed under the bride's genital area. After intercourse, the cloth is displayed to members of the groom's family as proof of the bride's virginity. If the groom refers to the sexual experience as "falling into a ditch," he may annul the marriage the next day.

## Men's Attitudes

There are conflicting accounts of Somali men's attitudes towards FGM. Although many men dismiss FGM as women's business, they refuse to marry an unmutilated woman. Fathers have an equally ambiguous outlook. "My father, like other fathers, pretended to be unaware the procedure was being done to me, although he paid for it. He did not visit me at all while I recuperated," Omer explains.

Virginity and chastity play a significant role in this perpetual practice. An infibulated woman is ensured to be chaste, clean and virginal, and therefore marriageable. Ironically, infibulated women can become infertile, and as a result are divorced by their husbands.

The rationales for FGM are as varied as the countries in which it is practiced. They include decreasing the risk of nymphomania, reducing female sexuality and masturbation, improving cleanliness, increasing fertility and rendering the genital area smoother, hence more appealing to men. It is also said to remove any obstruction to sexual intercourse, and to increase a man's pleasure by tightening the vagina.

## Childbirth for FGM Survivors

For many women, the greatest price of FGM is paid during childbirth. To make childbirth easier, midwives in Somalia cut the undamaged skin beside the previously stitched vulva area (anterior episiotomy). A lateral incision may also be performed along the sides of the perineum (medio-lateral episiotomy). These procedures were developed because Somali midwives found that a damaged perineum caused the loss of bladder control.

After giving birth, the women are stitched up to keep their

vaginal opening small. Thus, women who bear numerous children will be cut open and stitched repeatedly.

Because labour and delivery are difficult for an FGM survivor, many women die during childbirth. In addition, babies are often born brain-damaged or dead. The exact cause of the deaths remains unknown, as very little has been documented.

In Somalia, the maternal mortality rate is 1,100 per 100,000 births, compared to a rate of 24 per 100,000 births in industrial countries. In Ethiopia, including Eritrea, where about 90 percent of the girls are "circumcised," the mortality rate is 130 per 1,000 live births. In Ghana, where 20 percent of the girls undergo the procedure, the rate is 86 per 1,000 births.

### FGM in Canada
Is infibulation or other forms of FGM performed here in Canada? Since there are nearly 70,000 Somalis in Canada — 45,000 in Toronto alone — the likelihood exists.

Although the College of Physicians and Surgeons of Ontario banned genital mutilation in 1992, Mohamed says rumours of its continued practice persist. In its March 1992 press release, the college acknowledged that it "had received inquiries from concerned physicians being asked to perform this procedure." In addition, it has a policy paper which states, "In the event that a physician learns of a person performing female circumcision, excision or infibulation, the matter should immediately be brought to the attention of the college."

Medical professionals and the public alike need to be educated about the plight of FGM survivors. Omer urges health workers to be particularly sensitive to their needs. Intrusive questions such as whether or not orgasms are possible, or requests to display the patient's genital area to another colleague, are highly inappropriate. FGM survivors often experience shame and guilt due to their mutilated genitalia and would be further traumatized by such behaviour.

Physicians or other health professionals who are not familiar with the subject should do their homework before treating FGM survivors. For instance, when administering a pap test, physician should not insert a standard speculum as the vaginal opening is too small. A pelvic examination with a standard speculum can be painful for an FGM survivor since her pubic skin lacks elasticity.

When an infibulated women gives birth, many physicians insist on a Caesarean section. Omer, an experienced midwife, says an anterior or medio-lateral episiotomy is adequate.

As a counselor at the Toronto Birth Control Venereal Disease Clinic and an anti-FGM advocate, Omer answers inquiries and provides education material on the issue. She also counsels FGM survivors on sexuality, birth control and birthing. She says there is a need to establish an informal network of women who have undergone genital mutilation. This way, survivors would be able to share their experiences, lend one another support and channel information to health workers. To date, only the City of Toronto Department of Public Health has provided brochures on the issue.

In the past year, Mohamed has been working for Women's Health in Women's Hands, a community-based health centre for women in Toronto, which educates health professionals about FGM. Twelve community volunteers have been trained for this process and the group provides access to over 300 items of resource materials, including slides, books, tapes, articles and flip charts. As well, the Toronto Women's Health Network plans to

---

## BOUND BY BEAUTY

Many Westerners are quick to condemn practices such as FGM while ignoring equally questionable customs in their own culture. Women all around the world accept and encourage, pain, sickness and surgery as legitimate sacrifices for "beauty."

### Here are just a few examples:

| | |
|---|---|
| nose job | tummy tuck |
| tattooed eye make-up | high heeled shoes |
| eye lift | false nails with corrosive glue |
| bulimia | breast implants |
| tight jeans | face lift |
| collagen injection | face peel |
| electrolysis | hot waxing |
| anorexia | stomach staples |
| liposuction | suntanning |

---

continue educating health workers and midwives in the coming months.

"Female genital mutilation is criminal. It's a women's rights issue. It's a human rights issue," says Mohamed. "It's torture, and it should stop."

**VIRGINIA MAK** is a writer of fiction and non-fiction. Born in Hong Kong, she now makes her home in Toronto. In her spare time, Virginia sings unassumingly in an amateur choir and is a member of the *Healthsharing* editorial board.

# Episiotomy Unnecessary, Study Finds*

## Colleen Ferguson

One of the most common operations performed on women in Canada and the United States may not only be unnecessary, but disruptive and harmful as well, according to a new Canadian study.

Episiotomies, performed on 80 percent of women giving birth for the first time, includes a surgical incision along the perineum. Ideally, the procedure widens the vagina to prevent tearing and ease childbirth. However, stitches are needed to close the wound: stitches that might have been avoided if an episiotomy had not been performed.

The study, released this summer in a new computerized medical publication called the Online Journal of Current Clinical Trials, found that women who had episiotomies ended up with the same number of stitches as women who had minor tears. In some cases, episiotomies led to even more tearing than would have occurred without the incision.

The study included 703 pregnant women randomly divided into two groups. In one group, episiotomies were performed regularly, in the other, their use was restricted.

Researchers found that women who were giving birth for the first time received the same number of stitches whether they had an episiotomy or normal tearing during birth.

Women who had given birth previously, received significantly fewer stitches without an episiotomy than women in the same position in the other group. And, women who gave birth without any tearing and therefore without any stitches, fared the best and felt the least amount of discomfort after childbirth.

---

* Reprinted from *Healthsharing* vol. 13 no. 2 (Summer/Fall 1992): 7, with permission of the author.

An alarming finding of the study was that episiotomies may actually contribute to severe tearing. Out of 357 first births, 46 women who had episiotomies suffered severe tearing. By contrast, the restricted group had only one woman giving birth for the first time who suffered severe tearing.

Despite the findings of this study, many doctors continue to perform episiotomies routinely making the procedure the most common operation performed without consent on women in Canada and the United States.

# Don't Ask Your Gynecologist If You Need a Hysterectomy... [*]

## Zelda Abramson

A woman asking her gynecologist if she needs a hysterectomy is like a man asking his barber if he needs a shave. The answer is all too likely to be "yes" whether it is needed or not. Hysterectomy is the most common surgery performed on women in Canada today, in part because doctors fail to consider more conservative alternatives. This approach is deeply embedded in the history of gynecology.

The first successful hysterectomy, removal of the uterus only, was performed in Massachusetts in 1853. However, it was oophorectomy, the removal of ovaries or castration, which became the most popular gynecological surgery between 1880 and 1910. At this time, the field of gynecology provided treatment primarily for "female personality disorders." It was believed that a woman's ovaries controlled her personality and that any psychological problem — from irritability to insanity — should be treated by gynecological surgery.

Gynecologists also expressed deep concern over women's "uncontrollable" sexual desires and to cure this problem, castration was recommended and executed. Sexual transgressions, masturbation and orgasm were viewed as symptoms of women's mental disorders which in turn were regarded as a function of defective ovaries. Castration for treatment of so-called female personality disorders was still practiced as late as 1946.

Indeed, women's reproductive organs were held responsible for all female disorders such as headaches, backaches, sore

---

[*] Reprinted from *Healthsharing* vol. 11 no. 13 (Summer 1990): 12-17, with permission of the author.

throats, indigestion and even tuberculosis. Any symptom could easily provoke a medical attack on her ovaries.

Hysterectomy is the modern day replacement for oophorectomy. Approximately 90 percent of hysterectomies are performed for non-cancerous reasons. They are performed on women who have fibroid tumours, a prolapsed uterus, endometriosis, hyperplasia with abnormal bleeding, pelvic inflammatory disease, cysts or an obstetrical mishap. An estimated 25 percent of Canadian women have had hysterectomies compared to 30 percent of American women and 11 percent of English women. The rate in Canada is twice that of Europe. Close to 60,000 hysterectomies are performed in Canada each year. The majority are performed on women between the ages of 35 and 44. In fact 63 percent of all women having hysterectomies are under the age of 45. Removal of ovaries as well as the uterus is a procedure performed in about 50 percent of women over the age of 40.

It is estimated that up to half the hysterectomies performed in Canada are not medically necessary. In 1971, the Saskatchewan Ministry of Health commissioned a study examining whether hysterectomies were justified, as a result of a 72 percent increase in the number of hysterectomies performed between 1964 and 1971. The results of this study which audited medical charts of five hospitals found that between 17 and 59 percent of hysterectomies performed were unnecessary. An interesting side effect of this study was that the rate of hysterectomy in Saskatchewan subsequently dropped dramatically.

Between 1975 and 1977, the U.S. House of Representatives held hearings on unnecessary surgeries. Three major surgeries were evaluated to determine whether their prevalence was justified: appendectomy, prostatectomy and hysterectomy. The report concluded that the appendectomy and prostatectomy surgeries were justified, however, over 40 percent of the hysterectomies performed were unwarranted. A further study reported by the U.S. Department of Health and Human Services in 1983 found that in 48 percent of the 1,851 hysterectomies studied it was not confirmed that the uterus was diseased.

The Canadian rate of hysterectomy varies significantly from province to province. If you live in Newfoundland you have a 61 percent greater chance of having a hysterectomy compared to a woman living in Saskatchewan. The rate of hysterectomies performed in eastern Canada (including Quebec) is significantly greater than the rate in western Canada (including Ontario). Not only do rates vary between provinces, they also vary within provinces.

There are no simple answers to account for the dramatic differences between regions. However this data can be used to test various hypotheses that have been suggested to explain such differences.

One hypothesis is that the rate of hysterectomy corresponds to the rate of cancer of reproductive organs. This is clearly not the case in Canada. In fact the provinces with the highest hysterectomy rate, Newfoundland, Nova Scotia and New Brunswick, have the lowest rate of cancer of the reproductive organs while the provinces with the lowest rate of hysterectomy, Manitoba and Saskatchewan, have the highest rate of cancer.

A second hypothesis is that there is a direct correlation between the number of gynecologists and the number of hysterectomies performed. Again, this is clearly not the case in Canada. Indeed, the opposite is true. Eastern Canada has fewer gynecologists per capita than western Canada, yet hysterectomies are performed at a higher rate. For example, every year in eastern Canada, between 562 and 615 women out of 100,000 receive hysterectomies. This compares to a range between 377 and 480 out of 100,000 in Canada's western provinces. This means that in Newfoundland a gynecologist performs on average 75 hysterectomies per year while the national average for a gynecologist is 44 (in itself an astounding number).

Other hypotheses that have been offered to explain regional variations based on income, education, religion and medical fee structures do find support in the Canadian data. Some research has shown that women with lower levels of income and education have a higher hysterectomy rate. For example, a 1986 study of 2000 women in Pittsburgh found that black women with low incomes and education had twice as many hysterectomies as white women who tended to be better educated and have higher incomes.

Eastern Canada is indeed poorer than western Canada. The Atlantic provinces have the highest percentage of families with low incomes. In terms of education, a higher percentage of the population of eastern Canada has less than grade nine education and a lower percentage is in university compared to western Canada.

Religion may be a factor. It is believed that Roman Catholic women have a higher rate of hysterectomy, and there is a higher percentage of Roman Catholics in eastern Canada than in western Canada. One reason why Catholics may have a higher hysterectomy rate is because of their socio-demographic profile.

Compared to other religious groups in Canada, Roman Catholics have on average fewer years of schooling, a lower average income and higher unemployment rate. A second possibility to consider is that sterilization by hysterectomy is considered a legitimate form of birth control by this population.

With regard to fee structure, other research has shown that more hysterectomies are performed by fee-for-service physicians than salaried physicians. Medical care in Canada is overwhelmingly provided on a fee-for-service basis. Each province has independent billing schedules, and rates for hysterectomy procedures vary from province to province. If we compare the number of hysterectomies per 100,000 in each province to the amount paid to the physician per hysterectomy we find a negative relation: that is, the provinces with the higher rates of hysterectomy pay their physicians the least amount of money for this procedure.

Does financial motivation play a role in terms of numbers of hysterectomies? One physician quoted in the *New York Times Magazine* in September, 1975, said that since there is a decline in the birth rate, "some of us aren't making a living, so out comes a uterus or two each month to pay the rent."

If indeed financial motivation is a factor, one solution is to restructure the fee schedule so that more conservative treatments are financially rewarded. Currently, for example, a surgeon receives less money for a myomectomy (the removal of benign fibroids in or on the uterus), a more complex, time-consuming surgery than for a hysterectomy which removes the entire uterus. Logically, most surgeons opt for the best-paid, most straightforward solution — hysterectomy.

Although at this point we can only speculate about why regional variations exist, the very fact that they do allows us to conclude that the decision whether or not to have a hysterectomy for non-life threatening reasons, in the majority of cases, is based on the discretion of the attending physician.

Many diseases of the pelvic region are painful and uncomfortable. Pain and bleeding are often the first two signals of a problem needing medical assistance. Frequently physicians recommend hysterectomies as a cure for these symptoms. However hysterectomies do have serious negative physiological and psychological consequences which women must consider. Hysterectomy is major surgery. The recovery period is lengthy, on average 13 months, compared to four months for other abdominal surgeries (e.g. removal of gall bladder).

In 1984, a study examining the risks and benefits of hysterectomy in Manitoba reported that four percent of women experienced serious complications requiring readmission to hospital within two years following their hysterectomy. Furthermore, the study noted that although these women visited their gynecologists less often for gynecologic related problems following their surgery, they required medical intervention more frequently than other women for psychological problems, physiological problems and menopause.

Urinary tract problems appear to be a common complaint women have following a hysterectomy. This is indeed ironic as prevention of bladder problems, attributed to fibroids, is one of the most frequently used justifications to recommend a hysterectomy. Other common side effects following a hysterectomy are gastrointestinal problems such as cramping and bloated feelings. Also, internal scar tissue known as adhesions can lead to chronic pelvic pain. Adhesions occur in approximately 50 percent of women who have had pelvic surgery.

Post-operative depression is two to three times greater among women who have had hysterectomies than among those who have undergone other pelvic surgeries. One study which examined women four years after surgery noted that women who have had hysterectomies are referred to psychiatrists at a rate three times greater than women in the general population. Moreover, the connection between depression and hysterectomy often goes unnoticed both by the woman and her physician for years after her surgery and therefore she may receive improper treatment or none at all.

The reasons for the high rate of depression in women who have had hysterectomies are not altogether clear. Depression is prevalent both among women who hoped to have children and did not and among women who do not wish to have more children. For many women the loss of their uterus represents their loss of choice to bear children. Negative changes in body image are common concerns especially when women make a strong connection between their uterus and their femininity.

Many researchers believe that the depression is largely due to neurochemical changes as a result of the hysterectomy. Recent research appears to connect the uterus to the functioning of the body's endocrine system. There is evidence to suggest that the uterus produces and releases estrogen as the ovaries do. Women who have hysterectomies appear to have lower levels of tryptophan. Tryptophan is an amino acid produced in the brain which seems, when levels are low, to trigger depression. Levels of tryptophan correlate with estrogen levels: as levels of estrogen increase levels of tryptophan increase; as estrogen levels decrease tryptophan levels follow.

Furthermore, it is believed that the biochemistry of the uterus contributes to the overall well-being of a woman's health and not only to reproduction. Although not scientifically confirmed it is speculated that the uterus produces prostaglandins which may protect against arthritic inflammation. Finally, the uterus may protect against coronary artery disease and therefore a hysterectomy may increase the risk of heart disease.

Women routinely ask what impact a hysterectomy will have on their sexuality. Usually these women are emphatically reassured that the removal of the uterus will in no way affect their sexual pleasure. This is often not the case.

Many women experience a loss of sexual desire following the hysterectomy. When this occurs many physicians attribute the change to depression. This is WRONG! It is not depression that causes unsatisfying sex, rather the loss of satisfying sex leads to depression.

There are physiological reasons why women experience difficulty with sex after a hysterectomy. Some women report pain because of a tightened vagina or because of scar tissue in the vagina as a result of having the cervix removed. Whether a woman's orgasm is due to clitoral or vaginal stimulation, the uterus itself plays an important role in sexual arousal and orgasm. As a woman becomes sexually aroused the uterus becomes enlarged and moves around. The uterus is a muscle and during orgasm it contracts at rhythmic intervals. Many women find these contractions pleasurable. Furthermore, blood vessels and nerves which may affect sexual sensation are cut when the uterus is removed.

Studies show approximately 30 percent of women report improved sex after a hysterectomy. Many of these women experienced severe pain during sexual intercourse before their surgery. Pleasure then was not a consideration. Removing the uterus results in painless sex and thus improved sex, but does not necessarily enhance the woman's ability to achieve orgasm or experience pleasure. These studies do not differentiate between these questions.

The closer a woman comes to the age of 40, the fewer alternatives to hysterectomy are made available to her. For most women under the age of 40, it is easy to persuade the physician to look into alternatives. It is not difficult for physicians to understand and empathize with women wanting children. However, these same physicians do not have the same sensitivity when it comes to a woman who is older, that is, over 40, and who prefers to preserve her uterus, and, if indeed a hysterectomy is warranted, to keep her ovaries.

One American gynecologist, Ralph C. Wright, in 1969 justified the increasing number of hysterectomies as follows: "The uterus has but one function: reproduction. After the last planned pregnancy, the uterus becomes a useless, bleeding, symptom-producing, potentially cancer-bearing organ and therefore should be removed." This view continues to be popular today among gynecologists.

We are all afraid of cancer. Ovarian cancer is particularly frightening. Because it is generally not diagnosed early, there is a poor survival rate. Realistically, the chances of a healthy woman developing ovarian cancer and dying from it is marginally over one percent. Furthermore, the risk of ovarian cancer does not increase if you choose to keep your ovaries when having a hysterectomy. Nevertheless physicians continue to justify the removal of the ovaries on the grounds that it prevents ovarian cancer.

The routine removal of ovaries in post-child-bearing women has serious implications for a woman's sexuality. Ovaries continue to produce hormones, specifically androgens, which play an important role in a woman's sexual desire and in her ability to become aroused.

A recent study from McGill University confirms the complaints of many women who have had a hysterectomy and both ovaries removed: decreased sexual desire and arousal. Ironically, physicians in the 18th century were correct in linking a woman's libido to her ovaries.

Women who have had their ovaries surgically removed, are routinely prescribed Hormone Replacement Therapy (HRT), the popular medical treatment for menopause. HRT "replaces" the hormones in the woman's body which the ovaries are no longer producing. This is ironic because the justification for removal of the ovaries in first place was because they were no longer needed! Moreover, HRT does not improve a woman's libido. To improve her sexual desire, testosterone (male hormone) is given in addition to HRT. This does increase sexual desire dramatically, but also causes negative side effects such as a deepened voice, increased growth of body hair and a larger clitoris. All this is a constant reminder that something is not quite right.

Until 1975 rates of hysterectomy were increasing. In recent years, in some but not all parts of Canada, rates have been marginally declining. In part, I believe this is due to women becoming increasingly knowledgeable about the abuse of this surgical procedure, as well as to significant gains in technology. Research has shown, as in Saskatchewan, that when hospitals are audited, the rate of hysterectomy decreases dramatically.

The most effective way to reduce the number of unnecessary hysterectomies performed is through active consumer participation in choice of treatment and in the development of public policies regulating health care. More public education and research is necessary to support this involvement.

If your physician recommends a hysterectomy for reasons other than cancer or hemorrhaging, your surgery is elective. Once your uterus and/or ovaries are removed there are no replacements. Take your time in deciding. Here are some suggestions:

EDUCATION — Understand your choices and know your alternatives; read books and articles; speak to women who have already had a hysterectomy.

**A SECOND OPINION** — Seek out second, third or fourth opinions if necessary. It is okay to be labeled "doctor shopper." A good consumer always shops around before making a purchase.

**COUNSELLING** — This can be helpful in identifying your feelings and concerns, at the same time supporting you in the decision making process.

**A RULE TO REMEMBER** — In deciding whether or not to have a hysterectomy, ask this question: "Is the treatment worse than the condition?"

Unless the reason for a hysterectomy is to preserve life, the most conservative treatment always should be explored first. Hysterectomy is the last alternative and only to be considered when all else fails.

## Further Reading

Ballweg, Mary Lou, and the Endometriosis Association. *Overcoming Endometriosis — New Help from the Endometriosis Association*. New York: Congdon and Weed, 1987.

Cobb, Janine O'Leary. *Understanding Menopause*. Toronto: Key-Porter Books, 1989.

Cutler, Winnifred B. *Hysterectomy Before and After*. New York: Harper and Row, 1988.

Hufnagel, Vicki. *No More Hysterectomies*. Markham: Penguin, 1989.

Lauersen, Niels H. *The Endometriosis Answer Book*. Fawcett Columbine, 1988.

Morgan, Susanne. *Coping With A Hysterectomy*. New York: Dial Press, 1984. (Out of print, but check your local library.)

Payer, Lynn. *How to Avoid a Hysterectomy*. Pantheon Books, 1987.

Strausz, Ivan K. *You Don't Need a Hysterectomy: New and Effective Ways of Avoiding Major Surgery*. New York: Addison Wesley, 1993.

**ZELDA ABRAMSON** is a women's health counselor in private practice in Toronto.

# Identifying and Challenging Notions of Disease

The articles presented in this section examine specific medical conditions and women's responses to "disease" and to the medical environment which frames it. As women, our responses are often very different from those proposed by the medical system, where typically, as Mary Louise Adams characterizes it, "cause 'x' leads to symptom 'y', which can be cured by 'z' treatment." Although we live within a society imbued with the values and assumptions of Western medical practice, women, both as patients and as health care providers, have struggled for many years for empowering alternatives: accessible information, women-centred researched, peer support models, non-drug therapies.

Jan Darby questions the medical preoccupation with establishing a link between cervical cancer and sexually transmitted diseases (STDs) with the moralistic implications of such a connection. The debate on this link continues, but few will dispute that punishments are often disguised as "health care" in the medical system's approach to the prevention and treatment of sexually transmitted diseases.

Articles by Pam Bristol and Darien Taylor give a voice to women living with two specific diseases which posed an increasing threat to the health of women: breast cancer and HIV/AIDS. They argue for the involvement of affected women in decision-making, from the choices that the individual woman makes about her treatment, for example, through to the provision of peer support and the creation of advocacy groups to guide hospital programs, research agendas and government funding.

Using the examples of candidiasis and Epstein-Barr Virus, Mary Louise Adams and Lorie Rotenberg expose a medical environment and a deteriorating physical environment which contributes to pervasive immune suppression. Their observations about the debilitated context within which health care takes place provide a window through which many medical conditions can be viewed.

These diseases, and especially the women who ask provocative questions and demand better answers to them, challenge the medical system to reconsider many of its basic premises.

# Sex and Punishment
## The Politics of Cervical Cancer[*]

### Jan Darby

Cervical cancer is one of the most common reproductive cancers among women worldwide. Women living in developing nations, poor women and women of colour are at greatest risk of dying from this disease. In Canada and other wealthy nations, women are subject to mass screening, intrusive diagnostic procedures and destructive treatments in an attempt to "prevent" the disease. Therefore, the question of what causes cervical cancer has profound implications for women's lives and health.

Medical research has found associations between cervical cancer and a variety of possible causes, such as smoking, oral contraceptives, talcum powder and the long-banned drug DES. DES is a synthetic estrogen prescribed to pregnant women to prevent miscarriages; it has been linked to the occurrence of a rare form of cancer in women who have taken the drug and in their children. In addition, feminist health activists have pointed out the potential role of other factors, such as Depo-Provera (a long-term injectable contraceptive) environmental and occupational carcinogens, nutritional deficiencies and tampon use. Within the medical literature, however, the risk factor which receives the greatest attention is that of a woman's sexual behaviour.

This research focus has a long history. Contemporary medical literature often refers to a study conducted in 1842 by Rigoni-Stern, who compared the incidence of certain types of cancer between cloistered nuns and women in the general population. This study is said to have demonstrated the absence of cervical cancer among "virginal" women, and has given rise to the prevailing theory that the disease is caused by women's "promiscuity."

[*] Reprinted from *Healthsharing* vol. 13 no. 2 (Summer/Fall 1992): 24-26, with permission of the author.

A great deal of effort has been expended by modern medical researchers in the attempt to substantiate this misogynist theory. Innumerable studies have been published which link cervical cancer to a woman having more than one (hetero)sexual partner or having intercourse before the age of 20. Liz, a white, heterosexual woman in her thirties, recounts her experience of being unwittingly recruited for one such study:

> When I went in [to the clinic], I was asked to fill out a form. And one of the questions that really shocked me was how many men I had had sex with. And I thought — I mean, obviously this is a question that is going to be used to do a study. And I thought, how dirty! They get you in here to treat you for cancer and then use you for data. And I sat there trying to figure out who I'd slept with, and thinking, this is ridiculous and this is invasive! And so I just simply didn't answer that part, I just left it blank.

Rhoda, a white lesbian, reported being asked similar questions about her sexual behaviour by the health professionals treating her for severe cervical dysplasia, a condition believed to lead to cervical cancer: "I go in there, and they ask me, 'Okay, how often do you have intercourse?' 'Well, I don't.' 'When was the last time you had intercourse?' And I have to think, 'Oh, ten years ago — once.' [laughter] And they still don't get it, they don't even consider it."

Having collected their data on the number of male sexual partners and age of first intercourse of women with cervical dysplasia and cancer, medical researchers not only use this information to support their claim that cervical cancer is caused by women's "promiscuity," they also cite this data as evidence that cervical cancer is a sexually transmitted disease (STD).

Over the years, medical researchers have first proposed, then accepted, and later rejected, a succession of sexually transmitted disease organisms as the probable cause of cervical cancer. Early research centred on the "classical venereal diseases," gonorrhea and syphilis. When evidence for the causal role of these organisms waned, researchers were nonetheless reluctant to give up their theory that cervical cancer is a STD. Other STD organisms presented as possible candidates include trichomonas, mycoplasma, cytomegalovirus and chlamydia, all of which have been dismissed as unlikely causal agents.

In the late 1960s and early 1970s medical researchers argued that HSV-2, the genital herpes virus, was responsible for the disease. Indeed, many doctors accepted the evidence linking HSV-2 to cervical cancer as conclusive. However, in 1976, a new theory was presented which suggested that human papilloma virus (HPV), the virus which causes genital warts, was the cause of cervical cancer. This theory gained wide acceptance in the 1980s, supported by numerous clinical studies.

Sarah, a heterosexual, Jewish woman who has been diagnosed as a DES daughter, found her doctors more willing to assume that her abnormal cervical cells were related to HPV than to DES: "Another thing, too, that they told me initially, was that it was sexually related, and that it was papilloma. But there was no papilloma. So afterwards, I said, 'Is this related to DES?' 'Well, no. It's sexually related.' 'Are you sure?' 'No.' And there was no papilloma at all. So what is it?"

In fact, the HPV theory was so strongly supported in the medical literature that even some feminist critics accepted HPV as the cause of cervical cancer. For example, Toronto journalist Alison Dickie, in an article entitled "Scraping the Surface: Politics and the Pap Smear," which appeared in a 1989 edition of *This Magazine*, stated, "both dysplasia and cervical cancer are caused by a virus transmitted by men. For at least 10 years the human papilloma virus (HPV) has been targeted as the cause of dysplasia and, ultimately, cervical cancer."

Yet, recently, the evidence supporting this theory has been re-evaluated by some medical researchers. Muñoz and Bosch, in a 1989 WHO (World Health Organization) report, argued that the existing studies linking HPV to cervical cancer "were not planned as full epidemiological investigations and so none of them satisfies the usual criteria of design and analysis which would ensure the control of bias, confounding and chance in their interpretation." Clive Meanwell, a Swiss researcher, makes similar methodological objections to these studies, claiming the evidence is "severely limited."

Medical researchers remain undaunted, however, in their quest for a sexually transmitted cause of cervical cancer. As the HPV theory comes under critical scrutiny, new research now suggests a link between cervical cancer and Epstein-Barr virus (EBV). While EBV is not normally considered a sexually transmitted disease, at least one research team has argued that "the demonstration that EBV replicates in cervical epithelium raises the possibility of venereal transmission." Having run out of candidate STDs, medical researchers investigating the cause of cervical cancer seem content to classify any organism found in cervical tissue as sexually transmitted.

The medical community's stubborn obsession with "promiscuity" and STDs as the root causes of cervical cancer is not only fruitless, but also detrimental to women's health in a number of ways. In the first place, this misogynist model suggests that women bring this disease upon themselves by violating social norms of sexual conduct. The disease thus becomes a badge of shame.

For example, Paula, a white, bisexual woman in her early twenties, did not tell her family that she had had an abnormal Pap test, because, as she explains: "I had an idea in my head that this was something that was my fault, something I'd done wrong. It was something linked to sex, which in my family is really repressed. So, it wasn't something to tell my parents about."

Similarly, Fran, a 23-year-old, white, lesbian, who had been heterosexually active at one time, stated: "I have an incredible guilt complex, because I was really promiscuous when I was a teenager. And he [GP] said this [abnormal cervical cells] commonly happens ... in young women who have had a lot of intercourse, or whatever. So, I felt incredibly guilty, and I felt like, 'Oh yeah, that's it, this is my sins being paid for, right — I'm going to die, I'm going to die for it.'"

These feelings of shame and guilt, as well as the self-imposed isolation which may result, put unnecessary additional stresses on the health of women trying to cope with cervical dysplasia and cancer. Furthermore, the medical model implicitly supports repressive patriarchal restrictions on women's sexuality, presenting women's sexual autonomy as a health risk.

The most dangerous aspect of this medical model, however, is its narrow focus. Some medical researchers have even attempted to explain the higher rates of cervical cancer among working-class women, women who smoke and women who use the pill, by claiming that these groups of women are particularly "promiscuous."

While the medical community has spent literally the last century and a half trying to prove the theory that cervical cancer is an STD, risk factors such as environmental carcinogens and contraceptive drugs have not been adequately researched. For example, Jean Robinson, a British women's health activist, presented compelling evidence in 1981 that linked cervical cancer to carcinogens in the workplace of both women and their male sexual partners. Medical researchers, however, have chosen not to pursue this area of research.

Similarly, the Vancouver Women's Health Collective, in their pamphlet, "A Feminist Approach To Pap Tests" point out that "Cervical cancer is the most common cancer among women in the Third World. Depo-Provera may be a factor for this occurrence." Although the World Health Organization studies indicate that Depo-Provera may double the risk of cervical cancer, few other medical studies on the effect of this drug exist.

Clearly, medical researchers need to broaden their approach to the causation of cervical cancer to take into account the complex social and environmental influences on women's lives. The current model, which portrays women as predominantly sexual beings, and labels our behaviour with moral terms such as "promiscuity," is based on misogynist assumptions about women, our bodies and our sexuality. While sexual behaviour may be a factor in the development of cervical cancer, it must be investigated in a non-judgemental way, and other possible factors must be given equal consideration.

JAN DARBY is a graduate student at York University. She has also been active in the anti-rape movement.

# The Politics of Breast Cancer[*]

## Pam Bristol

The more we learn about it, the more we fear it. We look to the media and the medical community for information on how to prevent it, detect it and if need be to cope with breast cancer. But we do not get many answers; and the answers we do get are often vague or contradictory.

For the one in ten Canadian women who will get breast cancer during their lifetime, answers are crucial. Like women in the United States, more Canadian women with breast cancer are becoming activists. They are questioning the direction of current research and the effectiveness of detection and treatment, the adequacy of funding and education. "AIDS activists have shown that the rewards are much greater if we speak out," says Pat Kelly of the Burlington Breast Cancer Support Services in Burlington, Ontario.

The incidence of breast cancer has been steadily increasing, according to data that dates back to the 1950s. Despite medical advances, the number of deaths per year has not declined and in 1991 reached more than 5,000.

Kelly and other breast cancer survivors expressed their concerns to a House of Commons subcommittee on the status of women which is examining breast cancer issues. It is expected to table its recommendations in parliament in the spring of 1992. The subcommittee provided the impetus for some of these women to join together to form a national advocacy group.

Called Breast Cancer Action — Write Now, the organization intends to make governments and the public more aware of breast cancer issues in the same way AIDS activists have forced the AIDS crisis onto the public agenda. The group is encouraging women to write their Members of Parliament demanding more action on

[*] Reprinted from *Healthsharing* vol. 12 no. 4 (Winter/Spring 1992), with permission of the author.

breast cancer; it is asking the National Action Committee on the Status of Women (NAC) to act as an advocate; and it is working to ensure that the subcommittee's report is taken seriously in the House of Commons and not lost in a shuffle of paperwork.

"We want to give the message that speaking out is not an indication of maladjustment to diagnosis," Kelly says, "We're not just trying to embarrass medical professionals; our complaints are legitimate." "Compared to men with AIDS, we've been incredibly passive about breast cancer," says Sharon Batt. She and other women with breast cancer are forming an activist group in Montreal. "It has to be politicized," says Paula McPherson, one of the women in St. Catharines, Ontario who have set up the Breast Cancer Information and Education Services to provide information, support and advocacy. Both Batt and McPherson have established contact with American activist organizations to help develop their groups. "I remember walking out of the hospital at one point and saying 'it feels like I'm the only woman who has breast cancer,'" McPherson recalls. "It's a mystery, but it doesn't have to be this way."

These two groups, and the Halton Women's Self Health Project (see *Healthsharing* vol. 12 no. 2, Summer 1991), are some of the few grassroots activist organizations operating in Canada. However, there are numerous support groups across the country affiliated with the Canadian Cancer Society. As well, the Canadian Breast Cancer Foundation has grown in influence since its creation in 1986 and has raised $400,000 toward research so far. With a board membership that reads like a Who's Who of Toronto's elite, it is not exactly a grassroots organization. But the Foundation is working effectively to raise both money and awareness.

### Research

One of the key areas under debate is research. In the past few years the medical community has increased its study of breast cancer. One Canadian researcher counted 4,561 articles listed in the international medical index in 1989 alone. But many important facts still elude us.

Although it is true that lung cancer kills almost as many Canadian women as breast cancer, more than 80 percent of these deaths are readily preventable. Research clearly shows smoking is directly responsible for these deaths. Nothing tells us how to prevent breast cancer.

We know it is a systemic disease that can eventually spread through the body if left untreated. But we do not know why or how it spreads. We do not understand why some women remain cancer-free for the rest of their lives after surgery, while others suffer a recurrence within a few years. We know there are certain risk factors, such as a high-fat diet, late child-bearing and late menopause. But, except for a direct family history of breast cancer, none of these risk factors has been definitely proven to contribute to the disease. Even a direct family link only increases risk marginally. In fact, three-quarters of women with breast cancer have none of the risk factors.

Judith Rosner-Siegel, diagnosed with breast cancer four years ago and undergoing treatment, is a patients' rights advocate and a peer counselor with the Canadian Cancer Society. She is angered by attempts to provide simplistic answers, especially in the areas of prevention. "The only way to prevent it is to chop off your breasts when you're 16," she says. "And even that doesn't work because it's a systemic disease."

Women contacted for this article expressed concern about the under-funding of breast cancer research. According to the National Cancer Institute of Canada, which administers about 60 percent of the country's cancer research dollars, they have reason to be concerned. Executive director Dr. David Beatty says Canada spends only one quarter the amount per person that the U.S. allots to cancer research and this holds true for breast cancer in particular.

However, Pat Kelly maintains that breast cancer does not receive its fair share of cancer research dollars. The Canadian Cancer Society spent about $45 million on cancer research in Canada last year, Kelly says, and about $2.5 million of that on breast cancer research. "Breast cancer represents 15 percent of all cancers; yet it gets a smaller percentage of the research budget." (Less than 6 percent.)

Kelly also believes that certain members of the medical establishment have too much control over which research projects are funded. "The Canadian Cancer Society is largely run by women volunteers who have no say on how the research money is spent."

Those contacted also questioned the direction of existing research. "So many groups are doing their own thing without talking to each other," notes Roy Clark, a breast cancer specialist with Princess Margaret Hospital in Toronto. "There's too much duplication between them."

Two areas especially need research. Despite several studies on the connection between high-fat diets and breast cancer, no link has been definitely established. However, it is well known that the incidence of breast cancer is much lower in Japan and other countries with low-fat diets. And when Japanese women move to a country with high-fat diets, their incidence rises.

It may take years before research discovers a definite link, but Clark feels common sense dictates that we lower our fat intake not only to reduce the risk of breast cancer but of other diseases as well.

The other area of research which could lead to a major breakthrough is the discovery of genetic markers. If we could pinpoint what inherited characteristics make certain women vulnerable to breast cancer, we could detect it much sooner than current methods allow and perhaps even prevent it.

Another complaint about research is that doctors often ignore its findings. Varying mastectomy rates across the country are the most graphic example of this. Since 1981 there has been solid evidence that lumpectomies (or partial mastectomies as they are sometimes called) provide the same chances of survival as mastectomies in the majority of cases.

A team of researchers from Princess Margaret Hospital and the University of Toronto, which included Clark, pioneered lumpectomy in North America in the late 1950s. Thirty years later 60 percent of breast cancer surgery in North America is lumpectomy. But this percentage should ideally be up to 80 percent or 85 percent, he says. In certain parts of Canada, such as Vancouver, mastectomies still outnumber lumpectomies. The reason, according to Clark: "Doctors get hooked on doing a particular kind of surgery." On the other hand, Rosner-Siegel expresses concern that some women are led to believe that a mastectomy is never necessary, and this is not the case.

## Support
Hundreds of women who have or had breast cancer volunteer their time for peer counseling through Canadian Cancer Society

groups such as Reach for Recovery or CanSurmont. However, these groups are unable to reach many women.

Some hospitals don't allow the volunteers to set foot in their wards, says Rosner-Siegel, who works with the Reach for Recovery program. They have qualms about including "non-professionals" in the treatment process. Other hospitals allow peer counseling only for women with mastectomies and not lumpectomies, which doesn't make sense, she adds. Rarely are patients told they can receive counseling support before surgery — a time when they are often the most confused and in need of reassurance from someone who has gone through it already.

"During treatment, need number one is peer support," Rosner-Siegel emphasizes. Some hospitals organize self-help groups for women who are recovering from surgery and undergoing chemo or radiation therapy. These groups, though helpful, are also flawed. Often they are organized without patient input. They are inflexible so if a woman misses the starting date she is unable to join.

However, stronger support seems forthcoming. After Rosner-Siegel and other cancer patients made their views known to the Cancer 2000 taskforce (whose mandate was to establish strategies for cancer management by the year 2000). The taskforce recommended the creation of a national cancer patient coalition. This coalition, expected to be organized by 1993, hopes to provide a telephone network for cancer patients across the country. This service will especially benefit those who don't have access to support groups or peer counseling. These people will be able to pick up a phone and be directed to someone who has undergone a similar experience with cancer.

Because breast cancer can be a long-term disease, support is needed after hospitalization. Rosner-Siegel recalls an incident that illustrates this need. When her cancer recurred two years ago, she felt there was no hope. "I felt like jumping in front of a subway train," she says. But soon after, through her counseling work, she spoke with a woman who had suffered a similar recurrence 16 years ago and has had no further difficulties. It is this kind of personal experience sharing that can save someone from despair. The Toronto branch of the Canadian Cancer Society plans to start the first long-term support group for women with breast cancer in the spring. If it is successful, more will follow.

Although the Canadian Cancer Society provides needed support services, its mandate does not include political advocacy activities which could best be handled by groups directed solely by activist-survivors. "I think there should be groups across Canada which are survivor-directed," McPherson says. Such groups could push more aggressively to raise awareness.

### Early detection

Early detection is key. About 80 percent of women survive the five-year mark if their cancer is caught in the early stages. But early detection is relative. Most breast cancer is now detected by women themselves, usually about five years after the tumor first appeared. Mammograms are said to detect tumors about two years after they form. Obviously, a method of earlier detection is needed.

Despite the controversy surrounding it, mammography is now our only medical resource and has been proven effective in women 50 years or older. It's hard to reject something when there is nothing to take its place. But, unfortunately, many groups have polarized on the issue. Some call mammography a miracle of technology while others label it an ineffective smokescreen for the lack of progress in treating breast cancer.

There are problems with mammography. Most Canadians involved in the treatment of breast cancer believe the United States has created many of these problems by over-promoting mammography's use. University of Toronto professor of preventive medicine, Cornelia Baines, disagrees with the promotion of mammograms for women under 50 by both the American College of Radiology and the American Cancer Society (ACS). The ACS recommends a baseline mammogram between the ages of 35 and 40 and subsequent tests every one to two years between ages 40 to 50.

This recommendation contradicts evidence to date which shows no benefit from screening women under 50 in terms of reducing breast cancer mortality. Mammograms often do not detect irregularities in breast tissue of women under 50 because of the density of their breasts. However, they do help to diagnose breast cancer after irregularities have been detected through physician or self-examination. Could the self-interest of American mammography equipment manufacturers and radiologists who charge up to (U.S.) $250 per examination have anything to do with targeting women under 50?

In Canada, women under 50 are usually not screened unless circumstances, such as a family history of breast cancer, warrant it. But, influenced by American media, many Canadian women are asking for mammograms at relatively young ages. And some Canadian organizations, such as the B.C. Breast Screening Program, support the testing of women in their 40s.

On the other hand, women age 50 and up, who could benefit from regular mammograms, are often difficult to reach. Dr. Judith Weinroth is the medical coordinator for the Ontario Breast Screening Program. Under this program, centres have opened across Ontario to ensure that women age 50 and up have access to screening. She estimates that if these centres can reach 70 percent of their intended clients, they can provide the early detection needed to reduce mortality in that age group by 40 percent.

Screening programs have sprung up across the country. British Columbia started the first program two years ago. Alberta, Saskatchewan, Nova Scotia and Yukon are now offering similar programs, and others are planned in Quebec and Manitoba. However, these screening programs have to fight against fears of cancer and anxieties about mammography. "A lot of women are really afraid," notes Weinroth. "Intelligent women finally come in with huge lesions in their breasts. There's a lot of denial."

It is Shebina Amlani's job to alleviate these fears with education. In her role as health promotion officer for the Metro Toronto Breast Screening Centre, Amlani attempts to educate different ethnic communities within her region. She speaks to women's groups, multicultural groups and public health workers. She also writes articles for ethnic newspapers. The Metro Toronto Breast Screening Centre provides translators for several languages.

Holly Dee of the Southeast Asian Centre serves on an outreach committee Amlani formed for the screening centre. When Dee speaks to groups in the Asian community about breast cancer, she proceeds with caution. "Breast cancer is taboo to many in the Southeast Asian community." She aims her information sessions at the young, who she feels are easier to reach than older women. Because of the closeness of many Asian families, Dee anticipates that younger members of the family will inform their elders and encourage them to visit a screening centre.

Ontario's screening centres do not concentrate solely on mammography but embrace a more holistic approach. A nurse examiner checks a client's breasts and then spends at least 20 minutes demonstrating the techniques of Breast Self-Examination (BSE). Other provincial screening centres teach BSE to varying degrees.

Unfortunately, women rarely receive comprehensive instruction on BSE. Where would they learn it? BSE is not taught in schools and many doctors either do not know proper BSE techniques or do not take the time to inform women. Yet monthly BSE is the best means of detecting breast cancer in women under 50 and is also necessary for women over 50.

Activist groups can play an important role in this regard. The Halton Women's Self Health Project teaches BSE to any group which requests its services. Paula McPherson's group in St. Catharines plans to work with teachers to introduce BSE instruction in high schools.

No woman, regardless of age, should rely exclusively on mammograms for two reasons. First, mammograms are estimated to be only 85 percent effective in detecting irregularities in women over 50. Second, the quality of mammography equipment and the qualifications of its operators vary. A woman has every right to check on the qualifications of both.

## Fighting Misconceptions

While women need information on breast cancer, we do not need the misconceptions that sometimes come with it. Rosner-Siegel is concerned about polarized views of the disease. The media often focus on either success stories or tragedies. The survival rate of 85 percent for breast cancer caught in its early stages is often quoted. But in reality survival rates are much lower.

As well, the fact that a women's life is permanently altered is not always made clear. Instead, we're often presented with "smiling celebrity" profiles of famous women who seem to be completely recovered. "We're talking about a chronic disease," Rosner-Siegel points out. "You're constantly monitored and facing the fear of it coming back."

Other aspects of the media's and society's treatment of breast cancer can be questioned. For instance, why are most articles about breast cancer accompanied by a picture of a young woman's breasts when the majority of women who get the disease are over 50?

Clearly, after years of neglect regarding women and breast cancer, we have achieved recognition of its seriousness. The next step is recognition of the need for more research funding and more support for women who are diagnosed with breast cancer.

**PAM BRISTOL** is the editor of a national food magazine and has volunteered with Women Healthsharing for several years.

# Candidiasis

## Beginning to Understand a New Disease Complex[*]

### Mary Louise Adams

I had extraordinary fatigue. I'd sleep for 10 hours, get up for two, then sleep for four. Getting up to go to the bathroom or make a pot of tea would exhaust me. Climbing stairs was a monumental task. I was very, very pale and I had headaches so bad that I just had to put my head down. I was also constipated and bloated and had terrible gas .... I went to a doctor and asked for tests ... for mono — and he said, 'There's nothing wrong with you, you don't need these tests. It's just a cold. Go home and rest.' I went back later and another doctor at the clinic told me the same thing, 'It's just a virus, everybody's getting it. Go home and sleep.' A week later I still felt awful. After talking to a friend, I went back and asked to be checked for parasites.

Candida albicans, a common yeast organism, known to cause vaginitis in women and thrush in infants, is challenging the traditional western approach to illness, an approach typified by the equation: cause "x" leads to "y" symptoms, which can be cured by "z" treatment. Candida is threatening assumptions that have allowed doctors to see their patients as little more than complex machines. In the past few years, as knowledge and understanding of Candida albicans has grown, and as it has been implicated in an ever-broader spectrum of illnesses, some people are beginning to question the simple cause/effect equation.

Chris Donnelly (not her real name) was lucky. It only took her three months of visiting a naturopath, a chiropractor and several doctors to find out that her increasingly deteriorating health was a result of Candida albicans. Some people search for years before

[*]  Reprinted from *Healthsharing* vol. 6 no. 3 (Summer 1985): 9-12, with permission of the author.

being diagnosed. Still others are never fortunate enough to receive the validation that comes with diagnosis.

Reluctantly, the doctor tested Chris, found that in fact she did have parasites and prescribed a drug for her. For two days she felt better, but then she became worse and it seemed the drug was making her sicker.

"I was trying to collect unemployment insurance at the time because I was too sick to work. UIC referred me to a new doctor." Dr. Kathleen Kerr analysed Chris's hair, urine and blood, did a comprehensive computer analysis of her diet and took a thorough health history. The results suggested that in addition to the parasites, Chris was suffering from an overgrowth of Candida. A past history of antibiotic use was the most important clue.

It is estimated that 30 percent of the population is susceptible to severe Candida infections. Women are affected more often than men. According to Dr. Orian Truss, one of the pioneers of Candida research, yeast proliferation can result in health problems as diverse as arthritis, premenstrual syndrome (PMS), depression, multiple sclerosis, migraines and schizophrenia.

Candida exists peacefully in the bodies of 97 percent of the population, entering infants during or shortly after birth. Its favoured locales are the mucous membranes and the gastrointestinal and genitourinary tracts. When our immune system is strong and when we have a healthy population of yeast-controlling bacteria, Candida is kept in check. But certain factors can combine to increase its growth. Those factors most often cited play a frequent, if not constant, part in many of our lives: antibiotics, birth control pills and diets high in carbohydrates — Candida's favourite food. Other factors include immunosuppressant drugs, i. e. cortisone, exposure to occupational and environmental chemicals, and various kinds of hormonal changes.

William Crook, author of *The Yeast Connection*, a layperson's book about Candida, lists a number of reasons why women are more susceptible to yeast-related illnesses:

- the hormonal changes associated with the menstrual cycle (and with adolescence) encourage yeast colonization
- the birth control pill encourages Candida growth
- teenage girls are often prescribed antibiotics (especially tetracycline) as part of long-term acne treatment

- the vagina, because it is warm and dark, is an excellent environment for Candida
- women are the main target of antibiotics because we tend to have more vaginal and urinary tract infections
- the hormonal changes associated with pregnancy encourage Candida.

Normally, bacteria in the digestive tract keep Candida under control. When those bacteria are reduced in number (or wiped out) by exposure to antibiotics, for example, the balance between them and the yeast is gone, leaving room for Candida to grow. Colonizing in the mucous membranes, it changes shape from a single cell into a form more like a filament, which encourages increased colonization. It becomes rooted in the membranes, sending out long filaments which perforate the membranes, allowing toxic byproducts to enter the bloodstream and travel to other parts of the body. Thus abnormal function in a tissue is not because of the yeast itself, but because of its various byproducts or toxins, 79 in total, which may enter the blood.

When the conditions which allow the initial yeast overgrowth continue, for example prolonged use of birth control pills, the immune system becomes so overwhelmed by accumulating toxins or antigens that it loses its ability to fight. It starts to tolerate the antigen. Such immune tolerance can leave you susceptible to disease and can increase your susceptibility to continuing yeast infections.

People working in polluted environments are continually exposed to toxins. Their immune systems become overburdened and begin to tolerate harmful substances. Furthermore a poorly functioning immune system makes one especially likely to be infected by Candida, which in turn acts to keep the immune system suppressed.

According to Chris' doctor, Kathleen Kerr, an understanding of how Candida works is relatively new. Five years ago, someone with a yeast-related illness would have been hard pressed to find anyone knowledgeable about its treatment. Although the situation has improved somewhat, Candida remains relatively unknown in the medical community, except as an occasional nuisance — the cause of vaginitis and diaper rash.

Candida does not fit easily into the traditional framework of medicine. Able to manifest itself in so many different ways, it is extraordinarily difficult to test for (although an American doctor is developing a blood test). Establishing its presence, which is possible, means nothing, since Candida lives in 97 percent of the population. A true diagnosis of a Candida infection is arrived at only after prescribing the appropriate treatment and observing the results in hopes of finding a reduction of symptoms. It is a somewhat uncertain course of events, one that sometimes takes months to show progress, a fact which hardly endears it to the proponents of both "quick-fix" healing and the "physician as god" mentality.

Given the serious depression and anxiety that are often a result of Candidiasis, people who suffer from it are often labelled as hypochondriacs, their ailments explained as psychosomatic. Few doctors have the humility to confess ignorance — if the physician can't name it, you're not sick. How many people have been referred to psychiatric care and all the dangerous drugs it involves because of an undiagnosed yeast infection?

Maggie Burston has had chronic Candidiasis for the last 20 years. A bladder infection led to prolonged use of antibiotics which set the stage for a buildup of yeast. The yeast weakened her immune system causing, among other things, a bladder infection. Maggie became locked in an unceasing cycle. Over the years her condition worsened. The bladder infection has never cleared. Maggie's immune system was weakened and she developed allergic reactions to almost everything — the drugs she was taking, plastic, tobacco smoke, paper, perfumes, petrochemical fumes and most foods. In the media her condition is commonly referred to as "twentieth century disease" or "ecological illness."

Searching for a diagnosis Maggie went from doctor to doctor. She was told repeatedly that there was nothing wrong with her.

> One specialist in infectious diseases said that, after all what on earth was I, a woman of my age, making a fuss about. I was over the hill and these symptoms were quite usual for 30 percent of the women that he knew my age, and why didn't I go home and learn to live with the symptoms."

One allergist told her not even to try and understand her illness: "You'll never be able to know, its far too complicated."

In spite of the fact that all Maggie's vital signs were normal, she was in constant pain and could hardly eat. But doctors, preferring to speak to her husband, insisted she was healthy. Maggie was isolated with the conflicting advice she received from different physicians — one rejecting with scorn the opinion of another.

Eventually a doctor in Ottawa put Maggie on the right track, telling her about Candida. It was an opinion Maggie's Toronto doctors refused to consider. So she herself researched the illness. At one point when she was too ill to read, a doctor friend gave her the tapes from a conference. From these she found out that the people who could be of most help to her were in San Francisco. Several months later she went to see them.

Maggie was so immune-threatened they prescribed a treatment called "transfer factor," injections of white blood products from the immune systems of healthy people. She was told she would need the treatment every two weeks indefinitely. But Maggie, for financial reasons, was unable to stay in California and returned to Toronto where the blood products are unavailable.

> My life may depend on those treatments. What are my rights as
> a citizen of this province? At the very least there should be some
> sort of investigation into both the condition and the treatment.

Maggie continues to search for a doctor who will petition on her behalf to import the blood products to Canada.

According to Devaki Berkson, a California chiropractor who works with people who have Candidiasis, traditional medicine, based as it is on men's bodies, tends to ignore the fact that women's hormonal fluctuations make our bodies somewhat more complicated. With more fluctuations, there is a greater chance of something going wrong. Fluctuating estrogen levels are linked to an overgrowth of yeast. We deal with toxins entering our bodies from outside differently if our hormones are out of balance. For example, women who are on the pill have increased amounts of estrogen in their bodies and some develop migraines and allergies. People not on the pill are exposed to estrogen in animal products. Certain foods in our diet — sugar, caffeine and meat — are known to increase our bodies' own production of estrogen, producing yeast-favourable conditions.

Candida itself interferes with hormone functions, thus helping to establish circumstances under which it can flourish. Although the hormones are produced as usual, body tissues do not respond properly to them. It's a situation that can lead to acne, rough, dry skin, menstrual problems, decreased fullness in the breasts, loss of sensitivity in the nipples, decreased libido, increasingly severe PMS, chronic vaginitis, irritability and depression, and sometimes endometriosis, infertility and miscarriage.

Hormonal changes are responsible for a pregnant woman's susceptibility to yeast overgrowth especially if she has a history of taking the pill. If a woman gets Candidiasis while she's pregnant, there are 79 different toxins/antigens which can cross the placenta. Her child could develop tolerance to the yeast before she or he is even born. After birth, yeast enters the baby's body; a single round of antibiotics could stimulate yeast growth.

Women become depressed for a variety of reasons in this society which fails to validate experiences not conforming to a heterosexual, white, middle class norm. Our complaints are often written off as "female hysteria" and treated with, at the least, mood-altering drugs. Depressed women are said to be maladjusted, attention-seekers. In light of this, Truss' findings with regard to Candida and psychological and emotional problems are worth noting. He tells of case after case of depressed and anxiety-ridden women who have responded positively to anti-Candida treatment. According to him, their emotional and psychological states are indicative of allergies affecting their brains, the result of interference with chemical and physiological reactions responsible for the expression of emotion. The interference in many cases is caused by Candida. Similarly he suggests that some cases of anorexia may be yeast-related.

The importance of discovering the "yeast connection" (as William Crook calls it) to such a variety of health problems lies in the potential for them to be treated. Chris now eats a yeast and mold free diet that is extremely low in carbohydrates and high in proteins. She takes nilstat (also known as nystatin), a yeast suppressing drug, and nutritional supplements to strengthen her immune system. As her immune system becomes stronger she will add foods to her diet, one at a time, to see if her body will accept them. She'll probably be on a severely restricted diet for at least a year, but her eating habits have changed for life. "No more living on yoghurt, salad and fruit, with toast and jam for break-fast. That's almost all sugar. I know now what I need to survive."

To maintain her health Chris is making a commitment of time, energy and money. She must prepare all her food from scratch and has to be careful to rotate the foods in her diet. "I had to buy a whole set of baking utensils along with the special foods. My supplements alone cost $150 a month." For many women the financial demands of this treatment would be too great.

Maggie Burston is still too sensitive to eat a great many foods. Even the smell of cooking can make her ill. She has a housekeeper who cooks for her in the recreation room of their apartment building. What happens to people without such resources?

How can we best reduce our vulnerability to Candida? Dr. Kathleen Kerr says the best thing to do — and perhaps the hardest for many people — is to regulate our diets. Restrict the carbohy-drates in your diet — especially sugar. Avoid yeast-promoting foods like cakes, cookies and breads, fruit juices, dried fruits, dried herbs and teas, chocolate, pickled and smoked foods. When possible avoid antibiotic drugs. If you must take them, there are some which are less yeast-promoting than others. Also be sure to supplement them with yoghurt to maintain the level of healthy, yeast controlling bacteria in your body. Don't take the pill. Try to reduce your exposure to chemicals which threaten the immune system. Work for better environmental and occupational health standards in your community and at work. Try to reduce the amount of stress you endure because it too can weaken your immune system.

Dr. Alen Levin, a specialist in immunology, allergy and envi-ronmental medicine, participated in a segment of CBC Radio's *Ideas* program devoted to ecological illness. He suggests that the average human alive right now has a body that is genetically different from the average human body of 1964. We are now seeing the first and second generations of people "who previously wouldn't have survived without sophisticated antibiotics and hospitalization and insulin and surgery, and things like that." We are also living in a time when the use of prescription drugs is remarkably high. Patterns of disease are changing. Jet travel means bacteria, viruses and parasites are now found in places where they were previously unknown. Environmental chemicals have given us a whole new list of ailments. Our bodies have been able to adapt to many of these changes. Someone with ecological illness has reached their limit.

The question now is whether traditional medicine can adapt, can assimilate this new understanding of disease. As Kathleen Kerr says, in spite of Orian Truss' success and supporting evidence from other physicians, she has yet to see any mention of yeast-related illness in a journal like *The New England Journal of Medicine,* the big-time of medical publishing. If, as Truss has said, yeast may be responsible for health problems as varied as schizophrenia, multiple sclerosis, and PMS, the ramifications of his findings are tremendous. They offer some hope to people suffering from previously "incurable" ailments. He admits how difficult it is to accept the view that so many remarkably different illnesses could be caused by a single agent.

In adding yeast-related illnesses to the body of medical knowledge, physicians will be forced to treat their patients as whole persons, not merely as the amalgamation of various joints and organs. They will be forced to listen to and to take into account their patients' views of their various symptoms, even those as intangible as depression or anxiety. In short they will be forced to take their patients seriously, to acknowledge them as the experts they are about their own bodies. It's a goal the feminist health movement has been working towards for years.

### Further Reading
Crook, Dr. William G. *The Yeast Connection.* Jackson, TN: Future Health.
Truss, C. Orion."The Role of Candida Albicans in Human Illness"
 *Orthomolecular Psychiatry* vol. 10 no. 4 (1981): 228-38.

**MARY LOUISE ADAMS** lives in Toronto and works for *Herizons* and *Resources for Feminist Research.*

# Winning the Battle
## Living with Epstein-Barr Virus[*]

### Lorie Rotenberg

No longer is the sky the limit nor the world my oyster. Through my experience with chronic Epstein-Barr virus syndrome (CEBV), I have come to learn the meaning of living with limitation. Although I have always been an introspective person, this illness has challenged me to look even deeper within myself to discover how to hear the messages of my body. I am much better now, which tells me that I have gained some understanding of the significance of the Epstein-Barr virus in my life.

### Links with my Father

On March 30, 1987, I received the diagnosis of Epstein-Barr virus from my physician. I was 37 years old at the time. On March 30, 1955, my father died of chronic nephritis (irreversible kidney malfunction) when he was only 37 years old. This striking coincidence seems an appropriate departure point for my journey into self-knowledge.

My father coped with terminal illness by living each day as if he believed he had many years yet to enjoy. This stance enabled him to survive 13 years after his fateful diagnosis was pronounced. Up until a few months before his death, he functioned normally to all outward appearances, with only two limitations: he had to adhere to a strict diet and avoid stress.

What does my father's illness have to do with me? When I was at my lowest point with Epstein-Barr virus, I often flashed on a mental picture of my father lying listlessly in his bed, overcome with fatigue. I sensed a commonality between his experience and the crisis I was grappling with. I feared that, like him, I too would be unable to live my life to its fullest. At that time I did not know

* Reprinted from *Healthsharing* vol. 10 no. 2 (Spring 1989): 20-25, with permission of the author.

that chronic fatigue, the key symptom of CEBV, is, indeed, not a symptom of nephritis. Nor was I aware that my father had actually only retired to his bed during the month prior to his death. The memory still so fresh in my mind is the five-year-old child's last image of her father as a sick parent devoid of energy. When I shared this memory with the counselor whom I was seeing for CEBV-related depression, she urged me to disassociate myself from it. Since my father was wearing pyjamas while at home sick, she suggested that I wear my street clothes during those days when I was too weak to get out of bed. His illness was not mine.

Ever since my father's death, I have equated illness with something very grave, portending disastrous consequences. One of my unconsciously held assumptions has been that each time I get sick, I risk never recovering. Flowing from this unacknowledged belief has been my tendency, when first becoming ill, to avoid hearing my body's message that I need to slow down and take time off work. In the past I never went to bed unless I was literally on the verge of collapse — unless my body forced me to. Witness my behaviour in the few weeks leading up to my diagnosis of pleurisy in November 1979. When I finally did get to my doctor's office, she expressed astonishment that I had not reported my symptoms sooner. It was as if I needed her to give me permission to take to my sick bed.

My denial of any illness which has not reached serious proportions, has meant, in fact, that I have failed to hear my body's warning signals and thus been unable to nip minor ailments in the bud. My own actions have made my illnesses more alarming than necessary.

Although I have known for years that I have difficulty ministering to myself at the first signs of sickness, I have not understood until now how this behaviour is linked to my childhood experience of my father's illness. To acknowledge illness in myself is to acknowledge the possibility of death. This insight feels both painfully obvious and also quite liberating. The challenge facing me is to come to grips with my fear of mortality.

## Coming Out with CEBV
Initially my way of dealing (or not dealing) with the Epstein-Barr virus was similar to the approach adopted by my father towards his disease. Like my father, I sought out alternative healing,

although in my case it has been through a naturopath. (I believe the homeopathic remedies which I have taken are, in part, responsible for my improved condition.) Other than homeopathy, my main coping strategy for many months entailed bargaining with the virus through denial. It was as if I were saying to the virus, "If I act like you're not really there and don't give you any attention, then you'll have to go away." I did not want most people to know that I had CEBV. It was a secret only to be disclosed to a chosen few. But even the chosen few, my close friends and family, were spared most of the details. I tended to constantly minimize the level of fatigue I was experiencing, thereby continuing to push myself. I seemed unable or unwilling to accept limitation as an ongoing and integral part of my life.

As was true for my father, most of the time I show little, if any, physical evidence of being afflicted with a disease. None of my most pronounced symptoms, which have included deep and pervasive fatigue (only detectable in my face and eyes by the experienced observer), tingling sensations and occasional numbness in my arms and legs, depression, low-grade fever, enlarged lymph nodes and problems with sleep, is immediately visible. Since what is exposed to others does not accurately reflect the inner reality, 1 have to constantly make a choice about whether, and to what degree, I wish to be known. Somehow this issue of being known seems central to my experience of this illness. Always the question presents itself: "Do I wish to pretend I am 'normal' or to acknowledge in an open way that I live with Epstein-Barr virus?" For the first five months following my diagnosis I honed my ability to 'pass' for 'normal,' although on a conscious level I did not understand nor would I have described my actions that way.

In September 1987 I read two articles which profoundly affected my interaction with my illness. Through the insights stimulated by these readings I have been able to transform my understanding of my self in illness and thus, over time, transform my experience of illness. "Learning to Live with It," an article by Ray Jobling, presents a detailed account of the author's life with chronic psoriasis. Jobling's description of his "passing," "impression management" and finally his "coming out" as a chronically ill person helped me to recognize my own cover-up mechanisms.

Shortly after reading Jobling I came across an article in *Health-sharing* by Betty-Ann Lloyd entitled "No Longer Silently Disabled" which helped me build on my new learning. Lloyd suffers from multiple sclerosis, but most of the time her disability is not evident. She speaks eloquently of her struggle to accept her difference, to "come out" as a disabled person and to raise consciousness of disability issues within the feminist community in Halifax. She tells of the embarrassment she feels about her actual or potential dependency. For her, "coming out" as a lesbian is usually less difficult than "coming out" as a disabled person.

Her experience resonated with my own. I realized that I was just as afraid of revealing my illness status to people as I am cautious about sharing information about my sexual orientation. Partly it is because of the intimacy and vulnerability which both forms of "coming out" entail. I came to understand how, each time I hid the fact that I have Epstein-Barr virus, I had been disconnecting from a significant part of my being. And I already knew from spending ten years denying my love for women, what psychic damage such repression can cause. I was dumbfounded to discover that I had been expending large amounts of energy in "stage managing" my illness, striving very hard to be accepted as an able-bodied person. But, of course, this often meant that I did not get the support and empathy I felt I needed from my intimates.

By the time I had finished Lloyd's article, I had made an important decision. My days of "passing" in terms of denying illness were over. No longer would I hide my exhaustion or my fear. I would try to redirect the energy formerly drained off into secrecy towards self-healing. If I believed it was psychologically and politically important for me to "come out" as a lesbian, then certainly the same held true for me as an Epstein-Barr virus sufferer. I began to accept the powerful need I have to be known and appreciated just as I am. This virus, like my lesbianism which is also invisible, demands that I reclaim my self not only in the private arena, but in the public arena as well — that I state explicitly who I am and how I am feeling at any moment in time.

As a result of my new understanding, I began to really let others into my world of illness, a world which had previously been barred to all except my partner. I felt a tremendous sense of relief at no longer having to carry the burden of secrecy. I began to arrange social commitments with the stated agreement that, depending on the severity of my symptoms, I might have to reschedule. My loved ones have certainly offered more support than they possibly could have when I was still "passing."

However, there has been some disappointment as well. In some ways I have found the reaction to "coming out" as an Epstein-Barr sufferer similar to "coming out" as a lesbian. Most of my intimates do not regularly ask me how the virus is behaving. I talk much more than I used to about what it means to live with chronic illness, to wake up most mornings feeling absolutely exhausted no matter how much sleep I have had, to know that, as yet, there is no cure for Epstein-Barr virus and that indeed I may have to live the rest of my life with some degree of limitation. They listen, with interest and concern. But, for the most part, they do not take the initiative in discussing illness with me. Before, I was unknown and invisible. Now, I am known, but in some ways, even more invisible.

It is fear, I think, that prevents them. Fear of acknowledging their fear that they might lose me or that they might develop a chronic illness themselves. Here the parallels with the reactions of heterosexuals to my "coming out" as a lesbian are unmistakeably clear. Perhaps it is also discomfort and a sense of impotence that prevents them from talking to me about the virus. My wanting to be fully known and appreciated does not mean that others desire to fully know and appreciate me.

## Symptoms of Femininity

Throughout the decade in which I repressed my love for women, I often felt unwell. I knew at some level, that I was sacrificing an important part of my personhood. However, I did not realize that this would also lead to repressing my Jewish identity, my feminism and my socialism. During this period, I experienced an array of "symptoms of femininity" (to use the phraseology of Miriam Greenspan in her book *A New Approach to Women and Therapy*), ranging from depression and chronic fatigue to claustrophobia and so-called psychosomatic pain (headaches, dizziness, nausea and low-grade fever). After reading Greenspan I began to reinterpret this lengthy period of ill-health, to see for the first time that most of the symptoms which finally drove me to psychotherapy in 1980 were, in reality, passive forms of female resistance to the culturally defined standard of femininity. My body was trying to tell me how unhappy it was to have to hide its sexual passion.

Regrettably, by that point I was so out of touch with my feelings that I was unable to pick up most bodily signals. In order to suppress my deep love for women, I had to suppress other heartfelt sentiments as well. I became emotionally controlled and distant. I threw myself into the world of work and achievement. My workaholism was fuelled by displaced passion. The real dilemma facing me as I took my first step into the world of therapy was whether I was going to accept the traditional female role with its concomitant heterosexuality

## Letting Go
In May 1987 I embarked on a sabbatical leave from my job as a senior trade union representative. This came none too soon after seven years of intense, emotionally demanding, energy-draining work in an environment where I did not feel that I could be all of myself. My lesbianism was hidden from all but a few of my closest colleagues and my feminism and socialism were often muted to avoid potential conflict. The masculinist world of paid work, with its emphasis on hierarchy, competition and goal orientation at the expense of process and relationship, did not allow for the expression of my "womanly" values. I realized that like my foremothers, Charlotte Perkins Gilman and Jane Addams, who had taken to their sick beds as misfits, I too was unable to make myself fit without incurring psychic injury.

That summer I spent three glorious months camping and hiking with my partner. I was able to slow down and get in touch with the part of me that feels deeply connected to nature. On returning home, I began to seriously contemplate my future working life. It seemed clear that I had but one option — to seek to create a new work situation which would not demand participation on masculinist terms. Eventually I did choose to make a radical career switch involving a return to university. It was while I was struggling with my decision about whether or not to leave my job and the labour movement that I first noted and reported to my naturopath the symptom of overwhelming tiredness.

I remember vividly my complete astonishment and bewilderment at finding myself ill while on sabbatical leave. Hadn't I been doing all the right things to change my life so it was not longer based on self-denial? After "coming out" as a lesbian and entering a committed love relationship, I had moderated my pace of living and working, becoming more rounded by developing new interests and friends, and even begun to let my vulnerability show on occasion. I had started to see a naturopath and, through hiking and swimming, finally felt physically fit. I had begun to work with a feminist counselor who was teaching me how to value myself. Just prior to the onset of the Epstein-Barr virus, I was someone who had never felt better in her life.

I have come to see that the timing of this virus' arrival in my life is an expression of my letting go after many years of having girded myself. It was only when I was away from my work-place environment, when I was no longer looking over my shoulder all the time to see if someone would discover Lorie the lesbian, that my body could finally succumb to the adrenal exhaustion it was experiencing. At a very basic level, my decision to change career paths has meant that I have been able to relax for the first time in my adult life. This has felt incredibly liberating and exciting. At last my body could yield to its own needs. And insist on making these needs known and felt by the emotional and intellectual components of my self.

## Listening to My Body

I am convinced that if I had not developed Epstein-Barr virus, I would have approached graduate school in exactly the same way I did undergraduate study and my work in the labour movement — that is obsessively and with definite workaholic tendencies. Somehow I think my body knew that just taking 10 months off work would not, in and of itself, ensure that I would seriously address my drive to perfectionism. Without illness, the most likely scenario is that I would have had a good rest and returned to work or school with renewed energy but no fundamental change in my pattern of living and, especially, of working. My body had to find some way to impress upon me the gravity of the situation. In that it certainly succeeded.

I now understand the virus as a self-regulating mechanism which ensures that I avoid overextending myself. When I was first exposed to the idea of illness as a metaphor, my instinctual reaction was to start humming the opening of Paul Simon's tune, *The 59th Street Brigade Song (Feelin' Groovy)*: "Slow down, you move too fast. You got to make the morning last." Through the language of illness comes a message from a deeper part of myself.

It is an entreaty to get out of the fast lane, to give up my need to achieve and control, to appreciate life in the present moment, to take time to savour life's gifts.

Epstein-Barr virus has, indeed, forced me to slow down the pace of my life. I found that if I did not get enough sleep or if I had too many social commitments, then my fatigue and general feelings of unwellness increased. Instead of becoming anxious, I listened to my body, pulled on the reins and reduced the tensions in my life. In this way I believe the virus allows the self to disengage from pressure so that it can withdraw and retreat to regain its strength.

Similarly, the virus has confronted my drive to perfectionism which I believe is intimately linked to my tendency towards overextension. I am still in the process of trying to discover the wellsprings of my psychic struggle for self-perfection so that I can change this unsatisfying way of functioning. Again, reading Miriam Greenspan gave me some valuable insights. She views perfectionism as an attempt by the victim of social oppression to gain what appears to be some degree of internal control in a world where external control is denied her. It is a strategy employed by those who are devalued by society. They try to obtain the approval of others through their accomplishments and by striving to be perfect in all that they do. But, since this method of gaining control involves an attempt to measure up to standards which are most often defined by the oppressor, it is, at root, externally based. So, in the end, compulsive perfectionism robs the oppressed of any remaining vestiges of self-acceptance or self-worth. It can also, as in my case, hurt the body and make one's life unbalanced by overemphasizing work at the expense of everything else.

As a woman, a Jew and a lesbian, I am an outsider in my own society. I have been, and continue to be, subjected to sexism, antisemitism, heterosexism and homophobia. To some extent I have internalized the negative messages this society propagates about people like me. However, I have come to learn that I will only feel like a misfit if I allow others to define me in that way. Since "coming out" as a lesbian and getting back in touch with my Judaism, my feminism and my socialism, I have begun to reclaim the locus of control of my self-worth so that more and more I find it residing within me. Through insisting on living my life as the person I am and through engaging in political action aimed at changing the discriminatory conditions under which I am forced to live, I am beginning to acquire a measure of control that is far healthier physically and psychically than my old "friend" perfectionism.

My difficulty in valuing myself may offer a clue to a deeper insight. The virus allows me to disengage from the prescribed female role of nurturing and taking care of others so that I can turn my attention inward. Perhaps there is another lesson here: the need to develop the capacity for self-nurturing and to accept nurturing from others. The virus provides an opportunity to learn how to use the energy I do have to take care of myself in a loving and appreciative manner. And it challenges me to ask for support from others when it is necessary.

## CHRONIC FATIGUE SYNDROME

Chronic fatigue syndrome is also known as post-viral neuromyasthenia or chronic Epstein-Barr-virus syndrome (CEBV). Although the cause is not exactly known, there may be a connection with a virus (possibly the Epstein-Barr virus) plus some other attack on the immune system.

Epstein-Barr is a member of the herpes family of viruses which include herpes simplex, chicken pox and human B lymphotrophic virus (HBLV). What these viruses have in common is that they infect B-lymphocytes and are with us for life. After their initial attack they remain dormant in our bodies and may erupt at any time under conditions of stress or immune system upset. The Epstein-Barr virus is everywhere, and is thought to be present in 90 percent of the world's population. The initial attack may come in childhood when it is very mild, or in adolescence when it causes infectious mononucleosis or "kissing disease."

Many patients with chronic fatigue syndrome have elevated levels of antibodies against the Epstein-Barr virus which led researchers to think the virus was the cause of the syndrome. However, the number of patients who have normal antibody levels has led to the controversy about whether the Epstein-Barr virus is the only cause. At present there is speculation about other co-factors including a depressed immune system or another virus being involved.

— Women Healthsharing

## Internal Harmony

My learning from living with chronic Epstein-Barr virus has led to dramatic changes in my relationship with my body. For most of my life I have subscribed to two common causal explanations of illness. First, I have conceptualized and experienced my body as an object, viewing illness as comparable to machine breakdown. My physician describes how I used to arrive for my appointments demanding that she fix the "problem" immediately so that I could continue to function without interruption. I saw my body as something divorced from the "real me" which prevented me from doing what I wanted. I did not trust it and refused to give its signals anywhere near the weight I allotted to those that emanated from the other parts of myself. I did little to maintain my own body in good shape nor would I allow it to experience much sexual passion. Secondly, since I saw illness as a punishment for failure to take care of my body, whenever I got sick, I would resort to moralistic self-blame, assuming that I had either failed to do something or done something wrong.

Shortly after being diagnosed with Epstein-Barr virus, I watched a television programme featuring Dr. Carl Simonton, the renowned cancer specialist. His discussion of the benefits of imagery and visualization as self-healing techniques for cancer patients inspired me. I realized that I had been fighting my body, seeing it as an enemy, rather than cooperating with it in its struggle to strengthen my immune system. I began to visualize my white blood cells as an army of Amazon warriors with thousands of spray cans full of antibodies designed especially to kill the Epstein-Barr virus. Visualization did not come easily to me. What worked best for me were brief flashes on the battle scene 20 times a day.

Too often in the early days virus-induced depression would overwhelm me and I would lapse into feeling wounded and sorry for myself. My attempts to normalize myself through "passing" only intensified my sense of isolation and despair. As I have gradually learned to hear and honour my body's messages I have begun to experience myself as less driven and more at peace with my body and, hence, my self. My body no longer appears to my emotional, intellectual and spiritual selves as the great controller. Internal harmony among my selves is becoming a reality.

On some very fundamental level, I see my prolonged involvement with illness as mirroring my struggle for authenticity. If I can reject external definitions of myself, and instead accept who I am and act on my need to be known as I am, then I believe full health will be mine again. This journey inward has increased my desire to savour the joys of the present, whatever my physical limitations, and given me courage to face the future.

## Notes
A longer version of this article was first written in December 1987 for a course taught by Ron Silvers at the Ontario Institute for Studies in Education.

## Further Reading

Jobling, R. "Learning to Live With It." In *Medical Encounters: The Experience of Illness and Treatment*, edited by A. Davis and G. Horobin. London: Croom Helm, 1977.

Lloyd, B. "No Longer Silently Disabled." *Healthsharing* no. 8 vol. 4 (Fall 1987): 26-28.

Greenspan, M. *A New Approach to Women and Therapy*. New York: McGraw-Hill, 1983.

Simonton, O.C., S. Matthews-Simonton and J.L. Creighton. *Getting Well Again*. New York: Bantam Books, 1970.

**LORIE ROTENBERG** is very much alive and well and living in Toronto. She will soon be starting work as a feminist therapist.

# Testing Positive [*]

## Darien Taylor

AIDS is a woman's issue. Gone are the days when we believed that we lived safely on the outside of this epidemic. We grieve and mourn the loss of friends and family members. We offer support and care. We educate and counsel. AIDS forces us to re-evaluate basic patterns in our lives, particularly how we express ourselves sexually. And increasingly, women are testing positive for exposure to the AIDS virus.

Who are these women and what is our experience of living with HIV, the human immune-deficiency virus which may lead to AIDS? How does our experience differ from that of HIV positive men, many of whom are gay? I want to examine these issues by focusing on a group for HIV positive women in the Toronto area. I will look at the implications of HIV to women's health and the services offered us in our struggle to live knowledgeably and responsibly in healthy bodies.

Since November 1988, a support group for HIV positive women in the Toronto area has met weekly. The group formed in response to a dramatic increase in the number of women who were testing HIV positive. The AIDS Committee of Toronto and Hassle Free Clinic jointly sponsor the group, which is the first support group in Canada exclusively for HIV positive women. (More recently, in Montreal, a city which is experiencing an alarmingly rapid increase in women testing positive to HIV, the Comité Sida à Montréal (CSAM) has started a similar group.)

Since it's inception, approximately 20 women have attended the Toronto support group, some continually, some once or twice. These women have concerns which are unique and existing support groups which are largely composed of gay men couldn't

[*]  Reprinted from *Healthsharing* vol. 11 no. 2 (Spring 1990): 9-13, with permission of the author.

meet their needs. But aside from testing positive to the HIV antibody, most of the women have little else in common.

These 20 women tell stories of lovers, wives, mothers, sisters, friends and daughters; of productive working lives, fulfilling relationships and rewarding studies. Stories of physical violence, sexual abuse and racism. Stories of poverty, addictions, eating disorders and destructive relationships. These stories remind us that the health of most women hangs in a precarious balance.

Most women who have attended the group were infected by a bisexual partner. In many cases they were unaware of their partner's bisexuality. Some women were infected by a heterosexual partner from an area where HIV infection is widespread. A smaller number of women trace their infection to injection drug use. They were sharing needles and also having sex with a partner who was also an injection drug user. (In this respect the support group does not reflect the predominance of injection drug use as a major cause of HIV transmission in women.) One woman was infected by a blood transfusion. A few women are not sure of the source of their infection.

Roughly one-third of the participants have male partners and a similar number have children, some as single parents. None of the women have partners of the same sex. In all cases where the woman's partner is HIV positive, he has an advanced infection. In the past few months, two of the women have lost their partners to AIDS. None of the women has a child who is HIV positive.

Three women of colour have attended the support group, all of them immigrants. Some of the group members are bisexual, but none considers herself to be a lesbian. Most participants are healthy and asymptomatic, though five women have significant symptoms of immune impairment, such as shingles, pneumonia, chronic diarrhea or significant weight loss. None of the women have died.

At first the support group served the very basic but extraordinarily important function of bringing HIV positive women together for the first time. Most women who receive a positive HIV antibody test ("AIDS test") do not know any other women in the same situation. As a result, they can experience an isolation much more profound than that experienced by a gay man who tests HIV positive. Lacking a community in which to share their fears and grief, HIV positive women remain isolated, secretive and fearful. In a society which does not produce or reflect accurate images of women living with AIDS, the existence of the support group is extremely important. It offers HIV positive women the reassuring opportunity to meet other HIV positive women, to hear their stories and to realize that they are not victims but survivors.

Many HIV positive women are not well-informed about their medical condition so they look to the support group to help them access this information. They are often not prepared for the positive test result and have not thought about the possibility of having AIDS. Isolated from a supportive community many of these women do not know how to manage the various aspects of their serious and unpredictable illness. They are often not provided with useful or accurate information by their physicians or health care workers, who may not perceive them as "at risk." Their symptoms of HIV infection are usually attributed to other causes and they are often discouraged from taking an HIV test.

The mainstream media also contributes to women's ignorance of their condition by representing HIV in women either with sensational accounts of sex trade workers, which incorrectly scapegoat prostitutes as "reservoirs of infection," or with sentimental stories of "innocent victims." Women who test HIV positive don't fit these stereotypes.

In the gay HIV community, a survival strategy which is extremely important is the grapevine of treatment information and personal anecdotes that circulate informally. This information is incomprehensible to the uninitiated, but a matter, literally, of life and death in the AIDS community. "I've been taking hypercin for three months now and my p24 antigen level is negative again," or "pneumovax is back in stock," or "here's the AL-721 home recipe." This is a haphazard, sometimes inaccurate and yet completely empowering involvement in an information network. And it has succeeded in enhancing and extending the lifespan of HIV positive gay men. Most HIV positive women are excluded from it however, because many don't socialize with gay men and aren't situated within the larger AIDS community.

HIV positive women have difficulty accessing information on HIV, but beyond this they face another serious problem: the lack of documentation and education about how HIV manifests itself specifically in women's bodies and women's lives. The clinical model of HIV disease is as an illness of gay men. In women, HIV appears differently — the symptoms are different and so is the development of full-blown AIDS. But as a result of the predominance of the male clinical model, women focus on the wrong symptoms. They watch for the appearance of Kaposi's sarcoma (KS), the purplish cancer lesions which are a common opportunistic infection amongst men with AIDS, or symptoms of the particular pneumonia associated with AIDS, PCP (pneumocystis carinii pneumonia). A woman with AIDS, however, is extremely unlikely to develop KS and more likely to develop a bacterial pneumonia before she develops PCP.

Discussion within the Toronto support group confirms what doctors are beginning to notice: one of the first ways that HIV manifests itself in women is through gynecological problems. Women experience persistent and virulent yeast infections, irregular menstrual periods and hormonal imbalances. Too often, women have learned to ignore these symptoms as the usual "women's problems." This attitude has unfortunate implications since recent treatment strategies suggest that HIV infection in women can be managed by early control of these gynecological problems.

Unwillingness to look at AIDS as a woman's disease means that women do not have the information that they need about safer sex, intimacy, childcare and their reproductive rights. We often don't ask questions about what safer sex means to a woman's sexual experience. Safer sex often describes a sexuality which is more comfortable to many women, sex that de-emphasizes penetration as the route to orgasm and replaces it with activities that stimulate the entire body and skin, and fantasies that stimulate the imagination. Yet most AIDS education pressures women to respond to safer sex either by abstaining or by using a condom. The condom makes penetration safer, but it doesn't question the primacy of penetration in heterosexual relations, which is an issue that needs to be examined in light of HIV.

Currently, a great deal of conflict is generated about women's reproductive choice. We must pay attention to how this struggle affects the reproductive choices of HIV positive women. Some statistics indicate that a healthy, asymptomatic HIV positive woman has about a 50 percent chance of having a healthy child, who won't go on to develop AIDS. All babies born to HIV positive women are born HIV positive due to the presence of maternal antibodies. However, after a period of time the child may or may not replace the maternal antibodies with HIV negative antibodies produced by her or his own immune system. This is the information around which HIV positive women's reproductive choices should be made. However, clinical drug trials, which are often the only access to treatment open to people living with AIDS and HIV, discriminate against women on the basis of their reproductive potential. Some exclude women altogether. Early drug trials in the U.S. demanded that women be sterilized in order to participate. Recent drug trials in Canada attach conditions relating to birth control procedures. The recent ddI (another experimental AIDS drug) trials in Toronto require that pregnancy tests be administered to women participants.

Though many of the women in the Toronto support group have chosen celibacy as their response to positive antibody status, HIV positive women need to be aware of their sexual and reproductive options. Women require support in whatever decisions they make with respect to sexuality and having children.

As long as HIV positive women are not provided with an accurate model of their infection, they will continue to ignore its symptoms and AIDS will diminish our lives unnecessarily. HIV positive women will continue to seek treatment later than gay men when significant damage to their immune system has already taken place. Women with a diagnosis of AIDS live a shorter time than do gay men. If we change the model of AIDS and AIDS education to include women, and if we begin to value women's lives, we prevent the spread of AIDS and for those women who do get it, we will know how to manage the illness better and survive longer.

Women in the Toronto support group are learning about the broad physical and social contexts of HIV and its management *and* their own experiences are voiced and validated. An atmosphere of mutual support and self-help has been nurtured.

As the confidence of HIV positive women grows, many women begin to see the need for more accurate representations of themselves. Some women in the support group now feel that it is part of their personal agenda to educate and inform various audiences about women's experience of HIV. Some have begun writing projects such as diaries, magazine and newspaper articles or correspondence with other support groups for HIV positive women. One woman has appeared on television and in an educational film identifying herself as an ex-prostitute living with AIDS. Others have spoken out publicly at forums, conferences and demonstrations.

This work is the beginning of a long and difficult process of representing women within the community of people living with AIDS and HIV illnesses. It is very important that the voices of HIV positive women are heard so that we do not remain unrepresented, underrepresented or misrepresented by others.

Every woman who has attended the Toronto support group for even a short period of time has shown a great willingness to put aside her personal beliefs, moral judgements and prejudices to listen to the stories of other HIV positive women and to offer sympathy, advice and support. Inevitably, even the greatest goodwill does not support women whose lives are in crisis or who feel marginalized by age, race, culture or lifestyle. HIV tends to bring women together but other circumstances of women's lives can set them apart. Thus an ex-prostitute, whose lifestyle is different from other women in the support group, stayed until her drug addiction pulled her away. An immigrant woman who may have felt uncomfortable because no one else shared her language, ethnic background or strong religious beliefs, attended until her childcare arrangements broke down. A battered woman left the group in the midst of her attempt to break with her abusive partner. All of these women faced problems beyond HIV. These are often difficulties that the support group is unable to contain.

Some women may feel more comfortable confronting HIV in a context which is culturally familiar to them, amongst women who share their lifestyle or speak their mother tongue. A number of community organizations exist for this purpose and provide education and support groups.

Patterns of membership and attendance in the Toronto support group for HIV positive women point to the need for a variety of outreach services for women. Certainly regular attendance at a support group by diverse HIV positive women would expand all members' views of what HIV means to women. But in practice, wide-ranging membership is difficult to maintain. The support group can not be responsible for breaking addictions or intervening in an abusive relationship. It cannot force women to confront issues which they are reluctant to face.

For many women a precondition to dealing with HIV is getting other areas of their life in order. HIV provides a very strong impetus to confront such things as alcoholism, addictions or abusive relationships. But it is not enough that women are ready to confront these issues. Our social services system must be ready to provide the services that will facilitate these changes. Yet it is still the case that there are too few daycare spaces available, too few beds in women's shelters, too long a list of people waiting for addiction treatment, too long a list to get into affordable co-op housing, and never enough money. These are problems central to women's lives. They are made more extreme by HIV. Though services exist to help women whose health is jeopardized in these ways, these services are overtaxed, underfunded and they are scrambling to· deal with the implications of HIV. Under these circumstances, some women with HIV find it difficult to cope.

Once these pressing needs of women can be met, then HIV positive women will be freer to explore alternative treatments like vitamin supplements, acupuncture and Chinese herbs. Or we may become involved in political issues as they relate to living with HIV. One woman may become interested in the relationship between macrobiotics and viral suppression and start to change her diet. Another might start exercising more. And another may represent an HIV positive woman's perspective within Aids Action Now!, an activist group organized around treatment strategy. Women will become more knowledgeable about non-drug therapies for enhancing their immune system and thereby decrease their dependence on what is too often a paternalistic medical system.

One of the members of the Toronto support group recently visited the offices of Positively Women in London, England. She brought back exciting news of an organization run by and for HIV positive women which offers counseling, a support group and publishes pamphlets which announce themselves proudly as "plain-speaking about AIDS and how it affects women, written for women by the experts — women." Such glimpses of an international picture of women responding to their positive HIV status offer encouragement and inspiration for the development of women's groups in Toronto and across Canada.

For Canadian women living with HIV it is a time of uncertainty and hesitation. It is a time of coming to terms with who we are and what we want as women and as HIV positive women. We will be stronger to demand those things that will help us to manage our HIV infection: education, outreach and informed medical response, daycare, support groups and other social services specific to women with HIV. HIV positive women will also benefit from greater integration within the AIDS community and from access to an increased number of groups which deal with HIV in a way which allows women to be included.

HIV positive women are moving out of their isolation to develop connections with each other and with other people living with AIDS. They speak and write about themselves as HIV positive women, promoting accurate and unsentimental descriptions of themselves. They are making important and caring decisions about the way they want to live and, should it happen, the way they want to die.

Here are some of the women who have attended the Toronto support group:

- A young woman, infected nearly ten years ago by one of her first boyfriends. She is currently enrolled in the clinical trial of ddI, a promising anti-viral drug. Her employers have noticed her physical deterioration and are complaining about her job performance. She believes that her job is the key to her survival but fears she may be fired without notice and lose her medical and insurance plan.

- An older woman from Eastern Europe whose husband recently died of AIDS at home amidst their extended family. When their adult children learned about what was happening to their parents, they purchased a large house so that they could all live together during this time of crisis.

- A diabetic woman caring for her partner, an ex-prostitute and injection drug user. They live on family benefits and she is responsible for managing most aspects of their daily life including waking her partner for his medication every four hours during the night.

- A health worker with three children who didn't know of her husband's bisexuality until he developed AIDS. She arranged for his admission to a residence for people with AIDS and moved with her children to Whitby.

- A young wife grieving for her husband who died of AIDS during the preparation of this article. Her two-year-old daughter is healthy, but was born since her mother has been HIV positive. This woman, who seldom speaks during group discussions, has written 85 pages of an autobiography detailing her experience of living with AIDS.
- A black woman from the West Indies infected during a blood transfusion who was initially told by her doctor that she was HIV positive because she came from Africa.
- A woman with AIDS Related Complex (ARC) who is an ex-prostitute and an injection drug user. She held a dinner for other group members at her apartment and then never returned to the group. After a clean year, she is back on the streets.
- A young student who tested positive during her first year of law school and who is about to begin practicing in a prestigious downtown firm.
- The woman who wrote this article.

**DARIEN TAYLOR** is a freelance writer and AIDS activist.

# Centre Stage

## Life as Little Miss Easter Seals[*]

### Lina Chartrand

The article which follows reflects Lina's experience as a child with polio. In 1949, at the age of 16 months, Lina developed polio; 11 years later she had the dubious honour of being one of Canada's "Miss Easter Seals." She was encouraged by Easter Seals campaign officials to use her crutches, even when she didn't greatly need them; her responsibility, was simply to "look crippled."

### Mother's Monologue

I nursed her till she was five months old but I never liked it so I put her on a bottle after that. They say a breastfed baby has more resistance to disease. It's a wonder I did it at all, I hardly breastfed the boys, just a few weeks.

She was strong. She was so smart, she could walk at 12 months and she was out of diapers. There was no holding her back, she was everywhere. She was a bit chubby, chunky little legs, she was so cute. My husband played with her, god how he played with that one.

I was lonely in Timmins. My husband had brothers and sisters here but I had no sisters, nobody here, just old Madame Blanchard, my mother's cousin. She was good to me. I can never repay her for what she did.

The year Lina got polio there was a big flu going around. At first I thought that's what she had. I called the doctor, Docteur Clairmont. He was being run off his feet with sick babies. I was sure there was more wrong with her than just flu.

It started like a bad flu, she slept a lot, she felt hot and feverish.

* Reprinted from *Healthsharing* vol. 6 no. 1 (Winter 1984): 12-15, with permission.

After three days she stopped walking, she couldn't hold her neck up.

This time I was crying when I called the doctor, the telephone operator wouldn't talk to me in French; in those days they weren't allowed to talk French even if they could. She kept saying the line was busy and I kept trying to say it was an emergency in English.

Finally I called the police and they came over with the doctor. He knew right away she had polio. We rushed her to Toronto by airplane.

She was afraid of everything. In Toronto, she wouldn't let them X-ray her. It took about six people to hold her still. She was afraid of that X-ray machine; it was big. She screamed and screamed like they were trying to kill her. I couldn't stand to hear it. She was impossible.

She just wouldn't calm down. Even after when she re-learned to walk, even though it took a long time, she crawled and skittered about so fast, she was always getting loose from me.

The polio paralyzed her. Slowly she got back the control over her muscles, but some stayed weak. The Toronto doctors gave me exercises to make her do in Timmins. She always refused to do them.

The doctor said it was important. Who knows, she might not have needed to have operations, she might not have gotten so crooked in the spine if I could have got her to do those exercises.

What could I do? She said it hurt and she was so hard to control.

I was dead, I was nervous, I had the big liver operation. I missed my mother that year.

I wonder why she got polio when she was such a healthy baby and I did everything good for her. I remember once I caught her eating peaches that hadn't been washed. I thought that might be how she caught it. She got needles and boosters, she had got them all. Other kids in town who got polio ended up in wheelchairs or blind, she was lucky to be able to walk.

## Over the Rainbow

In 1960 I was chosen to be little Miss Easter Seals and to go on a tour of the Porcupine area with Whipper Billy Watson. When the campaign was announced, he flew up to Timmins for a TV interview in our living room on Preston Avenue.

He sat beside me on the old green couch, beside my mother's beautiful big fern. The camera and sound crews were all over the room and pouring out the front porch.

The Whipper talked about giving the handicapped more opportunities for jobs and education. I did very well answering the questions about my age, school grade and how I felt grateful to Easter Seals. My foot was in a cast and my crutches leaned against the couch beside me. I was shy but proud, slightly precocious and I had a beautiful sweet smile.

The Whipper never spoke to me privately. We played our roles. No one ever told me what to say or how to smile.

Easter Seals funded the Kiwanis Club in Timmins. This organization paid the train fares for my mother and I to travel to Toronto for my operations. The Easter Seals campaign lasted several months, covering many events including a Christmas party, a tour of high schools, a banquet at the Empire Hotel.

The Whipper flew up to the Porcupine twice, first to do the TV interview to launch the campaign and several months later for a couple of days of speeches and banquets. I handled the other gigs on my own, assisted by my mother, Public Health nurse Miss Collins and Kiwanis volunteers. I never really had to do much but smile, answer questions about my age and grade and say something like "Please give to Easter Seals," or even just "Please give" was fine.

An event I especially remember is a Kiwanis-sponsored fund-raising variety show of local talent at the Dante Club. There were cute little girls tap-dancing, teenagers who played the violin or the piano, and a men's barbershop singing group. Each act had its own sets of backdrops, white benches, flowers. Everyone was English; I was French.

I made my first stage appearance with the Krakana Sisters. The three sisters wore identical long bouffant dark hair with an Annette Funicello flip and flared dresses. They sang a number of songs appropriate to sister singing groups like Sugartime and it was while they belted out "You've Gotta Have Heart" that I came on stage on my crutches and sat on the white bench near them. The Krakanas then moved to the other side of the stage and sang "Somewhere Over The Rainbow" to me amid multi-coloured light effects. It was a hit and the applause lasted a long time.

They never said a word to me backstage. Maybe they thought

I didn't speak English, that all I could say in English was "Please give to Easter Seals." I told them their singing was nice but all they said was "Oh, thanks."

## No Union

Tonight I put Maman on the train to Timmins and I walked away, out of the station, to my home in Toronto.

I walked out of Union Station, away from Gate 9, along the other departure gates, past the line-ups, up the ramp leading to the main part of the station, past the magazine kiosk, towards the big clock in the middle. The loudspeaker voiced the names — Gravenhurst, Noranda, Kirkland Lake, North Bay, Cochrane, Timmins.

Between Gate 9 at Toronto's Union Station and the Timmins train station, the world is transformed. In between is lots of darkness, sometimes rocky bedpans, motion sickness, chocolate bars. Early in the morning when I hear a long train whistle, I am back on that train between Timmins and Toronto, between home and Sick Children's Hospital.

On one of my first train rides, Maman was afraid of the black porters. She'd only seen one or two black people. We couldn't get hot water in our roomette so she buzzed for the porter. He ran the hot water for a long time feeling the temperature with his fingers. Maman was trying not to giggle. She imagined he was trying to wash away his blackness but he never got any whiter.

I was afraid. People stared at me when I walked to breakfast on my crutches. I wouldn't look at them. I tried to be quiet. Maman complained about how much the food cost on the train. It drew attention to us. I hated it.

I'm sleeping in an upper train berth. I can hear people walking back and forth on their way to breakfast. The night has been long. I can't tell if it's light or dark, no window up here. The butterscotch soft blanket keeps me cozy, the rocking keeps me snoozing. I'm in disguise. No one knows who I am. I'm an Eaton's catalogue model. I'm a child actress. I'm travelling by myself. If Maman talks to me, I won't answer her. She just wants to ruin my fun. If Maman wasn't here, they wouldn't know I'm French, they wouldn't know I'm from Timmins.

The train forms a tunnel between two realities for me now. Along the way there are shelves of experience leading out of the old way of life. It is a maze. You could end up right back where you started. There is little to see out the window: snow-covered trees, desolate huge empty lots frozen with dead cars, small cabins dilapidated so you don't want to look inside, shabby motels, rocky roadsides with blast scars. Cold, 50 below.

No union.

LINA CHARTRAND has been an administrator for Pelican Players for three years. She is currently writing a performance piece about her experiences as Little Miss Easter Seals, funded by Canada Council. She lives in Toronto.

## section nine

# Organizing Changes in Women's Health Care

*Healthsharing* was started by a group of educators and activists and the magazine itself has been a vehicle for organizing changes in women's health. From the first issue to the last, *Healthsharing* brought its readers news from the front lines — those organizations and projects which have been creative forces in expanding and reinventing a mandate for women's health.

The Centre de Santé des Femmes du Quartier of Montreal, the Vancouver Women's Health Collective, the Immigrant Women's Centre of Toronto, the Community Health Representatives of British Columbia's Native communities, the AIDS and Disability Action Project of British Columbia all creatively combine education and politics as they struggle to meet the wellness and sickness needs of their diverse communities. The Centre de Santé is still the only free-standing clinic for women in the country. This is a sobering thought at a time when many feminist health activists have been dismayed to see our demands for free-standing autonomous clinics taken up and repackaged by provincial health ministries as clinic adjuncts to existing hospital administrations. Yet it is equally sobering to see that those women's health institutions that have been able to remain autonomous are chronically underfunded. The Vancouver Women's Health Collective, of which Melanie Conn and Rebecca Fox were members (see their article "Undoing Medical Conditioning"), is an example. While some women's health projects or clinics may have an advantage of relatively autonomous operation and geographic separation from heavy-handed administrations and bureaucracies, this advantage is undermined by perpetual crisis caused by underfunding. "The Story of the Community Health Representative" describes how the severely underpaid paramedics of B.C. Native communities deal with the many chronic diseases effected by two hundred years of colonization. Besides their role as health care providers, they function as administrators, language and cultural interpreters, educators, activists and lobbyists.

In "Black Women Organize for Health," Makeda Silvera interviews Erica Mercer of Toronto's Immigrant Women's Centre about a U.S. conference on Black women's health. This article not only informs readers about Black women's perspectives on health issues, it also challenges the white women's movement to examine its ideological underpinning and the absence of race in its analysis.

In "AIDS and Disability Action Project," Ann Daskal and Beth Easton urge us to examine the AIDS and disability interlock. Not only are women with disabilities particularly vulnerable to HIV, but, as well, all persons with AIDS are living with a disability.

In "Resisting Psychiatry," Angela Browne introduces the term "psychiatric survivor," referring to individuals who have survived "mental illness" *and* its treatment. Like the other articles in this section, "Resisting Psychiatry" contains the premise that those most affected by specific health problems should be key players in organizing health solutions.

# Nurturing Politics and Health
## Centre de Santé des Femmes du Quartier[*]

Clara Valverde

Connie Clement

Looking for good health care services is often depressing. In Montreal, as in most other cities and towns, women in need of health services have few choices. Montreal has the usual range of physicians in private practice, hospital out-patient clinics, and a small number of alternative services such as herbalists, massage therapists, holistic healers and a women's self-help collective.

There are also government sponsored clinics (CLSC) which have been gradually set up throughout Quebec during the past five to ten years. Some CLSC's employ concerned and competent staff who work in a team setting rather than traditional hierarchical structures. This allows for greater support and innovation, reflected in the care received by consumers. The extent and quality of care found at CLSC'S, however, varies greatly.

In Montreal and other Quebec cities, women also have the choice of seeking care at popular clinics. Popular clinics are neighbourhood or community health centres located in working-class neighbourhoods. They are either run by or directly influenced by the users of the clinic. The growing number of popular clinics in Quebec contrasts with the very limited number of community health centres in other parts of Canada. The CLSC's were, in part, established to curb the growth of popular clinics throughout the province.

Even in the popular clinics which strive to provide quality health care according to the needs and desires of the people receiving the services, the specific needs of women may be overlooked. In Montreal, the Centre de Santé des Femmes du Quartier

---

[*] Reprinted from *Healthsharing* vol. 1, no. 1 (Winter 1979): 15-17, with permission of the authors.Text of Footnote

(Neighbourhood Women's Health Centre) provides health services for women by women.

## A Need for Women's Services

Why single out women as a sub-population which has difficulty procuring good health services? Nearly everyone, man and woman, feels at one time or another a sense of powerlessness before a doctor. For women, however, the imbalance of power between a doctor and a "patient" is coupled with the lack of social power which women as a group experience. Knowledge based on personal experience is not often validated by medical professionals. Neither is the day-to-day experience of women validated by most men.

Many women have long asserted that physicians take male complaints more seriously than female complaints. A recent California study provided data which backed up this complaint — doctors, when seeing women patients, are more likely to prescribe drugs, recommend major surgery and not follow up and test for reported symptoms than when they see male patients.

This situation is intensified on yet another level for Francophone Quebecoise women. In Montreal Francophone women often need to seek help from Anglophone health services where the doctors tend to be more liberal about sterilization, contraception and abortion criteria. For example, 80 percent of all hospital abortions performed in Quebec are done in Anglophone hospitals. This may be in part because Anglophone doctors have been exposed to the impact of the consumer and feminist health movements in the U.S. and English-speaking Canadian cities, and perhaps in part because they do not generally have a close association with the Catholic Church. Whatever the reason, the result is that Francophone women are often forced to go through the denigrating process of obtaining an abortion in the language of Quebec's ruling class.

## Centre de Santé des Femmes du Quartier

The Centre de Santé des Femmes du Quartier opened its doors in 1978. The centre provides a medical clinic, information and educational activities run by and for the women in the neighbourhood, and a focus for political action.

The centre is in the neighbourhood of Plateau Mont-Royal, a

working class area with Francophone Quebecois making up 90 percent of its population and immigrants 10 percent. Women using the centre also come from the St. Louis neighbourhood, adjacent to Plateau Mont-Royal. St. Louis is 40 percent Francophone Quebecois and 60 percent immigrant (Greek, Italian and Chinese), with a growing student population. Mostly unskilled workers live in St. Louis where many clothing factories employ immigrant women; more skilled workers tend to live in Plateau Mont-Royal.

Most of the women who come to the Centre de Santé des Femmes are Francophone Quebecoises. Most of the women using the clinical services are between 20 and 30 and are either working or attending school. The majority are single and have no children. The women using the educational services tend to be between 30 and 60. Most of them are married, have children and work in the home.

The attitude towards women which the centre embodies can be seen in the small details which make a visit to the centre less threatening and more supportive than women's visits to most traditional medical services. The main reception/work room at the centre is filled with comfortable couches, chairs and work tables. Several literature racks around the room display birth control, feminist and general medical literature. Posters and announcements of upcoming neighbourhood events are posted on a bulletin board on the wall across from a large banner which depicts various roles of women. There are toys for children to play with. Herbal and black teas, coffee and sometimes cookies are available. It is a relaxed place to chat with a neighbour as you wait to see a paramedic.

## Medical Services

The core of the centre is the clinic. At this time the services are limited to adult women and the focus is on gynecological services. Eventually the centre might be able to perform abortions, assist at non-problem births, provide services to children, and include more broadly based therapeutic and counseling care. However, at the present time with limited staff (both paid and volunteer) and funds, women seeking specialized care are referred elsewhere. Sterilizations, obstetrical needs and abortions, as well as general surgery or specified consultations, are all referred to specialists;

immunizations and services for children and spouses are referred to CLSC's.

The centre relies heavily on volunteer paramedics to provide its services. At present, three physicians work part-time at the centre. Each is paid through Assurance Maladie and turns over a portion of their payment from the government to the centre. These monies help pay for overhead, supplies and the salary for the one full-time paramedic/administrator. All other paramedics work on a volunteer basis for one or several half-day clinics per week. Paramedics work with doctors during physical examinations, IUD insertions, diaphragm fittings, etc. Otherwise paramedics work on their own to provide birth control information to clients, answer telephone inquiries, make referrals, maintain medical records, sterilize equipment, prepare laboratory samples, receive results back from the lab and keep the centre clean.

The care given women can be seen in the comprehensive, woman-oriented medical history, which women complete with a paramedic on their first visit. Each woman is encouraged to use a hand mirror during internal examinations in order to better understand her body and discuss her situation with the doctor or paramedic. Before any IUD insertion a woman is tested for infection by a paramedic; only if she appears clear of any sexually transmitted infection and pelvic inflammatory disease (PID) does the woman see a doctor for the insertion.

### Education

The centre's educational services are organized by the information committee, which is made up of interested users. The educational programme is geared towards and used mainly by housewives in the neighbourhood. Last spring women organized sessions about contraception, menopause, nutrition and weight problems, nervous depression and other topics.

This fall three middle-aged women in the neighbourhood have organized a series of ten sessions entitled "Woman and Her Body." The organizers set up the series to follow up a biology course they had recently taken through the University of Quebec with a feminist biologist. Four or five women, including the professor who taught the university course, have split up the "teaching" work load. They use videotapes and slides to approach basic anatomy, physiology, emotions and nutrition. The programme, however, is specifically geared to the women in Plateau Mont-Royal. At each session women talk together about the presentation and topic in the context of their daily experience and life in the neighbourhood environment. All sessions are held at the centre during the afternoons so that housewives can attend while their children are at school.

Another group organized this fall to follow up on interest expressed about depression during last spring's sessions. A collective support-therapy group is meeting at the centre weekly to discuss women's experience of depression, its possible causes and solutions. Some women attend weekly; others drop in when they feel the need. One of the paramedics from the centre and a psychologist are actively involved in the group. A second group may be started in the new year in response to the numerous inquiries which the centre has received.

## Political Action

The third aspect of the Centre de Santé des Femmes du Quartier is its political activity. The centre's coordination committee interacts regularly with other women's groups and popular organizations throughout Montreal and other parts of Quebec. Involvement ranges from simply posting a letter or announcement at the centre to actively organizing centre users and volunteers to attend a meeting or rally about better day care, housing or working conditions. Approximately one to three requests for help or support come to the centre weekly — each is seriously considered by the committee and acted upon or not depending on the issue.

The centre shares resources with other women's health groups in Quebec. Recently the centre helped women from Sherbrooke and Joliette set up two new women's health centres. Paramedics from the centre are called upon to help train CLSC staff about birth control (e.g., a session on diaphragm fitting) or provide outreach education programmes for CLSC's (e.g., a talk about menopause or a programme to help women be more assertive with their doctors). The centre is an active member of Quebec's National Coordination for Abortion on Demand, thereby working with other pro-choice groups in the province. Presently, the centre is working with an umbrella group to assess the impact of the closing of Montreal's rape crisis centre, and whether the centre can help fill this gap.

## Democratic Structures
The Centre de Santé des Femmes is democratically run so that women using the services have a large say in what services are provided and what form those services will take. The general assembly meets yearly to set all policy and establish the overall direction of the centre. All users are encouraged to participate and vote in the general assembly. The assembly elects a coordination committee which carries out policy between assemblies. The co-ordination committee meets once or twice a month, as needed, to hire doctors, decide upon interim policy and set long-range plans. The coordination committee is presently involved in assessing the future directions and goals of the centre.

Also reporting to the general assembly is the users' council, which meets every three months to evaluate the centre's pro-grammes and medical services. The users' council is open to all users and generally has a turnout of approximately 15 to 40 women.

Four committees report to the coordination committee. These are: the information committee, made up of users who develop educational activities; the medical committee, composed of para-medics and doctors who meet once a month to coordinate medical services and internal educationals; the abortion committee, made up of users who discuss and research the possibility of expanding to include abortion services; and the publicity committee, com-posed of users who run the publicity campaign for the centre.

The actual day-to-day work of running the centre falls primar-ily to the one paid paramedic/administrator. Until cutbacks last year, the centre employed two full-time staff. With only one staff, that staff person is presently very overworked. Volunteer para-medics are being encouraged to help take on more of the admin-istrative duties by working during non-clinic hours.

## Grass-Roots Impact
It is the combination of woman orientation and neighbourhood orientation which makes the Centre de Santé des Femmes du Quartier so vital. Most women's health centres in the U.S. draw upon women from a large area around their centre for their

client-base. Although some neighbourhood women may use these centres, many of the U.S. centres tend to cater to feminists already active in the women's movement or women's health issues.

Centre de Santé des Femmes du Quartier has the potential to involve women from the neighbourhood in an activating process which could propel them into greater involvement in other community, women's and health care struggles.

The centre is a fragile, but strengthening link between two relatively disparate movements — the popular movement for improved housing, cheaper food prices and better working conditions, which has traditionally been aligned with the workers' movement, and the women's movement, which, with few exceptions, has been relatively isolated from other struggles in Quebec.

The creation of woman-run centres is necessary if women are to begin to gain control of health services. By controlling neighbourhood health services women can focus on both collective and individual health. At the centre women can improve their own health and at the same time indirectly improve the health of their children, their lovers and husbands, and their friends. At Centre de Santé des Femmes du Quartier women nurture women, women nurture community and women nurture political conscience.

CLARA VALVERDE is a paramedic at the Centre de Santé des Femmes du Quartier.

CONNIE CLEMENT is the volunteer coordinator at Planned Parenthood Waterloo Region and is a member of Women Healthsharing.

# Undoing Medical Conditioning

## Melanie Conn
## Rebecca Fox

In this society, we undergo a good deal of conditioning in many areas of our lives. Through this process of conditioning we are taught, sometimes subtly, sometimes not-so-subtly, to view certain things as fixed, unchanging, not open to question. One example of this is sex-role conditioning, in which we are encouraged to measure maleness and femaleness according to certain norms: women are passive, men aggressive; women work in the home, men work outside it. Sex-role conditioning is now being challenged on many fronts, but there are other forms of conditioning, equally insidious, that mould our thinking in other areas of our lives, and that have only begun to be questioned. Perhaps the most powerful conditioning is that which we receive in the area of health care.

At the Vancouver Women's Health Collective we have in the past year begun to explore this fact of our medical conditioning. Our discussions on this topic were stimulated by a growing awareness of "alternative" treatments for abnormal Pap smears — tests to detect cervical cancer or early cell changes thought to be pre-cancerous. The alternative treatments we kept hearing about included the use of herbs, nutrition therapy and visualization (a type of meditation in which the healing power of the body is positively imagined). At first, we didn't pay too much attention to this new information, because cervical cancer is one of the few cancers with a good cure rate, and because the conventional treatments we already knew about — freezing the cervix, removing a section of it and hysterectomy — usually worked. Gradually,

*    Reprinted from *Healthsharing* vol. 1 no. 4 (Fall 1980): 10-12, with permission of the author.

it became important for us to look at our reasons for not paying much attention or giving equal credence to the new treatments that women were using to revert abnormal cervical cells back to normal. We had a number of discussions which led eventually to a series of public forums in which we explored our "conditioning around Western medicine" — how it happens, how it shapes our views on health, disease and the kinds of medical treatment we receive.

One of the most insidious and powerful influences in our medical conditioning comes from advertising. Through our daily lives we are bombarded with messages both direct and subtle on how to behave, how to took, what to buy. So it is no accident that we mechanically take aspirin for a headache instead of stopping to consider the source of the pain and perhaps deciding to try a relaxation technique instead. Often we cannot take the time for such consideration or medication, because the pace of our lives supports our reaching for the pill bottle.

Drug companies have spent millions of dollars on advertising so that when we notice that throb along our temples we think of acetylsalicylic acid. We are not the only ones who are prey to this conditioning: doctors' main source of information on drugs is also pharmaceutical companies. After all the direct-mail promotion, medical journal ads and free samples from drug company salesmen, it's not at all surprising to see that new drug on our prescription.

Most important is our vulnerability to the lack of accurate information on the safety and real effectiveness of these products. It is a step forward in our health consciousness when we start to ask questions, when we stop to look at what we're buying and why.

But when we do go after evidence to support a conventional treatment, we come up against "The Scientific Study." We grow up with the idea that medicine is an exact science, that proof positive exists for every treatment and procedure. When we take a closer look at the dynamics of medical research, however, we find it's not as simple as all that. Scientific studies, lo and behold, often contradict each other. Not all studies are of equal merit either; there are good, carefully controlled studies, there are sloppy, poorly conducted studies, and a whole range of studies in between. Studies can be biased by a number of factors, from the initial hypothesis to the methods of collecting the data to the way in which the data are presented. Studies which are funded by self-interested groups like drug companies are often biased at the outset.

An example of the vicissitudes of studies: for many years there was conflicting information about the diaphragm and its effectiveness as a birth control method. While women were being primed for the new "wonder" methods — the pill and the IUD (intrauterine device) — the diaphragm was being dismissed as outdated, "what our mothers used to use." In 1973 a good study was done at the Margaret Sanger Institute in New York showing the diaphragm to be 98 percent effective. The difference between this study and previous ones was that the women using diaphragms in the Sanger study were all well-fitted and carefully instructed, a time-consuming process. The only pregnancies included in the Sanger statistics were those where the women had actually used the diaphragm at the time of conception, in contrast to earlier studies.

We hear a lot about preventive health care as a potential alternative to conventional medical treatments. But the "health" industry's profits are much higher for treating illness than for preventing it. Conventional treatment almost invariably involves drugs, and often means filling hospital beds and the use of expensive equipment.

Screening has been conventional medicine's response to the demand for preventive health care. We have been conditioned to believe, for example, that an annual physical exam is our surest bet to continuing good health. But there is no clear evidence that annual check-ups positively affect the health status of any given population. The procedure reveals relatively little, since most diseases can be detected only after symptoms occur. In the case of some diseases, like lung cancer, early detection makes little difference in the life expectancy rate.

Furthermore, some forms of screening may be downright dangerous to our health. Mammography, or breast X-rays, was to be medicine's chief weapon against breast cancer, in preference to breast self-exam, an effective, cheap, woman-controlled procedure. Some studies now suggest that routine mammography of women who have no symptoms may actually increase their risk of contracting breast cancer.

The real hook in the conditioning we receive around screening is that we (and our doctors) genuinely believe that we re responsibly taking care of our health. In actual fact, we may be exposing ourselves to unnecessary procedures and ignoring other significant indicators of health and illness.

The politics that prevent the preventive health model from becoming more than an experiment extend deeply into our very perception of the meaning of health, and limit doctors' understanding of health as well. Doctors are not trained to assess our state of health or to assist its maintenance. Rather, they see us as our complaints and isolate the illness, focusing on the absence of health. We've learned to think of our everyday concerns — persistent vaginal infections, intermittent headaches and depression, low back pain — as trivial problems. We're embarrassed to take them to the doctor, who rarely sees them as part of the fabric of our total state of well-being.

But our conditioning around doctors is perhaps the most powerful, and the hardest to unlearn. We have grown up to trust them to make decisions for us, in the belief that they are skilled and dedicated humanitarians whose professional standing reflects their superior intelligence and years of technical training. The step from the doctor's office to some form of self-help can seem a rather large and intimidating one. One of the major breakthroughs of the women's health movement has been precisely in the development of self-help techniques, and in its emphasis on seeing ourselves as whole persons both in sickness and in health. We've learned to look at birth control, vaginal health and the menstrual cycle not as medical "problems" but as an integral part of our sexuality and whole being.

Another problem is our lack of practice in perceiving our bodies as basically healthy systems. We feel utter panic when something goes wrong. We can't imagine that we, our bodies, can co-exist with an infection or pain long enough to combat it without immediately calling in the troops: heavy doses of potent prescription drugs or surgery.

"Nature is a slow healer," the herbal books tell us. But we have become so accustomed to "fast, fast, fast relief," erroneously equating the disappearance of symptoms with the elimination of disease, that slower, gentler methods are hard for us to trust. In our own discussions at the Health Collective, we found that while we occasionally used or were prepared to try alternate remedies, such as herbs or visualization, we weren't willing to "fool around" when it was a question of our children's health or if we had a serious condition, such as cancer. We weren't willing to wait out the time necessary for the treatments, and our bodies, to deal with illness.

The familiarity of the conventional methods encourages their use. We may be amused by the cartoon anatomy in the TV ads, but the route they depict — mouth-stomach-bloodstream (where the medication radiates "relief") — dominates our perception of the healing process. Sipping tea or applying a poultice to the *outside* of the affected area seem strange, old-fashioned and ineffective approaches to curing our ills.

Furthermore, our dependence on conventional methods reinforces itself. In the case of antibiotics, we have become so used to routine treatment with them that in some cases we find ourselves less resistant to minor infections than we used to be. It then becomes necessary to use even stronger antibiotics that have more toxic effects. Strains of harmful bacteria, once easily controlled through antibiotics, are no longer affected by them.

Another issue related to the "fast powerful relief" message has to do with the source of the medicines we're used to taking. Although we have some degree of choice with over-the-counter drugs, we have been trained to believe that if we're "really" sick, we need "powerful" drugs. Our training further tells us that powerful drugs are those that are regulated by law, and dispensed by qualified professionals from licensed pharmacies, after being prescribed by a doctor. An herb that grows in the garden or a mixture that can be made for a few pennies simply doesn't have the weight of a conventional drug for most of us.

We've also learned to believe in the specific action of drugs: aspirins relieve pain, antihistamines dry up mucous membranes, birth control pills suppress ovulation. In comparison, the widely disparate claims for most herbs seem outrageous. How can the same herb, like comfrey, be good for vaginal infections, arthritic pain, respiratory infections and as a skin conditioner? As it happens, the whole notion of "side effects" is a semantic one; all drugs, like herbs, have a wide range of effects on the body. In fact, the so-called "major" effect of many conventional drugs was discovered by accident while researchers were investigating other effects. For example, the antihistaminic effect was discovered as a by-product of a sedative. But now we're told that drowsiness is a "side effect" of antihistamines as though it were a lesser effect, when in fact it's simply one that the drug company is choosing not to promote when it's selling us a "cold remedy." And as many women have bitterly learned, the suppression of ovulation is only one effect of the birth control pill. Oral contraceptives affect every system of our bodies in some way, and some of those effects are dangerous to our health.

So our conditioning dissuades us from trying remedies that seem to have too many applications to be plausible, encouraging us to dismiss them as "quack remedies" and the result of "old wives' tales." But that same conditioning obscures for us the action of conventional drugs on our bodies, and often misleads us about their toxic effects.

Health care has become a very private matter in our culture, and our isolation from each other reinforces our conditioning to accept conventional medicine. We're not around other people when they're sick, and they're not around us when we are. A vast communal body of knowledge of health and home remedies that once existed within families and communities is now largely lost. Parents don't teach their children about sickness and health because they simply don't know very much themselves. When you haven't been around a teething baby, you don't talk about it or hear different theories and remedies until your own child is crying in the night. What we have now is a vast array of "experts" like Dr. Spock, a poor substitute for a community of supportive and experienced neighbours.

Our intuitive sense about our bodies has also taken a beating from our medical conditioning. We've learned not to trust our own inner sense of what's right and wrong, even in small matters. At one of the Health Collective's public discussions a woman said that "in her heart" she knew her child's fever was the result of teething, but she called the doctor anyway to calm her worries. He prescribed antibiotics.

At the Vancouver Women's Health Collective we are beginning to integrate an effort at breaking this hold of our medical conditioning into our everyday work. In the process of examining our own attitudes and talking to other women, we've found a different, more positive view of "alternative" healing methods has emerged.

This doesn't mean that we recommend herbs to every woman who comes in the door. In fact, we reject the "practitioner" role of saying do this or that particular treatment. Instead we use the self-help model and apply it as widely as possible in our work. We try to help women make their own choices, and encourage them to look through our files, which include information on conventional treatments as well as herbs and nutrition. Our library now has standard medical texts and a good selection of books on herbs and self-help healing. We also do a lot of skill-sharing, such as teaching women to examine their own vaginal smears under the microscope.

A positive result of our discussions around "conditioning" is our eagerness to talk with women about their reluctance to consider less conventional treatments. Having explored our own scepticism and fears, we can understand exactly where they're at. But our goal is not to exchange one set of "sure cures" for another. What we strive for is to free our minds and hearts from the training that has prevented us from making genuine choices about our health.

**MELANIE CONN** and **REBECCA FOX** are workers at the Vancouver Women's Health Collective, which has organized self-help groups and other women's health activities in the Vancouver area since 1971.

# Black Women Organize for Health[*]

## Makeda Silvera interviews Erica Mercer

In 1983 Spelman College in Atlanta, Georgia, was the scene of what has been called the "Conference of the Decade." (Some 1,500 students are enrolled at Spelman. Founded in 1881, Spelman is an independently-funded black women's college offering a four year undergraduate program.) It was a weekend of workshops, speeches, films, self-help, demonstrations, exhibits and cultural and physical activities that brought together about 2,000 women from across the United States. The conference was sponsored by the Black Women's Health Project and the National Women's Health Network.

MAKEDA: The theme of the conference — "I'm Sick and Tired of Being Sick and Tired" — what does it symbolize?

ERICA: This saying is credited to Fannie Lou Hammer to whom the conference was dedicated. Fannie Lou was a founder of and delegate for the Mississippi Freedom Democratic Party which tried to unseat the "official" all white, all male delegation to the Democratic Convention in 1964. Although it did not get seated, the Mississippi Freedom Democratic Party forced the Convention to begin to take up Civil Rights issues. An activist, freedom fighter and "first lady of civil rights," Fannie Lou was often heard to say in her struggles to effect changes in Mississippi, "I'm sick and tired of being sick and tired." Yet in spite of her tiredness, she remained steadfast in her unwavering commitment and continued her activities for many, many years. The theme is rooted in our historical experience and represents the struggles of black

[*]   Reprinted from *Healthsharing* vol. 5 no. 2 (Spring 1984): 19-22, with permission of the author.

women. It is an expression that black women immediately identify with. I certainly did. I went to Atlanta "sick and tired," but I returned to Toronto with a feeling of renewed commitment.

MAKEDA: What were the objectives of the conference and what motivated the organizers to embark on such an undertaking?

ERICA: The conference brochures state four main objectives:
1. To educate black women about health care and health facts.
2. To present a cultural and historical perspective on health.
3. To instruct and provide guidance on self-care skills and promotion.
4. To increase awareness about public policies that have an impact on health access and the establishment of a network among black women.

The idea for the conference came into being after the organization of the Black Women's Health Project, a project developed around the model of mutual and self-help activism to empower women to make health care decisions and increase their awareness of reproductive health issues. The conference was perceived as being an integral part of charting a new activism in the quest for good health and well-being. As Byllye Avery, Director of the Black Women's Health Project, put it, the conference would give black female health consumers the opportunity for once to tell health care providers including white men and white women and black men to their faces what we want, need and demand.

MAKEDA: To what extend did low-income women participate in the conference?

ERICA: About 25 percent of the conference participants were low-income women who were able to attend only due to the extensive outreach and fund-raising effort of the BWHP. Many of the Southern rural women had done their own fund-raising and some of the groups had made attendance at the conference one of their goals and held activities around this goal. I think the conference organizers deserve special credit for making this an important item in the conference. They realized the added burden this put on them but felt that it had to be done.

This is something we should make note of. How often have

conferences been stages for special groups and you find "spokes-persons for" instead of representatives from the groups affected? And how often have conference organizers self-righteously con-demned a "lack of participation" and "lack of interest," when they never once considered that the time may be inconvenient or one simply could not afford the registration fee or the means of getting to the conference?

MAKEDA: Did you have any special expectations of the Confer-ence?

ERICA: My immediate interest was as a black woman. The idea of such a conference being held excited me so much that I talked to everyone. I could not possibly have missed such an event. What I expected when I stopped to think about it, was the chance to hear from black health care workers and consumers. I expected to compare and share with them types of activities and ap-proaches to problem solving. I hoped that I would return with lots of materials that I could share with my colleagues at the Immigrant Women's Centre.

MAKEDA: Could you talk about the workshops and presenta-tions? I understand that some were very dynamic and special.

ERICA: There were 60 workshops, and I thought, as I tried to make a selection, that this was madness. The best workshops seemed to run concurrently and it was impossible to attend all those that I was interested in. But I realized that what the organ-izers had done was to deal with all the issues so that they could accommodate as many interests, needs and viewpoints as possi-ble. The topics ranged from reproductive rights, to aging, self esteem and lifestyles. The workshops were facilitated by health advocates, practitioners and community activists. They were so well-structured that, although they were only one and a half hours long, there was enough time for discussion so that partici-pants really got into the topic.

MAKEDA: What about the presentations that were given? I recall you saying that they were also very powerful and moving.

ERICA: The opening session by Dr. Jane Jackson Christmas, Director of the Behavioural Science Program of the School of Biomedical Education, City College of New York on "Black Women and Health Care in the 80s" was powerful. The thrust of her presentation was directed to the United Nations Declaration on Health — the concept that "Health is more than the absence of disease; it is a state of positive well-being, physically, mentally, socially and spiritually in all its aspects." She defined the "triple jeopardy'" of oppression — racism, sexism and classism and how these interrelate under capitalism. Dr. Jackson called on us to learn the historical causes of sickness, the reasons why we are sick and tired, and to organize for change. She drew a standing ovation and thunderous applause when she called on black voters to make Reagan a one-term president.

The other plenary speaker, Dr. Alyce Gulattee, Administrator of the Alcohol and Drug Abuse and Addiction Program at Howard University (an independently-funded co-educational black university in the District of Columbia) talked on "The Politics of Substance Abuse." That was quite an experience. She talked a great deal on the risks and dangers in drug and substance abuse — the damage to mental functioning, the congenital and genetic abnormalities abuse brings to the reproductive system and how the life force of the black population could be destroyed in one generation. She dealt with issues of race and class, making the connection to drug use and the racism inherent in the way that statistics are compiled and disseminated. Again the message was how important it is for women to take control of our health as the first battle in the struggle to transform our lives and society. The atmosphere was that of a revival meeting — she brought us to our feet so many times. There were tears, cheers and a lot of stamping and banging. Outside of the chapel where the plenary session was held, I heard women nodding in tearful agreement that, had this been the only address they heard, this by itself would have made the weekend worthwhile. But there was lots more that made the weekend worthwhile for me.

MAKEDA: You mentioned experiences of a very personal nature, do you want to talk about that?

ERICA: Yes. This was a workshop "Black — What is the Reality?"

It was so popular it had to be repeated. The workshop was facilitated by Lillie Allen of the Department of Health Education at the Morehouse School of Medicine. She very skillfully guided a sister to share very intimate and deep-seated feelings that she had held for years. I was very skeptical of what she would achieve with this because I don't trust those soul baring, let-it-all-hang-out sessions that seem so popular with women's groups. That is why what happened in that room was so incredible, why it was such a moving experience for me. There was such an outpouring of love and empathy that I found myself in tears. I cried for me, my mother, my sisters, my friends I left behind in Toronto. We were instructed to hold the person next to us who was in tears. Of course I was not going to hold anybody, I don't like strangers touching me, but as I was crying, I felt these arms around me and I felt warmth and understanding and I felt secure.

The other workshops in Stress Reduction and Burnout Avoidance, Black Women and Sexuality, the Black Adolescent and her Pregnancy were all very dynamic and worthwhile.

MAKEDA: What about abortion? How was that issue addressed?

ERICA: I can tell you how it was addressed by giving the title of the workshop — "Abortion: Choice or Genocide?" That in itself is revealing of the concerns and problems that pervade that issue.

MAKEDA: Can you be more specific? On other occasions we've talked about the attitudes of white women — the fact that they say the black women benefit from the fight for freedom of choice but are not active in that struggle.

ERICA: Yes, that is a sore point with me as you well know. I am talking about the difference not only in perception, but also in standpoint. Black women and other women of colour support a definite distinction between being pro-abortion and being for abortion rights. As black women, we have had our reproductive rights curtailed, beginning with slavery when our children were taken from us as free labour. Some of us aborted and others even killed their children rather than see them grow up as slaves. But choosing between death or slavery for our children was no choice. We support abortion rights because we know only too well the consequences of their denial. We are the ones who have to resort to the back street abortions and the often fatal consequences. The pro-choice campaign, as articulated by "the women's movement," comes from a very middle-class white perspective which assumes that *all* women can make choices as to how they will develop their potential, advance their careers, have children or not, be able to provide for the children they have. But for black women, for Third World women, for women of colour who form the majority of poor women, there are no choices. We are battling for our economic survival — combatting low wages, high unemployment, housing and so on — which interferes with any notion of choice in the matter. Pro-choice has not addressed our reality.

MAKEDA: In the past the women's movement has also been criticized for not speaking to the needs of black women, particularly because of the high incidence of sterilization among poor black women.

ERICA: As far as sterilization goes there is a difference between the situation in the United States and in Canada, even in so far as the extent of the sterilization abuse practices in the States. Here in Canada this does not seem to have occurred to the same extent, although there are reports of sterilization abuse of Native women and among the developmentally handicapped.

There is a more fundamental issue that goes beyond abortion rights. It has more to do with attitudes coming from a class perspective. It is in keeping with the fact that the composition of the white women's movement, although experiencing oppression because of sex, is actually in a position of dominance. This blinds the movement to the real concerns and priorities of the women they presumably set out to help. Unless the women's movement undertakes some critical analysis of itself and the ideological underpinnings of the movement, I think we will continue to have the problem of them badgering us to take the "correct" position and we all continue to criticize them for being classist and racist. I know of some progressive elements in the women's movement here in Canada who are trying so I don't think we all remain at that impasse.

MAKEDA: Since we are on the subject of racism I understand that some white women who attended some workshops were asked to leave. What are your feelings on that and why were they asked to leave?

ERICA: I was in a workshop on "Black Women and Sexuality" where women asked for the white women to leave. It was not billed as a black only workshop. Not all the women agreed that the white women should leave, but I voted with the others because I appreciated the sentiments expressed about not revealing one's most intimate self to strangers. The facilitator, sensing the disappointment and anger of the white women, asked them not to regard the exclusion as rejection. I do agree that it should be made clear from the outset which workshop was exclusively for black women, but we all have to continue to make these separations, given the tradition of mistrust that exists between us.

MAKEDA: And what about feminism?

ERICA: The question was not raised. In fact, I don't think I heard the word feminism once. Yet it was obviously a very feminist undertaking. What could be more feminist than women organizing themselves to talk to each other and everybody else about their health concerns? That by its very nature is feminist. In Atlanta I was among sisters, among family. It was as though I were at home just waiting for my room to be fixed up. And that is sisterhood, the essence of feminism.

MAKEDA: Were your expectations of the conference fulfilled?

ERICA: My expectations were fulfilled in more ways than I could have ever imagined. There were some beautiful experiences. I also got a lot of information and materials that I brought back with me. The renewed commitment that I referred to earlier came from seeing the displays of the self-help groups and listening to the women talk about the different ways they organize themselves around specific issues. It gave the concept of self-help new meaning. I was able to see, in a way that I had not perceived before, the potential and power of such groups. I immediately began to envision the groups that could be formed around a number of health issues and the resources that could be unleashed. Though most of the groups remained basically oriented to health issues, the analytical and critical work they engaged in is bound to take them beyond health as such.

MAKEDA: When you came back from Atlanta you said that the general feeling of black women present was that they were at war. What exactly does that mean?

ERICA: They are "Women at War;" they are unarmed combatants fighting against the economic policies of the Reagan administration that seems hell-bent on annihilating them. There were chilling statistics that showed the effect of budgetary restraints and cutbacks in federally funded programs. According to the National Health Law Program, in 1981, infant death rates increased in eight states: Alabama, Alaska, Kansas, Michigan, Missouri, Nevada, Rhode Island and West Virginia since Reagan's election. There was a strong undercurrent of urgency around the situation of blacks in the U.S. today. In just about every workshop, in every presentation, women were being called upon to prepare themselves physically and mentally to take on the struggle, to prepare to return to their communities and, if not involved in community action, to start immediately. That is a war cry.

MAKEDA: What would you say was the most significant thing about the conference for black women? Would you say it was in methods of organizing around general health care or was it around a particular health concern, for example, high blood pressure?

ERICA: I would say both areas were significant. *Network News*, the newsletter of the National Women's Health Network, featured the Conference and discussed some of the particular health concerns raised. Black women have double the rates of high blood pressure, infant mortality, diabetes, teenage pregnancy, cancer and lupus as the rest of the population. Of all the factors that account for the health differential between blacks and whites, high blood pressure and related diseases make the greatest contribution. One of every four black adults suffers from hypertension, as opposed to one out of every six white adults. Not only is it more frequent among blacks, it also develops earlier in life, is often more severe and causes higher mortality at an earlier age. Deaths from high blood pressure before the age of 50 are six to seven times more common among blacks than whites (*Network News* June 1983).

According to Dr. Gerald E. Thomson of the Harlem Hospital Centre in New York City, for all ages of black women, the incidence of high blood pressure tends to be either equal to or higher than that of black men, depending on the survey reported (*Network News* June 1983). Some of the contributing factors of particular importance to black women whether they are hypertensive or know someone who is, are heredity, obesity, salt intake, birth control pills and smoking. High blood pressure is considered by many to be the greatest health threat to blacks in the U.S. For every black who dies from sickle cell anaemia, an estimated 100 die from high blood pressure-related diseases. What must be noted as well when we talk about hypertension, is the incredible stress of being black and poor in a racist society. We talked earlier about black women being at war — no population at war can expect not to suffer heavy casualties.

MAKEDA: Do you think it's possible to have a similar type conference for black women, sponsored by the Immigrant Women's Centre for example?

ERICA: Wouldn't that be wonderful! But I'm afraid such a conference is not something that can be organized in the immediate future. Let me list the many reasons why. First we have to get rid of a lot of stuff that gets in the way of organizing ourselves as black women in order to give us the kind of clout we need to demand our rights from the state. We first have to deal with our diverse backgrounds in a constructive way. This is not a major problem but our differences are exploited by the people whose interest this serves. So instead of getting down to brass tacks we find ourselves arguing over who arrived on Air Canada or who came with the underground railroad and which group has the right to make demands on the state and which group should be grateful to be present. Until we get rid of that garbage we can only come together as small, separate, weak groups.

There also has to be a heightening of consciousness around health care as an important issue around which to organize women. Women's health care has been on the back burner, left for later when other matters are taken care of. Unless we ourselves recognize that fact and begin to change our perspectives, then such a conference is not possible.

We should not consider holding a conference without allowing the time needed to plan properly, to strategize so that we get the outcome we want. Too many national conferences have left me wondering about the outcome when the last resolutions had been written. I don't think we can afford the expense of time and resources. We learned some valuable lessons in Atlanta that we should heed.

**ERICA MERCER** was one of the founders of Toronto's Immigrant Women's Centre where she presently works as a counselor. She has been working around health and other issues of concern to the black and immigrant communities for a number of years.

**MAKEDA SILVERA** is a writer and community activist in the Black and immigrant communities. Her first book, *Silenced*, a collection of oral interviews with West Indian domestic workers, will be published early in 1984.

# Resisting Psychiatry [*]

## Angela Browne

A few years ago, the Canadian Mental Health Association in conjunction with the Ontario government launched a major ad campaign to raise public awareness of barriers which exclude the "mentally ill" from the community. Such ads typically featured a school-aged boy expressing concerns that his father, who had been recently discharged from a psychiatric facility, might be shunned by neighbours and co-workers as if he were "still sick." Though the ads were meant to invite people to become involved in the association as volunteers, the terminology reinforced a medical model which perpetuates negative values and stereotypes about psychiatric survivors.

In the winter of 1986, a homeless woman was found frozen to death in the back of an abandoned truck. She was later identified as Drina Joubert and an inquiry was called into her death. Submissions to the inquest and recommendations that followed, painted a picture of the social services system as fragmented, inefficient and unresponsive to the needs of the neediest. Service workers were quoted as saying that if there were better coordination of services, Ms. Joubert would be alive today. However, the reality of a whole social system of poverty and homelessness was not addressed.

Shortly after the Joubert inquest was completed, a man living in a psychiatric boarding home died. Although John Dimun was being supervised by a physician and an adult protective service worker, no one noticed that he had developed a severe lung infection. The jury's verdict following an inquest into his death concluded that Dimun died by "natural" causes induced by a self-chosen inappropriate lifestyle." (See "Boarding house tragedy," *Phoenix Rising*, June 1987.) The social and economic context of his life was ignored.

[*]   Reprinted from *Healthsharing* vol. 11 no. 2 (Spring 1990): 17-21, with permission of the author.

More recently, a housing group, in its bid to house nine former inmates of psychiatric institutions, was faced with bitter opposition from people residing in the proposed neighbourhood. In its coverage of the story, the *Toronto Star* included a photograph of men, women and children holding signs bearing the words, "One more is too many." If the housing group tried to relocate the project elsewhere, similar opposition could be expected.

For every public outcry on the need to redirect more funds to the community, there is a louder, more vocal call to send the dollars and the people back to institutions. While male inmates are portrayed as likely to become violent if allowed out even for a day, women are portrayed as victims, as in the case of Drina Joubert. Public interest articles in newspapers give the message that if the institutions weren't there, former psychiatric inmates would either become violent, suicidal or deteriorate living on the streets.

Although both men and women psychiatric survivors are portrayed falsely, women are more likely to be described as dependent, weak and vulnerable. This image reinforces the philosophy of most social service agencies that tend to "do for," instead of "do with" the people they work with. This philosophy reinforces the notion that such individuals are sick, rather than victims of poverty, spousal abuse, working in the pink ghetto or devalued in some other way. Most of these agencies carry with them the notion that most or all so-called mental illnesses are biochemical/genetic in origin, even though most of the evidence continues to be speculative (see Penfold and Walker, *Women in the Psychiatric Paradox*, Montreal: Eden Press, 1983).

For various reasons, women become depressed more often than men. They also seek help more often and are prescribed more psychotropic drugs, which can have a negative effect on health. Because of this, many more women feel the need for, and seek out community support services.

Most community-based services, especially those run by hospitals or major charitable organizations (e.g. most branches of the Canadian Mental Health Association), were developed using the traditional charitable model. Giving help is usually a unidirectional action — the "well" party is expected to give help, while the "sick" party is expected to receive it and appreciate what is given to her. This creates a subtle power imbalance and prevents women from becoming involved in solving their problems.

There are many reasons for this adherence to the charitable model. Governments and community health funding bodies prefer to fund projects that are both professionally administered and supervised. Most such administrators come from backgrounds which prevent them from being aware of the day-to-day issues that affect those they "serve." They tend to be white, middle-class and frequently male. Most of the staff hired to run these programs are from a social services background and very few have been through the mental health system themselves.

Many former participants of such programs became frustrated in their attempts to deal directly with the power imbalances within, so they formed their own groups (e.g. On Our Own, Phoenix Rising). These groups are critical of the hierarchical structures and paternalism that exists in most traditional community mental health organizations. It is their view that the self-help approach in a democratically-organized structure is more effective at providing the mutual support that people need to regain control of their lives. Unfortunately most of these groups are poorly funded and almost as powerless as the individuals within them.

Their leaders have worked hard at advancing the interests of the self-help groups and have gained a few powerful allies such as Ontario MPP David Reville and Ontario New Democratic Party health critic, Carla MacKague, both of whom were once "treated" in the system themselves. One group, On Our Own, developed a drop-in centre, second-hand goods store and quarterly journal, *Phoenix Rising* (see D. Weitz, "On Our Own: A Self-Help Model," *Pheonix Rising* Spring 1983). *Phoenix Rising* has since become independent of On Our Own and continues to be operated entirely by former psychiatric inmates, as they prefer to call themselves.

Some service providers have begun to realize that the concept of "doing to" or "doing for" is no longer acceptable, due to increased criticisms from the newly formed self-help groups. Some responded to these criticisms by developing a new approach called "empowerment through partnership" (see *From Consumer to Citizen*, Canadian Mental Health Association, 1987).

Although a few organizations have achieved this, most are still struggling with a hierarchy that does not want to give up control.

A popular example of this innovation is the clubhouse model, currently practiced at Progress Place in Toronto and at an increasing number of branches of the Canadian Mental Health Association.

The clubhouse format is simple. Members and staff meet at the start of each day to choose tasks to perform. Tasks include clerical, statistics, maintenance, writing reports, sweeping the floor, washing windows and many other things. Lunch and sometimes supper is provided for, and by the members working in the cafe unit. At the end of the day, staff and members meet again to review the events of the day, give compliments and make small changes to the program.

Though this program seems to be egalitarian on the surface, there are many other issues that still remain to be addressed. When someone wishes to join a clubhouse, they must attend an interview conducted by a staff member who then decides on the candidate's suitability for the program. This usually includes the humiliating process of the candidate having to admit, either verbally or in written form, that she has been mentally ill. In contrast, staff automatically become members of the clubhouse upon being hired and in most jurisdictions it is illegal to ask a prospective employee about her psychiatric background.

Since this type of job attracts applicants with a social service training background, it is unlikely that such applicants approach the clubhouse to get help from the other members. By virtue of definition, paid staff are more likely to see themselves as giving help rather than receiving it. It becomes clear that not all members are equal and only some members get paid for their contributions.

Another problem barely addressed is the scope of decision-making allowed for members at the daily meetings. They can decide to bar an unruly member but they cannot discipline staff. They can make Thursday nights euchre nights instead of bowling nights but they cannot decide on directing more money into one activity or another. Final program decisions and personnel matters are out of the hands of clubhouse members. Unless there is a generous supply of program users on the agency board of directors, the clubhouse is not run by its members.

Most discussions and meetings take place with staff present.

Personal issues, such as the budgeting of one's own money or finding a room to live in are discussed, but rarely spoken of are general problems of poverty and oppression. Members are expected to adjust to a bad society and stay on their prescribed medication. Problems arising from poverty or discrimination are thought of as being the fault of the woman or her "illness."

Vocational training has become more popular with all community mental health programs, but it usually comes in the form of supported work placements or transitional employment programs. Transitional employment programs (TEPs) are usually added as an advanced component of clubhouse programs and offer benefits to both employer and potential employee. The employer is guaranteed that a position will always be filled and the employee obtains much needed job experience, without undergoing the problems associated with a job interview.

But TEPs do have their problems. Clubhouse members are expected to seek only low-stress, entry-level positions, such as clerical work, restaurant help and cleaning. Most of these jobs pay minimum wage and offer little advancement. If a clubhouse member already has skills or a university or college degree, she may now only get a job that is significantly below her personal aspirations.

The employer, like most members of the general public, likely lacks knowledge and understanding of mental health issues. Although they are told only that the workers are involved in the TEP program, they could assume that you have been labeled as having mental or emotional problems. They may treat such employees differently by being patronizing or nervous. This can create an uneasy feeling in some women, especially if her employer is a man.

Another popular empowerment measure that some agencies use is the members' council. The member/clients of an agency elect their own executive and report to staff with recommendations for program changes and activities. The council may also be in charge of operating social activities in the evenings and may publish their own newsletter. However, the council work of the members is supervised by staff and/or designated volunteers, who are always present during activity nights. If members publish anything controversial, such as challenging the biochemical model, in their own newsletter, the staff can act as final editors and choose to censor such articles.

The council also has no final say in program changes, budgeting, personnel and long range goals. These decisions are made by the agency board or executive committee. While most boards are now admitting consumers (as they are often called), their small numbers don't produce a sense of representativeness and variety of viewpoints. The result is that less vocal individuals don't feel comfortable to seriously challenge certain assumptions made by other board members about what is "best for the mentally ill."

Placing a *significant* number of service users on boards and decision-making committees will not only add credibility to the consumer voice, but can also raise the level of self-respect among many who have lost it through the undermining processes of becoming a patient. With more input from their users, services will also become more relevant and responsive.

Recently, the national office of the Canadian Mental Health Association published several papers addressing shortfalls within the mental health system. They also examined how their own organizational structure involves consumers (as psychiatric survivors are called there) at all levels of decision-making and in self-directed advocacy. The national office recently opened their board to such interested persons and created a task force to facilitate more constructive participation by consumers. This task force is not directly under the auspices of the Canadian Mental Health Association and the formation of an independent national network is among its many goals.

A few smaller agencies have broken away from the traditional mode of simply doing for the "mentally ill." In seeing a need for a real partnership between those who help and those who turn to mental health agencies for support, Friends and Advocates Etobicoke formed in 1977. Shortly thereafter, Friends and Advocates began new programs in North York and Peel that are run with a similar philosophy to the Etobicoke chapter. Responsibility for the budget, personnel, programs, researching of social issues, the publication of their quarterly newsletter, *Reflections*, and other functions are carried out through the agency's various committees, all of which are run, primarily, by psychiatric survivors. Recommendations come from these committees which are then brought to the general membership meetings, where program users, staff and volunteers each have one vote. Many of the staff and volunteers have previously been through the system and all participants are encouraged to take on a helping role, as well as receive support from others. Activities include discussion groups, member-run social and recreational events, a quarterly newsletter and social support networks. The Friends and Advocates program has been shown to be effective in reducing hospitalizations among those who belong to the organization. The agency demonstrates that it is possible to develop a partnership between community members and those that have received psychiatric treatment.

Friends and Advocates Etobicoke is currently assisting with the development of an Ontario provincial network of current and former psychiatric survivors. The first task of this group is to create a network of interested persons who wish to attend an upcoming national conference in Montreal. The network will also assist in the development of organized advocacy efforts for and by psychiatric survivors. This network is operated almost exclusively by psychiatric survivors and offers some hope of connecting people who live in remote areas of Ontario.

But, including more psychiatric survivors on the boards of decision-making bodies and agencies is not in itself enough to resolve the central issue of how people can help themselves. Psychiatric survivors need organizations run exclusively, or almost exclusively, for and by themselves. As mentioned earlier, the quarterly journal *Phoenix Rising* is run only by individuals who have directly experienced the system. A new political action group in Toronto, Resistance Against Psychiatry, is also completely ex-inmate controlled.

There are also a number of self-help groups run by psychiatric survivors that tend to be less radical and more accepting of the medical model, such as manic-depressive associations. They have also been fighting for greater representation for their members on decision-making bodies.

In November of 1989, representatives from across Canada attended a national conference on "mental health alternatives" in Montreal. The conference itself was meant to be a networking device as participants were mostly psychiatric survivors. Workshop topics included local organizing, dealing with agencies, obtaining funding, living with or without medication and women and psychiatry. This conference could facilitate the development of a national psychiatric survivor-run organization.

These organizations will not entirely solve the issues affecting women facing these problems, but they are a positive step forward. Increased participation by those who directly experienced the mental health system can give women more control of their lives and will also facilitate the development of more appropriate services.

Mental health self-help groups should also form coalitions with various organizations formed to fight other issues, such as incest, wife abuse, poverty, sexism, heterosexism and racism. Female psychiatric survivors can borrow from the women's shelter movement and develop local projects that enable other women in crisis to seek refuge in a shelter with high levels of emotional support. In her book, *On Our Own: Patient Controlled Alternatives to the Mental Health System*, Judi Chamberlain wrote about her positive experience while visiting Vancouver's Emotional Emergency Shelter, which was then operated by the Mental Patients' Association.

Similar agencies could be developed to deal with related issues of racism, sexual abuse and poverty. Cooperative workplaces and businesses (with the added benefit of child care facilities) could be formed to assist women in getting out of the traditional pink ghetto.

These issues must be resolved for the benefit of both men and women. If we then discover that a small fraction of those labeled "mentally ill" do indeed have clear neurological, biological or nutritional imbalances, we shall attempt to work with them in much the same way. We must oppose potentially harmful treatments, often administered to people in the name of so-called biological psychiatry. Those we refer to as "mentally ill" should have the same rights as everybody else.

## Further Reading

Canadian Mental Health Association. *From Consumer to Citizen.* Toronto: 1987.

Canadian Mental Health Association. *Women and Mental Health in Canada: Strategies for Change.* Toronto: 1987.

Chamberlain, Judi. *On Our Own: Patient Controlled Alternatives to the Mental Health System.* New York: McGraw-Hill, 1978.

Penfold, Susan, and Gillian Walker. *Women and the Psychiatric Paradox.*

Montreal: Eden Press, 1986. An excellent book on psychiatry's particular assault on women.

Weitz, Don. "On Our Own: A Self-Help Model." *Phoenix Rising* (Spring 1983).

**ANGELA BROWNE** is a sociology student, self-help group activist, freelance researcher and writer who also sits on numerous committees and community boards dealing with mental health and poverty issues.

# The Story of the Community Health Representative*

## Rita Manuel

Community health representatives (CHRs) are primary health care workers in Native communities. Most of us work on Native reserves and a few work in urban areas. Our role parallels that of the "foot doctors" in China — we are front-line health service providers.

Each province and territory in Canada has community health representatives but most are located in British Columbia where we have at least 200. This may sound like a lot of positions but they are sparsely scattered throughout the province in half-, quarter- and full-time positions. The Medical Services Branch of Health and Welfare Canada divides British Columbia into four zones: Northeast, Northwest, South Mainland and Vancouver Island.[1]

The CHR program has been in existence since 1960. It was set up to meet four major needs. First, the need for greater involvement of Native people in their own health program, and greater participation by them in the identification and solution of their health problems. Second, there is a need for greater understanding between the Indian people and the Medical Services staff at Health and Welfare Canada. Third, the desire to improve cross-cultural communication between the Native community and the providers of health care. And fourth, the need to increase basic health care and instruction in Native homes and communities.

CHRs have proven to be "made to order" health resources in our communities. Our roles are very diverse because each CHR responds to the particular needs of her or his community. There

* Reprinted from *Healthsharing* vol. 13 no. 1 (Spring/Summer 1992): 31-2, with permission of the author.

are many factors which affect our roles: the age and size of the population, the location of the community (e.g., rural, urban, or isolated), the awareness of community members of health concerns, the availability of employment, the creation of Native-operated schools from pre-school to colleges/technical institutes level and the availability of health institutions such as clinics and hospitals.

## Band Control versus Medical Services Control

Of the 200 CHRs in B.C., there are five of us, working in Merritt, Salmon Arm and Kispoix, who are still employed by the Medical Services Branch. At one time the federal government, through Medical Services, employed all the CHRs and determined their job descriptions. Over the years however, the Native Bands have agreed to the transfer of the CHR program from the federal government to the Bands. This has its pros and cons.

Native Control of health care can promote self-determination which is very important for our communities. To be successful, a transfer like this requires much preparation. A Band needs to learn how to meet their own health care needs and they also require sufficient dollars to be able to do the job efficiently. Unfortunately, sometimes the transfer happens without enough preparation or proper funding. This makes the CHRs job extremely difficult.

With the transfers, CHRs' working conditions and benefits have sometimes declined. For example, little or no benefits accompany some transfer agreements with the Bands. Pension plans are included in some agreements and not in others, leaving some CHRs wondering what will happen when they retire.

In B.C., there are two Health Boards that have signed transfer agreements with the federal government for control of their entire health care programs. These are the Nisga Valley in New Aiyansh and Nuu-Chah-Nulth in Port Alberni. The situation of the CHR in these communities is more secure in that their jobs are not threatened with the change in Band leaders, which occurs in a few instances, and benefits are an integral part of their contracts.

## A Varied Vocation

Job descriptions for CHRs vary. Our job is focused on prevention rather than treatment. Ongoing programs we administer include providing complete health services to our Band Operated Schools, conducting pre- and postnatal visits, heightening AIDS awareness (including dispensing condoms), serving high-risk children from birth to three-years-old and house visits. Flu clinics, baby and elder clinics, follow-up on chronic patients, diabetic in-service and follow-up, collecting of water samples, medic-alert and Vial of Life Programs are encouraged where possible.

CHRs may also act as liaisons and possibly interpreters to the Band members in dealing with health personnel or finding resources. Many CHRs attend Band meetings to give reports on their work and to get support for the community's health programs.

Often, especially in isolated areas, the CHR is required to arrange for patient transportation to hospitals, clinics, or a specialist. This may be by air ambulance, boat, bus or private vehicle. In remote areas, such as the Nemiah Valley where there is no telephone communication, the CHR would communicate with a c.b. radio.

There are preventive health care programs planned for the communities. However in situations where the CHR is the sole health resource person for the Band, this often gets put on the back burner. They are so busy dealing with critical issues that little time is left for program planning.

Where neither Band nor Medical Services has a community health nurse or resource centre nearby, the nearest health resource for these CHRs would be the provincial health nurse and health unit. This applies to CHRs working on reserves in Penticton, Oliver and Squamish, who not only have to perform their health services duties but have clerical responsibilities as well.

The most extreme situation exists where the CHR has neither federal nor provincial health nurses and is the sole health resource in her/his community. This exists in the communities at Oweekeno, River's Inlet, Bella Bella and Nemiah Valley. The responsibilities that fall on these CHRs are enormous. Regardless of their work hours and statutory holidays, they are on call 24-hours-a-day. The word "overtime" has no significance. There's no such thing as payment for overtime worked.

As public servants and CHRs we do support what we believe in. When the Public Service Alliance of Canada Union went on strike in September of 1990, we supported the strike and walked off our jobs. For CHRs the strike was unsuccessful. However in

April 1991, a decision was rendered by the Human Rights Commission that CHRs, as members of the Hospital Services Group in the Public Service Alliance of Canada, qualified for a reclassification effective from 1987. This was good news for us. It has not happened yet, but when it does, we hope that both government and Band-employed CHRs will receive the same benefits this reclassification will provide.

## Training

CHR training has been a mixture of everything. Medical Services Branch initially allocated training to their "health educators," who did so to the best of their abilities given the short time they had. Generally, training ran from several weeks to several months and occurred in provinces outside of British Columbia.

Today, there is ongoing training for CHRs through various educational institutions throughout Canada. In some instances, CHRs train new CHRs. Medical Services has a contribution agreement with a private educational institution that is concentrating on standardizing the CHR training. Recognized accreditation is the ultimate goal. Perhaps one day a CHR will be able to use her or his training as the first step towards further training to become a registered nurse, public health nurse or other health care worker.

Our work as CHRs is challenging and sometimes rewarding. Too many times CHRs are the victims of "burn-out;" we are constantly on call because the majority of us reside in the same community we service. Throughout my 20 years as a CHR, I have seen many positive changes in our roles in our communities, in our job descriptions and in our daily responsibilities. It is this change that keeps you going.

**Note**
1. Two articles written by CHRs from these zones were part of *Healthsharing*'s special report on B.C. and Alberta; they follow this article.

**RITA MANUEL** is a community health representative with the Medical Services Branch, in Merritt, B.C.

# Community Health Representatives

## A Report from the Northwest Zone[*]

### Diane Brown

My career as the community health representative (CHR) for
Skidegate, Haida Gwaii, British Columbia began in March 1970
when I attended a six-week Family Aid training program in
Prince Rupert. There were 15 of us from the northwest zone. The
only stipulation made by Medical Services was that those taking
the course had to be over 25 years old. That was the first rule I
broke. I was much younger, but I won't say how much.

We were taught St. John's Ambulance First Aid treatments, the
fundamentals of home nursing, basic sanitation and general
guidelines for improving family health by maintaining proper
nutrition.

We had the same nurse in Skidegate for 40 years. She was a
registered nurse, but more like a doctor. She delivered almost all
the babies born in Skidegate; she nursed people through flu
epidemics and pneumonia when there were no antibiotics. I had
quite an act to follow as the elders thought I was a nurse as well.
Because I was so young I was teased a lot. I wasn't prepared for
what awaited me. I was called for all emergencies, all accidents,
dealing with sick babies to sick elders, seven days-a-week, 24
hours-a-day and $70.00 a month. I was supposed to be working
half-time, but it was more like time-and-a-half.

When I began working on the reserve over 20 years ago, many
of our elders did not speak English and had no confidence in the
medical system. I had to liaise between the doctors and my people
— often translating from Haida to English. I worked out of a small
room in my own home. A Medical Service nurse flew in once a

---

[*]   Reprinted from *Healthsharing* vol. 13 no. 1 (Spring/Summer 1992): 34-5,
    with permission of the author.

month from Prince Rupert to immunize infants. We had a different nurse every month and that in itself made things very confusing.

Back in 1971 when I first began this work, I realized that a dentist hadn't visited the reserve for over two years. The major problem in those days was toothaches and some elders needed dentures. I made home visits to every house in Skidegate and examined everyone's teeth. I wrote down exactly how many cavities each person had, if they needed dentures, etc. and sent the letter to the zone office. Somehow my letter got to Ottawa because I received a reply from Monique Begin who was then Federal Minister of Health. Shortly after, a dentist came to Skidegate and relieved our dental problems for awhile.

It is interesting that the main health problem then was dental. Now, 20 years later, it is alcohol, drug abuse, diabetes, heart conditions and arthritis, in that order. Skidegate's population in 1970 was 279; today it is 525. Of those 525 people, 125 have a chronic illness and 35 are diabetics who have many other chronic diseases. Our most recent area of concern is sexual abuse.

In 1976, I received a letter from the zone office saying there was Nechi training (Nechi is a Cree word which refers to an alcohol and drug training program offered to and designed for Native counselors) available for community health representatives. I knew nothing about Nechi but went anyway. I arrived in Vancouver with a huge hangover and went to the first session where I found out that the training was for alcohol and drug counselors. I told the group that I felt I was definitely in the wrong place. They told me to stay for three days and if I felt the same way I could go home. I stayed for the full six-week program and have not had a drink since. In 1977, we put in place our first alcohol and drug program in Skidegate.

The main role for CHRs is to promote a healthy lifestyle and to educate people to take care of themselves. With the heavy workload in Skidegate, we are just barely managing to keep up and care for our chronically-ill patients. My co-worker completed her CHR training three years ago and came home with great insights into the causes of our community's health problems. She was able to see what I could not — that our people were too dependent on the CHRs or Band Council. We both see now that it was the history of white society pushing their values on us that has led to many of the illnesses that plague us now. For 200 years we have heard that our traditional values are wrong and that our language was not to be spoken; we have seen our sacred ceremonies stopped and our way of living in harmony with Mother Earth ended. Then came the Department of Indian Affairs making all decisions in every aspect of our lives. All of this, along with the repercussions of the residential school (when children at ages five or six were removed from their homes to be "educated" by church-run residential schools), has had devastating effects on First Nations People. When all your power has been taken away for 200 years, your spirit begins to die. You do many things to avoid the pain — drinking, taking drugs, inflicting self-abuse, overeating. I feel this is where we are at today.

One of the major tasks for caregivers is to empower people. This is a slow process, after all it took 200 years for us to get this way. We are at the beginning of this process of self-empowerment. The spiritual, physical and mental aspects all have to work together, at everyone's individual pace. My co-worker and I can see this starting. However, in order to get the healing started, we need trained therapists. There are some available, but no funding to hire them. If Medical Services provides the funding, they have a long list of rules attached.

If you asked me six months ago if I had hope, I would have said "No!" But today, I am very hopeful that there will be some changes for our people. The suffering has gone on long enough. I see a future where our children will be singing our songs and speaking the Haida language with pride.

**DIANE BROWN** is the community health representative for Skidegate, Haida Gwaii, British Columbia

# Community Health Representatives

## A Report from Vancouver Island[*]

### Charlotte Williams

The Cowichan reserve is a combination of eight villages, which make up the Cowichan Band population of approximately 2,609. Our community is located on Vancouver Island, in the heart of the Cowichan Valley. Our area is considered urban, as we have a hospital, medical and dental facilities, schools, shopping centres and human services within a few miles of our villages. The reserve skirts the city of Duncan, as our boundaries surround the town. Approximately 75 percent of our population is under the age of 24.

The Cowichan people are known for the famous Cowichan sweaters. This cottage industry forms a large part of our peoples' livelihood — knitting sweaters, toques, socks and scarves.

The Cowichan Band employs about 85 of our people in all areas of service to the community, but there are still a large number of people unemployed. Forestry and farming are seasonal work for many. Recently with the introduction of the natural gas pipeline to the island, additional jobs have been provided. There are also a number of our families that are self-employed, owning their own businesses.

Many of our people live off the reserve either due to land or housing shortages or overcrowding. There are five urban Native housing projects in this area, under the Makola Housing Society.

There are currently three full-time community health representatives; each of us has our own geographic area to service. We work with nurses in maternal and child health and in chronic care and elder programs. We do regular CHR duties and specialize in

* Reprinted from *Healthsharing* vol. 13 no. 1 (Spring/Summer 1992): 37, with permission of the author.

different areas of the health care program — such as hospital liaison, workshop facilitation, interpretation or translation, and home care. I supervise the CHRs and serve on the Band's management staff as a supervisor.

One of our key projects is Project C.H.I.L.D. (Cowichan Holistic Intervention and Life Development), a four-phase education and awareness program which focuses on issues of child sexual abuse and the impact such abuse has on our community. Three phases of the project have been completed, focusing on training, heightening community awareness, research and developing materials specific to the people in our area. We are now in the final phase of the project which will provide a community workshop for our Band Council.

Another program is the Kwunatsustul Counseling Services. Staffed with four counselors and one supervisor, Kwunatsustul Counseling Services runs several programs such as the children's program. This is a six-week program offered to our families with children between the ages of nine and 12 which concentrates on the physical, mental and spiritual growth of our children. The children participate in group activities developing their own problem-solving techniques, communication styles and social skills. Elders are invited to participate in the program by telling stories and teaching the customs of our people to the youth and their parents. The children's program has proved to be an excellent program for our young people.

Our lifestyles have changed over the years. Women are becoming the main support for their families. A sedentary lifestyle has led to more diabetes amongst our people. The change of eating habits to more processed foods instead of the traditional food preparation of the past has had a significant impact on the health of Native people. The stresses of every day survival causes a lot of mental health concerns as well.

We live in a bi-cultural society today. Natives and non-Natives have different values and systems. For our people this means always trying to adjust to two worlds. Our children face the strongest demands by going to school daily and learning new things. As parents we have to bridge the gap and somehow bring that world into ours.

As a CHR, I often see our work as having a bridging function as well — helping our people and non-Natives to live side by side and to better understand each other.

**CHARLOTTE WILLIAMS** is a community health representative on Vancouver Island, British Columbia.

# AIDS and Disability Action Project[*]

## Ann Daskal
## Beth Easton

Women with disabilities are particularly vulnerable to HIV and sexually transmitted disease (STD) transmission. Visual and hearing impairments, physical, learning, psychiatric and mental disabilities or chronic illness can lead to circumstances which put them at risk. Despite their presence in all communities, women with disabilities remain some of the most physically, socially and emotionally isolated among us, adding to their vulnerability. They tend to be seen as sexually inactive and disinterested, without potential to be otherwise. This further deprives women with disabilities who live in a society where standards of beauty, sexuality and acceptable sexual expression are rigid, stifling the diversity of the sexual needs and interests of women with disabilities. Sexual rights, sexual information and sexual health education, including AIDS information, is often not provided.

In response, the AIDS and Disability Action Project (ADAP) was created by the British Columbia Coalition of People with Disabilities, a cross-disability organization committed to promoting self-help and independence. Funded in part by the Health Promotion Directorate of Health and Welfare Canada and the VanDusen Foundation, one of the main tasks of the project was to develop educational materials with and for the different disability communities that addresses basic AIDS information needs, using content and formats that are accessible. This was done by committees, comprised of members from disability communities and some service providers. These working committees also helped develop distribution and promotion strategies, and played

[*] Reprinted from *Healthsharing* vol. 13 no. 1 (Spring/Summer 1992): 17, with permission of the author.

a crucial role in enabling project members to gain permission for speaking engagements and AIDS educational workshops.

The reluctance of many disability organizations, be they peer or professional, to address AIDS, parallels that of non-disability organizations. In addition, the tendency of service providers, caregivers and family to deny or overlook the needs, rights and activities of people with disabilities, especially regarding taboo areas such as sexuality and drug use, makes it especially difficult to make changes within organizations and institutions. AIDS education, even in peer-based disability organizations, is slow to be implemented or not seen as necessary. This is why appropriate materials and trained resource people within the community are crucial.

The material created by the AIDS and Disability Action Project reflects the interests and input of all the working committees. For example, the booklet created by the Deaf and Hard of Hearing Working Committee raises their concern for the general lack of sexually-transmitted disease information in their often residential-school-educated community. Their booklet, as well as being written with American Sign Language-style grammar and having many graphics, has extensive STD information. The pamphlet for the physically-disabled community provides standard information with an additional section about transmission via contact with personal caregivers. A low literacy version and audio tape were also created. The Blind and Visually Impaired Working Committee, after reviewing materials read to them, selected several existing pamphlets and a national resource list of AIDS organizations to be translated into Braille and put on audio tape. The Psychiatric Working Committee requested a printing of the pamphlets for people with physical disabilities, minus the caregiver section. Working with the Committee for People with Mental Handicaps, a set of materials was created that includes two booklets, "Let's Talk About AIDS," "Let's Talk About Condoms" and an eight-page Support Worker's Kit.

Because of funding limitations and the importance of establishing ongoing community-based activities, the AIDS and Disability Action Project encouraged the creation of networks for AIDS information dispersal and links to AIDS-related organizations, while educating the latter about the issues and needs of disability communities. One outstanding development is the beginning of a Deaf Outreach Project based at AIDS Vancouver, similar to the one at the AIDS Committee of Toronto. It will provide AIDS prevention education and support services to the local Deaf, Hard of Hearing and Deaf/Blind communities.

ADAP has always operated from the assumption that AIDS is a disability and that shared concerns, discrimination and the protection of rights necessitates a close working relationship and sense of mutual support between all disability groups. As part of the project, a joint conference "AIDS as a Disability" was held last October in Vancouver, and was well attended by both people living with AIDS and people from the "traditional" disability communities.

Our concern is that fear of AIDS and lack of appropriate information will foster a return to the promotion of restrictive sexual, social and physical environments for people with disabilities, especially women. The best resources are those which help make all people's sexual environments safe for maximum independence and choice.

**ANN DASKAL** was a staff member of the AIDS and Disability Action Project and has been active in women's issues for over two decades. She continues to be involved with AIDS and other disability concerns, especially chronic environmental illness.

**BETH EASTON** is the coordinator of the Women and AIDS Project, and a volunteer member of the Vancouver Women and HIV/AIDS Network.

*postscript*

# Saying Goodbye to Healthsharing[*]

## Amy Gottlieb

Like saying goodbye to a loved one, I struggle with the loss of *Healthsharing* magazine. I was part of the third wave of women involved in the magazine. It says something that we were around long enough to have three waves, but I feel angry that successive women will be robbed of this precious resource. And this is so clearly a collective loss. For whether we read, wrote, edited, designed or illustrated the magazine, there was a connection that will be missed and a resource that we will yearn for.

I alternate between feeling guilty that we weren't able to save the magazine, and feelings of rage that despite our achievements we couldn't survive Tory deficit-cutting attacks on working people and progressive and feminist movements in Canada. I keep coming back to the fighting spirit of the *Healthsharing* project, remembering the energy and commitment that women poured into the magazine and the thousands of readers who felt connected.

*Healthsharing*'s serious financial troubles began in 1989, when our federal funding was cut by 15 percent. But the bigger blow, and the one which we never really recovered from, was in 1990 when $2 million was cut from the Secretary of State Women's Program which then eliminated funding to three national feminist magazines including *Healthsharing*, over 100 women's centres and drastically cut funds to several national women's research

---

[*] Reprinted from *Canadian Woman Studies/les cahiers de la femme* vol. 14 no. 3 (Summer 1994), with permission of the author.

and advocacy groups, including the National Action Committee on the Status of Women. It was clear that this was a political cut, designed to silence critics and demobilize our movements. Response to the cuts was quick and militant. Women's organizations across the country campaigned to stop the government cuts. We were successful but our victory was limited. While our actions forced the government to back down and reinstate funding to the 100 women's centres, funding to national women's groups and publications was never restored.

We need to be clear that there have been very serious long-term costs to the women's movement as a result of these cuts and those that have followed. The Tories were able to redefine the limits of government funding and shift the emphasis and focus away from stable operational funding to more limited project-based funding. And despite its rhetoric, the federal Liberal government is in no rush to reinstate or expand funding to groups that have traditionally been denied access to power in this society.

The current crisis in funding for women's groups is more accurately described as a struggle about who has the social responsibility to address and change the systemic inequalities that women face. The continued cuts to public funding for women's organizations suggest that this work should and is being privatized, that it is no longer the responsibility of the federal government. Funding cuts mean that our tax dollars are not being spent on the programs and services that are essential to fight all forms of discrimination against women. While there are clearly dangers that accompany public funding in the way that governments then try to set our agendas and dilute our militancy, we do have the right to demand that our tax dollars be spent on redressing the sexism, heterosexism, racism, poverty, ableism that are a permanent feature of our society. The move towards privatization makes me very angry, because it essentially means we must carry our organizations on our own backs — we work for less money, donate more money, put in more unpaid time. The denial of public funding means that our organizations are more often than not operating on a crisis footing, with very fragile infrastructures.

Publishing an alternative feminist magazine like *Healthsharing* became untenable without some ongoing operational support from the federal government. It is not possible to apply the logic of free enterprise to alternative magazines given the economy of the market, though the federal government cynically pushed us to do so.

When all is said and done, one of the lessons of the *Healthsharing* closure is that the women's movement has not been able to stem the tide of privatization, despite our attempts. Public funding is now at risk of disappearing altogether.

Since the devastating cuts of 1990, *Healthsharing* had survived on a small and overworked staff, lots of volunteer labour, loyal and supportive readers and a project grant from Health and Welfare to anchor the work of building a Canadian Women's Health Network. But in our search for more permanent public funding we came up empty handed, falling between the cracks of not being a service and therefore not eligible for much of the health-based funding or for arts funding at either a provincial or federal level.

Of course, to begin with, *Healthsharing* was very privileged to receive federal funding, when compared to many other groups organizing at the local and national level, particularly among working class and poor women, among disabled women, among rural women, among African, Asian, Arab, First Nation, Latin American women and among lesbians. But when I say that *Healthsharing* was privileged that doesn't mean we didn't deserve the funding, just that others did as well.

What I will miss most about *Healthsharing* is its radical message, found in the stories, analysis and advice from women who were activists and women struggling with their health and the health of their communities. Most of these women were not professional writers. *Healthsharing* attempted to reflect the radical roots of feminist health activism and broaden the traditional concept of health. For *Healthsharing*, women's health issues were not just reproductive issues, not just about diseases which affect women more than men. For *Healthsharing*, feminist health activism was about looking at women's lives as a whole, about the impact of women's oppression, poverty, racism, class bias, homophobia, ableism, ageism on our lives — it was and still is about making fundamental changes to our medical system so that it addresses all of who we are.

I have heard stories for years about how an article on how to choose a therapist, on hysterectomy or on body image has been passed from friend to friend like a precious talisman. During the closing of *Healthsharing* I have heard even more of these stories, illustrating how much a lifeline the magazine was to the women who read it and passed it around.

But, while *Healthsharing* was a really important lifeline and resource for women across Canada, it wasn't as good as it could have been. The magazine was constantly struggling with issues of representation. Located in Toronto and attempting to be a Canadian publication, *Healthsharing* struggled to be representative of regional specificities and differences. We laboured over the past five years to make *Healthsharing*, which had represented primarily white middle class women, into a publication which belonged as well to women of colour, working class women and women of diverse cultures. And always we struggled with making the information and analysis accessible and readable. My balance sheet is that *Healthsharing* had the potential to be much more inclusive than it was, much more powerful, much more radical and reach a hell of a lot more women than it did.

But that is not to take away from the remarkable things that *Healthsharing* did achieve over its fifteen years. Over that period, the magazine transformed itself, responding to different struggles and developments within our communities and taking on the mainstream medical system. The magazine touched individual women, bringing them information and analysis that then assisted them in making crucial decisions about, or taking new approaches to, their health. At a broader level, *Healthsharing*, along with feminist health activists across the country has had an impact. I'm not talking about a revolution, but rather an acknowledgement within mainstream organizations and at some levels of government that there are some very serious health concerns that women have and that the diversity of women's voices must be integrated when developing health policy and research programs. We see these changes not only reflected in the growth of free alternative health magazines and resources, but also in some provincial government initiatives. Preventive health programs have more support, because they cost less money and help trim health care budgets, but also because the groundwork has been laid by community and feminist health activists to break the health care system of its focus on curing or controlling disease. At the same time as *Healthsharing* maintained a critical stance, it provided support to people working for change within these institutions and to mainstream practitioners with an alternative vision.

Unfortunately, within mainstream publications and organizations, this reflection of women's health issues, is more often than not, "whitewashed" and focused on more respectable middle class concerns. My fear is that with the closing of *Healthsharing*, we are losing one of our strongest voices to counter this burying of the radical content of feminist health activism. Any movement loses some of its vitality, fighting spirit and grass roots mobilization when its left wing is cut off. Fiscal restraint and backlash mean that in practical terms concrete changes are harder to come by, though not impossible. Now, more than ever before, we need a *Healthsharing*.

One of the things that calms me in this period, is the knowledge that local organizations with powerful visions, working around a myriad of women's health issues, are alive and kicking. The closing of *Healthsharing* isn't about giving up, its about recognizing that the publication couldn't survive as it was in the current climate. And while that hurts, it doesn't signal that the politics of *Healthsharing* are dead. Far from it.

The project that *Healthsharing* was a part of over the past ten years and anchored over the past three, the Canadian Women's Health Network, is another source of hope. This project has a long history and is taking some concrete shape.

And finally, there is nothing like going out with a bang. And that spirit will be reflected in the book, *On Women Healthsharing*, which will both keep our memories of *Healthsharing* alive and push us to act with others to transform our notions and practice of health care in this society.

AMY GOTTLIEB is a former managing editor of *Healthsharing*. She is an artist and activist committed to radical social change.

# current biographies of contributors

**ZELDA ABRAMSON** is a women's health counselor in private practice in Toronto. She is a member of the Toronto Women's Health Network who is actively lobbying to reduce numbers of hysterectomies performed on women in Ontario.

**MARY LOUISE ADAMS** is a writer and teacher who lives in Toronto. She is currently working on a book about sexuality and sports.

**PAT ARMSTRONG** is currently Director of the School of Canadian Studies at Carleton University. Since "Where Have All the Nurses Gone?" appeared in *Healthsharing* in 1988, Pat has co-authored two books on health care work: *Vital Signs: Nursing in Transition* and *Take Care: Warning Signals for the Canadian Health System*.

**ROBIN BARNETT** is a health promotion consultant working at the Women's Health Centre in Vancouver. She also works with the Vancouver Health Department on social marketing campaigns promoting condom usage for young heterosexual adults.

**CECILIA BENOIT** is an associate professor in sociology at the University of Victoria, B.C. Her primary interests are in work, occupation and professions, health care systems, family and gender. She is the author of *Midwives in Passage*, has published articles on comparative health care systems, midwives and clients in the *Canadian Journal of Sociology*, *Canadian Review of Sociology and Anthropology*, *Current Research on Occupations and Professions* and *Sociology of Health and Illness*; and has contributed book chapters to *Delivering Motherhood* (1990), *Health and Canadian Society*, third edition (in press), *Considering Women in Newfoundland and Labrador* (in press) and *Western Geographical Series* in press.

**BHOOMA BHAYANA** is a family physician currently in private practice. Her practice consists largely of maternal child care, and the largest demographic is the new immigrant population in London. She formerly worked at the Intercommunity Health Centre and the South Riverdale Community Health Centre and is a former board member of the Riverdale Immigrant Women's Centre.

**MADELINE BOSCOE** is a longtime staff member at the Women's Health Clinic — a feminist community health centre for women in Winnipeg — where she coordinates their advocacy program. She is involved in organizing networks and action on health concerns for women. She is still very involved with midwifery activities and is struck by how prophetic "Birthing Options" turned out to be. Madeline is part of the organizing committee for the Canadian Women's Health Network — ensuring that *Healthsharing* never really stops!!

**PAM BRISTOL**, after spending a year in Europe as a freelance writer, has moved back to her home province of Saskatchewan to work as a writer for the provincial Department of Health.

**DIANE BROWN** is still with Skidegate Band Council as a community health representative. She is a member of the Haida Nation Eagle Clan. She has a husband, Dull, and two children, Jud and Lauren.

**ANGELA BROWNE** continues her involvement with the disability, anti-poverty, community economic development, and social planning communities through both her work as executive director of a community economic development project for psychiatric survivors and with the broader community through her management consulting firm, Browne Consulting & Research (Corbloc Postal Outlet, 80 King Street, Box 24099, St. Catharines, ON, L2R 7P7).

**LINA CHARTRAND** wrote the play *La P'tite Miss Easter Seals*; it was performed in 1988 by the Theatre Français de Toronto at the Du Maurier Theatre, in 1990 on CBC Radio's "Morningside," in 1993 by the Company of Sirens at the Tarragon Theatre, and was published in 1991.

In the years since "Centre Stage: Life as Little Miss Easter Seals" first appeared in *Healthsharing*, Lina also wrote many theatre pieces, short stories, a novel, two feature length screenplays, as well as several short screenplays including *Princess Margaret*, aired on CBC TV, and *In Limbo*, produced and launched by the Canadian Film Centre in 1994.

Lina died on April 2nd, 1994, due to complications from liver disease. Lina's friends and family have established a fund for the annual Lina Chartrand Poetry Award in honour of Lina's literary works.

**DONNA CILISKA** founded the Beyond Dieting program for the National Eating Disorder Information Centre, while a doctoral student at the University of Toronto. She is currently an Associate Professor at McMaster University, Faculty of Health Sciences, and a Clinical Nurse Consultant for the Hamilton-Wentworth Department of Health Services.

**CONNIE CLEMENT** stayed ten years at Women Healthsharing. She now works in health promotion and advocacy for the Toronto Department of Public Health. She's been a member of numerous health activist and feminist coalitions and organizations. Much of Connie's energy goes toward being a mother (which she loves) and toward saving the Toronto Island community (where she lives).

**KATSI COOK** is an Aboriginal midwife from Akwesasne First Nation and is Principal Investigator and Program Director for the Akwesasne First Environment Communications Program. She is an Instructor in the Department of Environmental Health and Toxicology at the University at Albany School of Public Health, and is a member of the Ecosystem Health Work Group of the Science Advisory Board of the International Joint Commission which oversees the quality of the boundary waters between the U.S. and Canada. Katsi's work in ecosystem recovery focuses on socio-cultural systems and human health issues. As a traditional practitioner, Katsi works intimately with the cycles of life and development, providing for the care of pregnant mothers and infants, and maintaining the activities of the Mohawk agricultural calendar. She is working on a book on Iroquois birthing traditions called *Daughters of Sky Woman*.

**MELANIE CONN** currently works in Vancouver with WomenFutures to deconstruct the dominant version of economics and to support women- and community-centred strategies. She still takes anti-histamines from time to time, although she relies much more on golden seal and echanacea.

**JAN DARBY** holds a Master of Arts Degree in the field of women's health from York University in Toronto. Her written work has also appeared in *The Womanist, LACES* and the *Canadian Journal of Human Sexuality*.

**ANN DASKAL** still works periodically at the AIDS and Disability Action Project (B.C. Coalition of People with Disabilities AIDS and Disability Action Project, #204-456 West Broadway, Vancouver, B.C., V5Y 1R3, Canada), which survives despite an uncertain funding climate...in case you wish to order materials.

**DR. CAROLYN DEMARCO** obtained her medical degree from the University of Toronto in 1972 and since that time has specialized in women's health. She has been a pioneer in natural childbirth and in raising public awareness about the overuse of drugs and surgery in women's health care. She has lectured on women's health throughout Canada and the U.S., and has frequently appeared on radio and television. Dr. DeMarco is the author of the recently revised book *Take Charge of Your Body: Women's Health Advisor*, which is available by calling 1 (800) 387-4761.

**MARGARET DE SOUZA** is a Uganda-born Canadian of East Indian origin who works as a Clinical Resource Nurse for the Family Life Program. She is the co-ordinator of the "menopausitive" workshops and founder of the Artificial Premature Menopause Self-Help Group at the Women's Health Centre at St. Joseph's Health Centre in Toronto. Margaret has also written "Premenstrual Syndrome," *Healthsharing* vol. 12 no. 2 (Summer 1991): 10-13; and the pamphlet *Being Menopausitive* (1994) for low literacy women and St. Joseph's Health Centre.

**JOANNE DOUCETTE** is no longer on welfare, but, given the lack of progress since she wrote "Welfare: Far from Well" in 1988, expects she may be unemployed and part of "the system" again. "Restructuring" isn't changing the power structure of our society. It blames the poor women for poverty and comforts the middle class. Joanne lives and works in Toronto as a writer. She is exploring the relationship between human beings and the environment through leading hikes, walks, canoe trips and other activities.

**ENAKSHI DUA** is an assistant professor in the Department of Sociology, Queens University. She writes on race, class and gender as well as Third World development. She joined the editorial collective of *On Women Healthsharing* to help document the legacy of *Healthsharing* magazine. *Healthsharing* informed and challenged Ena and her friends as they struggled to experience their health and illness in a more progressive way.

**BETH EASTON** is the Coordinator of Women's Programs, AIDS Vancouver where her responsibilities include program development, implementation and evaluation. In this capacity, and as a volunteer, she works with the Positive Women's Network. Coordinator of the former Women and AIDS Project, Vancouver, Beth has been doing women and AIDS work since 1991. Beth had sone AIDS and development work for the United Nations Development Program, and is a North American representative to the International AIDS Society's Women's Caucus.

**COLLEEN FERGUSON** is a teacher, freelance writer and editor. She currently teaches adult immigrants and refugees English as a second language and hosts "By All Means," a feminist radio show on CIUT in Toronto.

**MAUREEN FITZGERALD** teaches at the University of Toronto. She is a former managing editor of Women's Press. She says she got involved in this project because she loves to make books, she loves Amy Gottlieb and she had total amnesia about how long it takes to put a book together.

**REBECCA FOX** has used her U.S. training as a physician assistant to work in clinical research in the areas of both infectious disease and, presently, interventional cardiology at the Vancouver Hospital and Health Sciences Centre. She is also studying for a Masters of Science in Epidemiology at the University of British Columbia. Since writing "Undoing Medical Conditioning," she has had two children. In 1989, she became a founding member of the Positive Women's Network, a B.C. support organization for HIV Positive Women and their families and remained active on the board of directors until 1994.

**LINDA GARDNER** is the HIV/STD Program Coordinator at the Bay Centre for Birth Control, Regional Women's Health Centre, affiliated with Women's College Hospital in Toronto. She is a longtime grassroots activist and has worked extensively with the Ontario Coalition for Abortion Clinics, March 8th Coalition and more recently with AIDS Action Now! Currently, she is the co-chair of the board of directors of the Community AIDS Treatment Information Exchange, and a member of the Gay Asian AIDS Project's Advisory committee and the Hassle Free Clinic's board of directors.

**PATRICIA GIBSON** is a freelance journalist living in Vancouver. She is a former editor of *Kinesis*.

**AMY GOTTLIEB** is an editor, artist and activist and a former managing editor of *Healthsharing*. She is currently editing *Parallélogramme*, a magazine of the artist-run movement across Canada and is still in love with magazine publishing and Maureen FitzGerald.

**NORAH HUTCHINSON** is a social worker who co-founded the Elizabeth Bagshaw Women's Clinic in Vancouver, an abortion-providing health clinic operating since 1989. She is a board director of the clinic's Adjunct Society and is employed as a counselor at the clinic.

**PATRICIA KAUFERT** is a full professor in the Department of Community Health Sciences at the University of Manitoba.

**DIANNE KINNON** has worked as an independent consultant in social and health issues for the last seven years. She has completed several research and writing contracts related to sexuality and reproductive health, and has remained a volunteer at Planned Parenthood Ottawa.

**CATHLEEN KNEEN** continues to co-publish *The Ram's Horn*, a monthly newsletter of food system analysis, with her husband, Brewster Kneen. She has also edited Brewster's first three books, including *From Land to Mouth: Understanding the Food System* and *The Rape of Canola*.

As Executive Coordinator of the Assaulted Women's Help Line in Toronto, Cathleen is a well-known public advocate on issues of violence against women. She sees a strong relationship between this and the violence done to the land and people in our industrial food production system. As part of her commitment to healing from violence, she is currently editing *Eating Bitterness: A Vision Beyond the Prison Walls* by Native elder Art Solomon.

**BONNIE LAFAVE** is a current affairs producer with CBC's "Prime Time News."

**B. LEE** is a longtime reproductive rights and AIDS activist who has worked in the Ontario Coalition for Abortion Clinic for ten years, AIDS Action Now! since 1989, and is currently also on the board of the Community AIDS Treatment Information Exchange.

**CHRISTINA LEE** is currently manager of the Justice Policy Unit, Policy and Research Branch, Ministry of Citizenship.

**SHEILA JENNINGS LINEHAN** is presently on leave with her four-month-old son, Cormac, born at home with the assistance of two Ottawa midwives. Sheila has published in the legal and reproductive health fields.

**LINDA LOUNSBERRY** has quit typesetting since writing "The All Pervasive Ache" for *Healthsharing* in 1985. Linda now works as a Registered Massage Therapist in Toronto.

**RHONDA LOVE** is an associate professor at the University of Toronto in the department of Behavioral Science, Faculty of Medicine. She has taught on women and health as well as gender and health for many years. She teaches issues of violence against women to medical students and other health professionals and has made three teaching films on wife abuse. Rhonda was part of the advisory group for *The Healthsharing Book*, the Chair of the Status of Women Committee at the faculty association at the University of Toronto for several years, and on the Ontario Confederation of University Faculty Association's Status of Women committee for two years.

**JANET MAHER** is the co-ordinator for the new National Action Committee on the Status of Women Ontario Community Economic Development Community. She also works with the National Action Committee on the Status of Women on health and social policy and is the chair of the City of York Social Planning Council.

**VIRGINIA MAK** is a writer and photographer. In 1994, Virginia had two photography exhibitions at the Visual Arts Centre in Bowmanville and the Market Gallery in Toronto. Her photograph of guitar-maker Linda Manzer was published in the 1995 Woman's Day Book. She still sings with the Ryerson Oakham House Choir.

**RITA MANUEL** is still employed with Health Canada. She is on a DAP-Assignment with Occupational and Environmental Health Services, Health Canada until the end of the fiscal year 1994/95. Twenty-two years ago, Rita completed her training at the B.C. Institute of Technology in Burnaby, B.C. to become a Public Health Inspector. She worked for two years with Health Canada as an Environmental Health Officer and is anticipating returning to a full-time position pending her success on the DAP-Assignment.

**KATHLEEN MCDONNELL** is a Toronto writer with a number of books, plays and children's stories to her credit. Her most recent book is *Kid Culture* (Second Story Press, 1994).

**MARY NEILANS** is currently living in Vancouver with her four-year-old daughter, Emma. While instructing classes of adults in business communications and computer software, her creative side has been reawakened and she vows to live up to her former biography following her *Healthsharing* article "Midwifery: From Recognition to Regulation."

**HAZELLE PALMER** is the former managing editor of *Healthsharing* magazine. She has just completed her first collection of short stories *Tales from the Gardens and Beyond*, to be published in 1995 by Sister Vision Press. She is currently editing an anthology of writings by black women and women of colour entitled *...But Where Are You Really From: Writings on Identity and Assimilation*. Hazelle lives in Toronto with her daughter Ashae and partner Alfred.

**ARUNA PAPP** was born in India and emigrated to Canada in 1972. She earned her Masters degree in Sociology at York University in 1989. Ms. Papp founded three organizations in Canada to assist victims of wife abuse. Her service achievements have been widely covered by the media, including CBC's "The Journal" and "Canada A.M." Her work has also been recognized nationally including a YWCA Woman of Distinction Award (1991) and a Government of Canada's 125th Anniversary Commemoration Medal for Community Services (1993). She is a member of the board of governors of Centenary Hospital and Centennial College in Toronto; she participates on various task forces and government committees; and she is in demand as a consultant and workshop leader of organizations such as the National Panel on Violence Against Women, Ontario College of Physicians and Surgeons, the National Judiciary Institute, public and separate school boards in Toronto, the London (Ontario) Family Clinic and the Metro Housing Authority.

**CARLA RICE** is a counselor and writer who has been working with the Regional Women's Health Centre in Toronto to develop an innovative program for girls and women around body image problems. She is Chair of the Embodying Equity Working Group at the Toronto Board of Education and one of the founders of the

Body Image Pilot Project for children and youth. She is currently working towards a PhD in Women's Studies at York University.

**LORIE ROTENBERG** is a feminist therapist and anti-violence activist. She no longer suffers from the symptoms of Epstein-Barr virus. Since writing "Winning the Battle: Living with Epstein-Barr Virus," Lorie has uncovered memories of childhood sexual abuse. In order to survive this trauma, she had to suppress her pain, terror and rage. This repression contributed significantly to her physical and emotional dis-ease.

Subsequent to publication of Lorie's article "Winning the Battle," *Healthsharing*, a longer version was published in *Healing Journeys*, edited by S. Drake and C. Klopstock (South Surrey, B.C.: Pinecrest Publishers, 1992).

**MAKEDA SILVERA** is an African-Caribbean-Canadian writer. She has lived in Canada for over 25 years. Her writing explores themes of identity and language from a lesbian feminist perspective. She lives in Toronto.

**DARIEN TAYLOR** is the co-author of the international anthology *Positive Women: Voices of Women Living with AIDS* (Second Story Press, 1992) She is one of the founders of Voices of Positive Women, a Toronto-based organization directed by and for women living with HIV/AIDS. She continues to be involved with the issues of people living with HIV/AIDS in many ways, especially through the activist organization AIDS Action Now! which she sees as her home, even if she no longer attends every single meeting.

**MAGGIE THOMPSON** left the Vancouver Women's Health Collective in 1988. Since then, she has worked as a program co-ordinator with the Canadian Cancer Society and as Executive Director with the B.C. Schizophrenia Society in Victoria. In September 1994 Maggie was appointed to B.C.'s first Advisory Council on Women's Health. She currently operates CLADDAUGH HOUSE, a Bed and Breakfast business in Victoria, with her daughter Caila.

**CLARA VALVERDE** is a nurse working in health education. She has worked in women's health since 1975 and has a strong background in psychosocial aspects of health. Currently Clara trains health professional is Barcelona, Spain. For the four years prior to that she did health promotion for the James Bay Cree in Montreal.

**VICKI VAN WAGNER** has practised as a community midwife in Toronto since 1980. She has been an active participant in the Association of Ontario Midwives working toward the legal recognition of midwifery in Ontario. Currently Vicki is the program director of the Ryerson Midwifery Education Program.

**KAREN WEISBERG** left the legal clinic where she represented injured workers in their Workers' Compensation Board claims and subsequently worked in women's services. She is now an elementary teacher in Toronto.

**SUSAN WORTMAN** is now a psychodrama therapist in private practice. She is living happily on a farm, outside of Hamilton, Ontario.

**LISA WYNDELS** is a mother and a lawyer. She is currently working as staff lawyer at Kensington Bellwoods Community Legal Services, where she does work principally in the areas of immigration and income security. She has been a member of the Social Issues Manuscript Group at Women's Press for five years, and has one son, Chester, who is four years old.

**LORNA ZABACK** is now living on Vancouver Island where she is pursuing her continued interest in plant and human (particularly women's) health. She plans to study homeopathy.